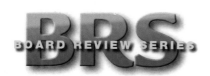

BOARD REVIEW SERIES

D1346768

Microbiology and Immunology

SIXTH EDITION

Louise Hawley, PhD

Professor and Chair
Department of Microbiology and Immunology
Ross University School of Medicine
Dominica, West Indies

Richard J. Ziegler, PhD

Professor of Microbiology
Department of Anatomy, Microbiology, and Pathology
University of Minnesota Medical School-Duluth
Duluth, Minnesota

Benjamin L. Clarke, PhD

Associate Professor
Department of Medical Microbiology and Immunology
University of Minnesota Medical School-Duluth
Duluth, Minnesota

 Wolters Kluwer | Lippincott Williams & Wilkins
Health

Philadelphia · Baltimore · New York · London
Buenos Aires · Hong Kong · Sydney · Tokyo

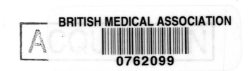

Acquisitions Editor: Sirkka Howes
Product Manager: Catherine Noonan
Vendor Manager: Bridgett Dougherty
Senior Marketing Manager: Joy Fisher-Williams
Manufacturing Coordinator: Margie Orzech
Design Coordinator: Holly Reid-McLaughlin
Compositor: S4Carlisle Publishing Services

Sixth Edition

351 West Camden Street
Baltimore, MD 21201

Two Commerce Square
2001 Market Street
Philadelphia, PA 19103

Printed in China

Library of Congress Cataloging-in-Publication Data

Hawley, Louise.
 Microbiology and Immunology / Louise Hawley, Richard J. Ziegler, Benjamin L. Clarke. — 6th ed.
  p. ; cm. — (Board review series)
 Rev. ed. of: Microbiology and immunology / Arthur G. Johnson, Richard J. Ziegler, Louise Hawley. 5th ed. c2010.
 Includes bibliographical references and index.
 ISBN 978-1-4511-7534-9 (alk. paper)
 I. Ziegler, Richard J.   II. Clarke, Benjamin L.   III. Johnson, Arthur G. Microbiology and immunology.
IV. Title. V. Series: Board review series.
 [DNLM: 1. Microbiological Phenomena—Examination Questions.   2. Immune System Phenomena—Examination Questions. QW 18.2]
 QR46
 616.9'041076—dc23

2013012309

DISCLAIMER
Care has been taken to confirm the accuracy of the information presented and to describe generally accepted practices. However, the authors, editors, and publisher are not responsible for errors or omissions or for any consequences from application of the information in this book and make no warranty, expressed or implied, with respect to the currency, completeness, or accuracy of the contents of the publication. Application of this information in a particular situation remains the professional responsibility of the practitioner; the clinical treatments described and recommended may not be considered absolute and universal recommendations.

The authors, editors, and publisher have exerted every effort to ensure that the drug selection and dosage set forth in this text are in accordance with the current recommendations and practice at the time of publication. However, in view of ongoing research, changes in government regulations, and the constant flow of information relating to drug therapy and drug reactions, the reader is urged to check the package insert for each drug for any change in indications and dosage and for added warnings and precautions. This is particularly important when the recommended agent is a new or infrequently employed drug.

Some drugs and medical devices presented in this publication have Food and Drug Administration (FDA) clearance for limited use in restricted research settings. It is the responsibility of the health care provider to ascertain the FDA status of each drug or device planned for use in their clinical practice.

To purchase additional copies of this book, call our customer service department at **(800) 638-3030** or fax orders to **(301) 223-2320**. International customers should call **(301) 223-2300**.

Visit Lippincott Williams & Wilkins on the Internet: http://www.lww.com. Lippincott Williams & Wilkins customer service representatives are available from 8:30 am to 6:00 pm, EST.

9 8 7 6 5 4 3 2 1

*The authors dedicate this book to their many students who have been
a source of stimulation over the years, and to their many colleagues
whose research and insight has resulted in the knowledge described herein.
We particularly want to thank Dr. Arthur Johnson, who has retired
from both his leadership role as senior author/editor and authorship
of the immunology section.*

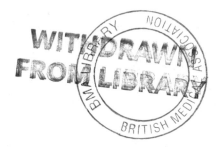

Acknowledgements

The authors are grateful for the excellent organizational and secretarial skills of Wendy Schwartz, who aided in the preparation of this edition. And very importantly, we want to thank our spouses and kids for their continued support and patience during the rewriting period.

How to Use this Book

This concise review of microbiology and immunology and its online resources are designed specifically for medical students to successfully prepare for Step 1 of the United States Medical Licensing Examination (USMLE), as well as other examinations. This newest edition remains a succinct description of the most important microbiological and immunological concepts, as well as a review of critical details needed to understand important human infections and the immune system's function and malfunction.

ORGANIZATION

Facilitates Use by Either a Bug Approach or Systems Approach

The book is divided into 12 chapters, starting with basic information and then leading the student quickly to the level of detail and comprehension needed for Step 1. For each major category of microbes (e.g., viruses), there is a fundamental chapter (two for the bacteria) followed by an organ-systems infectious disease approach with critical signs/symptoms, epidemiology, etiology, pathogenesis of infections and immune diseases, and the mechanisms for preventing infection and means of identifying and diagnosing the causative agent. Then an updated Chapter 11 (*Clues for Distinguishing Causative Agents*) presents the diseases a second time, this time utilizing an organ systems-based approach presented by text and great graphic flow-charts starting with symptoms frequently mentioned in case-based questions. Included also are tables listing agents associated with different types of rashes. New to the 6th edition are detailed summary tables of the characteristics and details of the different agents causing meningitis, encephalitis, upper and lower respiratory infections, and pneumonias.

Because many medical schools have switched to a fundamentals block followed by organ system modules, we have created an-online 6th edition *Systems-Based Table of Contents/ Guide* which facilitates use in a system-base course by listing both the pages of reading and chapter question-numbers for these courses. This aids faculty using the book in a system-based course and gives the reviewing student options for how they want to organize their review.

The outline format facilitates rapid review of important information. Each chapter is followed by review questions and answers, with explanations that reflect the style and content of the USMLE. These questions are available online as well and can generate systems-based or taxonomic self-quizzes. We have added four separate comprehensive examinations at the end of the book. Each has the same general sub-subject distribution generally found on Step 1 and so may be used as a practice exam and self-assessment tool to help students diagnose their weaknesses prior to, during, and after reviewing microbiology and immunology. The *Comprehensive Exam* questions (accessible online as well) are not mixed with the chapter questions so they can be saved for use after initial study.

Suggestion for increasing your retention: use two cover sheets (one to move down a page and a top one to move left to right) on tables and diagrams to see if you can predict what it is going to say in each section before reading the section.

KEY FEATURES

- Dual approach (bug and system) in one small book along with new online resources allows flexibility in study and self-testing to improve retention.
- An expanded, resource-rich Chapter 11 which has new System Summary Tables at the end.
- Updated four-color tables and figures summarize essential information for quick recall.
- End-of-chapter review tests feature updated USMLE-style questions.
- Four USMLE comprehensive exams with explanations are included in blocks of similar size to USMLE Step 1.
- Updated and current information is provided in all chapters.

We wish you well in your study and exams!

Louise Hawley, PhD
Richard J. Ziegler, PhD
Benjamin L. Clarke, PhD

Contents*

Systems-based Table of Contents/Guide is available online.

5.   VIRUSES   112

6.   SYSTEM-BASED AND SITUATIONAL VIRAL INFECTIONS   145

12. IMMUNOLOGY   238

chapter 1

General Properties of Microorganisms

I. THE MICROBIAL WORLD

A. **Microorganisms.**
  1. Belong to the Protista biologic kingdom.
  2. Include some eukaryotes and prokaryotes, viruses, viroids, and prions.
  3. Are classified according to their structure, chemical composition, and biosynthetic and genetic organization.

B. **Eukaryotic cells (Table 1.1).**
  1. Contain organelles and a nucleus bounded by a nuclear membrane.
  2. Contain complex phospholipids, sphingolipids, histones, and sterols.
  3. Lack a cell wall. (Plant cells and fungi have a cell wall.)
  4. Have multiple diploid chromosomes and nucleosomes.
  5. Have relatively long-lived mRNA formed from the processing of precursor mRNA, which contains exons and introns.
  6. Have 80S ribosomes and uncoupled transcription and translation.
  7. Include **protozoa** and **fungi.**
     a. Organisms in **kingdom Protozoa** are classified into seven phyla; three of these phyla (Sarcomastigophora, Apicomplexa, and Ciliophora) contain medically important species that are human parasites.
     b. Organisms in **kingdom Fungi:**
        (1) Are **eukaryotic** cells with a complex carbohydrate cell wall.
        (2) Have ergosterol as the dominant membrane sterol.
        (3) May be **monomorphic,** existing only as single-celled **yeasts** or multicellular, filamentous **molds.**
        (4) May be **dimorphic,** existing as **yeasts or molds depending on temperature and nutrition.**
        (5) May have both asexual and sexual reproduction capabilities. Deuteromycetes, or Fungi Imperfecti, have no known sexual stages.

C. **Prokaryotic cells (see Table 1.1).**
  1. Have no organelles, no membrane-enclosed nucleus, and no histones; in rare cases, they contain complex phospholipids, sphingolipids, and sterols.
  2. Have 70S ribosomes composed of 30S and 50S subunits.
  3. Have a cell wall composed of peptidoglycan-containing muramic acid.
  4. Are haploid with a single chromosome.
  5. Have short-lived, unprocessed mRNA.
  6. Have coupled transcription and translation.

table **1.1** Components of Microbial Cells

Structure	Composition	Cell Type					
		Fungi	Gram-Positive Bacteria	Gram-Negative Bacteria	Mycoplasmas	Chlamydia*	Rickettsia*
Envelope capsule	Polysaccharide or polypeptide	− or +**	+ or −	+ or −	−	−	−
Wall							
Chitin	Poly-N-acetylglucosamine	+	−	−	−	−	−
Peptidoglycan	Poly-N-acetylglucosamine-N-acetylmuramic acid tetrapeptide	−	+	+	−	−	+
Periplasm	Proteins and oligosaccharides	−	−	+	−	+	+
Lipoprotein	Lipoprotein	−	−	+	−	+	+
Outer membrane	Proteins, phospholipids, and lipopolysaccharide	−	−	+	−	+	+
Appendages							
Pili	Protein	−	+ or −	+ or −	−	−	−
Flagella	Protein	−	+ or −	+ or −	−	−	−
Cell membrane	Proteins and phospholipids	+ (plus ergosterol)	+	+	+	+	+
Cytosol							
Organelles	Protein, phospholipids, and nucleic acids	+	−	−	−	−	−
80S ribosomes	Protein and RNA	+	−	−	−	−	−
70S ribosomes	Protein and RNA	−	+	+	+	+	+
Genetic material							
Nucleus	Protein, phospholipids, and nucleic acids	+	−	−	−	−	−
Nucleoid	Protein and nucleic acids	−	+	+	+	+	+
Plasmids	DNA	+ or −	+ or −	+ or −	+ or −	+ or −	+ or −
Transposons	DNA	+	+	+	−	+	+
Spores							
Reproductive spores	All cellular components	+	−	−	−	−	−
Endospores	All cellular components plus dipicolinic acid	−	+ or −	−	−	−	−

*Obligate intracellular pathogens.
**Cryptococcus neoformans is the only medically important fungus with a capsule.

7. Include **typical bacteria, mycoplasmas,** and **obligate intracellular bacteria.**

    a. Typical bacteria:

        (1) Have a **cell wall.**

        (2) May be normal flora or may be pathogenic in humans.

        (3) Do not have a sexual growth cycle; however, some can produce asexual spores.

    b. Mycoplasmas:

        (1) Are the smallest and simplest of the bacteria that are self-replicating.

        (2) Lack a cell wall.

        (3) Are the only prokaryotes that contain **sterols.**

    c. Obligate intracellular bacteria include **Rickettsia** and **Chlamydia.**

        (1) Rickettsia are incapable of self-replication and depend on the host cell for adenosine triphosphate (ATP) production.

        (2) Chlamydia are bacteria-like pathogens with a complex growth cycle involving intracellular and extracellular forms. They depend on the host cell for ATP production.

D. Viruses.

    1. Are not cells and are not visible with the light microscope.

    2. Are **obligate intracellular parasites.**

    3. Contain no organelles or biosynthetic machinery, except for a few enzymes.

    4. Contain either RNA or DNA as genetic material.

    5. Are called **bacteriophages** (or **phages**) if they have a bacterial host.

E. Viroids.

    1. Are not cells and are not visible with the light microscope.

    2. Are **obligate intracellular parasites.**

    3. Are single-stranded, covalently closed, circular RNA molecules that exist as base-paired, rod-like structures.

    4. Cause plant diseases but have not been proven to cause human disease, although the RNA of the hepatitis D virus (HDV) is viroid-like.

F. Prions.

    1. Are infectious particles associated with subacute progressive, degenerative diseases of the central nervous system (e.g., Creutzfeldt-Jakob disease).

    2. Copurify with a specific glycoprotein (PrP) that has a molecular weight of 27 to 30 kDa. They are resistant to nucleases but are inactivated with proteases and other agents that inactivate proteins.

    3. Are altered conformations of a normal cellular protein that can autocatalytically form more copies of itself.

II.   HOST-PARASITE RELATIONSHIP

A. Normal flora consist mainly of bacteria, but fungi and protozoa may be present in some individuals. They can provide useful nutrients (e.g., vitamin K) and release compounds (e.g., colicins) with antibacterial activity against pathogenic bacteria.

    1. They reside in the skin, mouth, nose, oropharynx, large intestine, urethra, and vagina.

    2. Normal flora may produce disease if they invade normally sterile areas of the body or are not properly controlled by the immune system.

B. Microbial pathogenicity refers to a microbe's ability to cause disease, which depends on genetically determined virulence factors. A microbe's pathogenicity is related to its:

    1. Entry

    2. Colonization

    3. Escape from host defense mechanisms

    4. Multiplication

    5. Damage to host tissues

C. **Virulence factors** are chromosomal and extrachromosomal (plasmid) gene products that affect aspects related to an organism's:
1. Invasion *properties*
2. Adherence and colonization
3. Tissue damage induced by toxins, immune system reactions, and intracellular growth
4. Eluding host defense mechanisms
5. Antibiotic resistance

III. STERILIZATION AND DISINFECTION

A. Terminology.
1. **Sterility**—total absence of viable microorganisms as assessed by no growth on any medium.
2. **Bactericidal**—kills bacteria.
3. **Bacteriostatic**—inhibits growth of bacteria.
4. **Sterilization**—removal or killing of all microorganisms.
5. **Disinfection**—removal or killing of disease-causing microorganisms.
6. **Sepsis**—infection.
7. **Aseptic**—without infection.
8. **Antisepsis**—any procedure that inhibits the growth and multiplication of microorganisms.

B. Kinetics of killing.
1. Killing is affected by the medium, the concentration of organisms and antimicrobial agents, temperature, pH, and the presence of endospores.
2. It can be exponential (logarithmic); can result in a killing curve that becomes asymptotic, requiring extra considerations in killing final numbers, especially if the population is heterogeneous relative to sensitivity.

C. Methods of control.
1. **Moist heat** (autoclaving at 121°C/250°F for 15 minutes at a steam pressure of 15 pounds per square inch) kills microorganisms, including endospores.
2. **Dry heat** and **incineration** are both methods that oxidize proteins, killing bacteria.
3. **Ultraviolet radiation** blocks DNA replication.
4. **Chemicals:**
   a. **Phenol** is used as a disinfectant standard that is expressed as a phenol coefficient, which compares the rate of the minimal sterilizing concentration of phenol to that of the test compound for a particular organism.
   b. **Chlorhexidine** is a diphenyl cationic analog that is a useful topical disinfectant.
   c. **Iodine** is bactericidal in a 2% solution of aqueous alcohol containing potassium iodide. It acts as an oxidizing agent and combines irreversibly with proteins. It can cause hypersensitivity reactions.
   d. **Chlorine** inactivates bacteria and most viruses by oxidizing free sulfhydryl groups.
   e. **Quaternary ammonium compounds** (e.g., **benzalkonium chloride**) inactivate bacteria by their hydrophobic and lipophilic groups, interacting with the cell membrane to alter metabolic properties and permeability.
   f. **Ethylene oxide** is an alkylating agent that is especially useful for sterilizing heat-sensitive hospital instruments. It requires exposure times of 4 to 6 hours, followed by aeration to remove absorbed gas.
   g. **Alcohol** requires concentrations of 70% to 95% to kill bacteria given sufficient time. Isopropyl alcohol (90% to 95%) is the major form in use in hospitals.

Review Test

Directions: Each of the numbered items or incomplete statements in this section is followed by answers or completions of the statement. Select the ONE lettered answer that is BEST in each case.

1. A pharmaceutical company has developed a new compound that is well tolerated by the body and inhibits the sterol ergosterol synthesis. Screening of anti-infectious agent activity should be directed toward

(A) Bacteria
(B) Chlamydia species
(C) Fungi
(D) Rickettsia species
(E) Viruses

2. 50S ribosomal subunits are found in

(A) Bacteria
(B) Fungi
(C) Prions
(D) Protozoa
(E) Viruses

3. The normal flora of the large intestine consists mainly of

(A) Bacteria
(B) Fungi
(C) Protozoa
(D) Viruses
(E) No microbial agents

4. The minimal concentration of alcohol necessary to kill bacteria and enveloped viruses is

(A) 30%
(B) 40%
(C) 50%
(D) 60%
(E) 70%

5. Human obligate intracellular pathogens that depend on the host cell for ATP production are

(A) Bacteriophages
(B) Mycoplasma species
(C) Prions
(D) Rickettsia species
(E) Viroids

6. Dimorphism is a characteristic of

(A) Bacteria
(B) Fungi
(C) Prions
(D) Rickettsia species
(E) Viruses

7. A new infectious agent has been isolated from deer ticks. It lacks a cell wall but has 70S ribosomes. This agent is most likely a

(A) Bacterium
(B) Chlamydia species
(C) Mycoplasma species
(D) Rickettsia species
(E) Virus

8. The infectious agent associated with Creutzfeldt-Jakob disease is extremely hardy, but can be inactivated by

(A) Catalases
(B) Hyaluronidases
(C) Nucleases
(D) Phospholipases
(E) Proteases

9. Quaternary ammonium compounds inactivate bacteria because they

(A) Alter metabolic properties of membranes
(B) Bind irreversibly to DNA
(C) Denature proteins
(D) Inactivate 50S ribosomes
(E) Oxidize free sulfhydryl groups

Answers and Explanations

1. **The answer is C.** Fungi have ergosterol as their dominant membrane sterol. Mycoplasmas are the only prokaryotes with sterols in their cytoplasmic membrane, but they do not synthesize their own sterols.

2. **The answer is A.** Bacteria have 70S ribosomes composed of 30S and 50S subunits. Fungi and protozoa have 80S ribosomes, and prions and viruses do not have ribosomes.

3. **The answer is A.** Bacteria form the majority of the normal flora of the large intestine. Other types of human infectious agents are not usually present except in time of disease.

4. **The answer is E.** An alcohol concentration of 70% to 95% is necessary to kill bacteria.

5. **The answer is D.** Chlamydia and rickettsia are obligate intracellular pathogens because they depend on the host cell to provide them with ATP.

6. **The answer is B.** Certain species of pathogenic fungi are dimorphic (i.e., existing as yeast or mold forms depending on their environment).

7. **The answer is C.** Mycoplasmas are the only microbes that lack a cell wall, but they do have 70S ribosomes.

8. **The answer is E.** The infectious agent of Creutzfeldt-Jakob disease is a prion which is inactivated by proteases.

9. **The answer is A.** The hydrophobic and lipophilic portions of quaternary ammonium compounds react with the lipid components of the bacterial membrane so that it can no longer perform its normal metabolic and permeability functions, thus killing the cell.

I. BACTERIAL STRUCTURE

A. **Shape.** Along with other properties, shape is used to identify bacteria. It is determined by the mechanism of cell wall assembly.
   1. Bacterial shape usually can be determined with appropriate staining and a light microscope.
   2. **Types:**
      a. **Round** (coccus)
      b. **Rod-like** (bacillus)
      c. **Spiral**
   3. Cocci and bacilli often grow in doublets (diplococci) or chains (streptococci). Cocci that grow in clusters are called staphylococci.
   4. Some bacterial species are **pleomorphic,** such as *Bacteroides.*
   5. Antibiotics that affect cell wall biosynthesis (e.g., penicillin) may alter a bacteria's shape.

B. **Nucleus.** In bacteria, the nucleus generally is called a **nucleoid** or **nuclear body.**
   1. The bacterial nucleus is not surrounded by a nuclear membrane, nor does it contain a mitotic apparatus.
   2. **Composition.** The nucleus consists of polyamine and magnesium ions bound to negatively charged, circular, supercoiled, double-stranded DNA; small amounts of RNA; RNA polymerase; and other proteins.

C. **Cytoplasm.**
   1. Bacterial cytoplasm contains ribosomes and various types of nutritional storage granules.
   2. It contains **no organelles.**

D. **Ribosomes.** Bacterial ribosomes contain proteins and RNAs that differ from those of their eukaryotic counterparts.
   1. **Types.** Bacterial ribosomes have a sedimentation coefficient of 70S and are composed of 30S and 50S subunits containing 16S, and 23S and 5S RNA, respectively.
   2. Ribosomes engaged in protein biosynthesis are membrane bound.
   3. Many antibiotics target ribosomes, inhibiting protein biosynthesis. Some antibiotics selectively target the 70S ribosomes (e.g., erythromycin), but not 80S ribosomes.

E. **Cell (cytoplasmic) membrane.**
   1. **Structure.** The cell membrane is a typical phospholipid bilayer that contains the following constituents:
      a. Cytochromes and enzymes involved in electron transport and oxidative phosphorylation.
      b. Carrier lipids, enzymes, and **penicillin-binding proteins (PBP)** involved in cell wall biosynthesis.
      c. Enzymes involved in phospholipid synthesis and DNA replication.
      d. Chemoreceptors.
   2. **Functions:**
      a. Selective permeability and active transport facilitated by membrane-bound permeases, binding proteins, and various transport systems.
      b. Site of action of certain antibiotics such as polymyxin.

F. **Mesosomes** are controversial structures that are **convoluted invaginations** of the plasma membrane.
   1. **Septal mesosomes** occur at the septum (cross-wall); **lateral mesosomes** are nonseptal.
   2. **Function:** participate in DNA replication, cell division, and secretion.

G. **Plasmids.**
   1. Plasmids are small, circular, nonchromosomal, double-stranded DNA molecules that are:
      a. Capable of self-replication.
      b. Most frequently extrachromosomal but may become integrated into bacterial DNA.
   2. **Function:** contain genes that confer protective properties such as antibiotic resistance, virulence factors, or their own transmissibility to other bacteria.

H. **Transposons.**
   1. Transposons are small pieces of DNA that move between the DNA of bacteria and plasmids; they do not self-replicate.
   2. **Functions:**
      a. Code for antibiotic resistance enzymes, metabolic enzymes, or toxins.
      b. May alter expression of neighboring genes or cause mutations to genes into which they are inserted.

I. **Cell envelope** (Figs. 2.1 and 2.2).
   1. **General structure.** The cell envelope is composed of the macromolecular layers that surround the bacterium. It includes:
      a. A cell membrane and a peptidoglycan layer except for mycoplasma.
      b. An outer membrane layer in Gram-negative bacteria.
      c. A capsule, a glycocalyx layer, or both (sometimes).
      d. Antigens that frequently induce a specific antibody response.
   2. **Cell wall:**
      a. The cell wall refers to that portion of the cell envelope that is **external to the cytoplasmic membrane** and **internal to the capsule or glycocalyx.**
      b. It confers osmotic protection and Gram-staining characteristics.
      c. In **Gram-positive bacteria** it is composed of:
         (1) Peptidoglycan
         (2) Teichoic and teichuronic acids
         (3) Polysaccharides
      d. In **Gram-negative bacteria**, it is composed of:
         (1) Peptidoglycan
         (2) Lipoprotein
         (3) An outer phospholipid membrane that contains lipopolysaccharide

Gram-Positive Cell Envelope

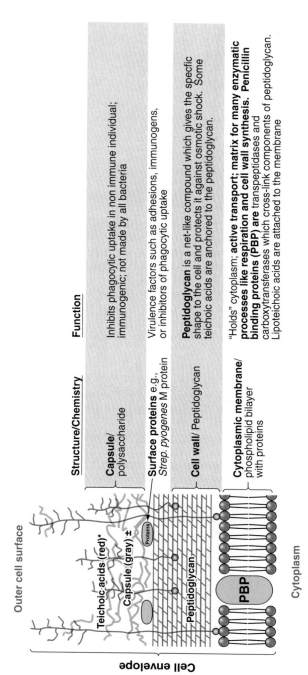

Structure/Chemistry	Function
Capsule/polysaccharide	Inhibits phagocytic uptake in non immune individual; immunogenic; not made by all bacteria
Surface proteins e.g., *Strep. pyogenes* M protein	Virulence factors such as adhesions, immunogens, or inhibitors of phagocytic uptake
Cell wall/ Peptidoglycan	**Peptidoglycan** is a net-like compound which gives the specfic shape to the cell and protects it against osmotic shock. Some teichoic acids are anchored to the peptidoglycan.
Cytoplasmic membrane/ phospholipid bilayer with proteins	"Holds" cytoplasm; **active transport; matrix for many enzymatic processes like respiration and cell wall synthesis. Penicillin binding proteins (PBP) are** transpeptidases and carboxytransferases which cross-link components of peptidoglycan. Lipoteichoic acids are attached to the membrane

*Teichoic acids (shown in red) are found only in Gram-positive cells.

FIGURE 2.1. Gram-positive cell envelope showing structures and describing their chemistry and function. (Updated from Hawley LB. *High-Yield Microbiology and Infectious Diseases.* 2nd ed. Baltimore, MD: Lippincott Williams & Wilkins; 2007.)

Gram-Negative Cell Envelope

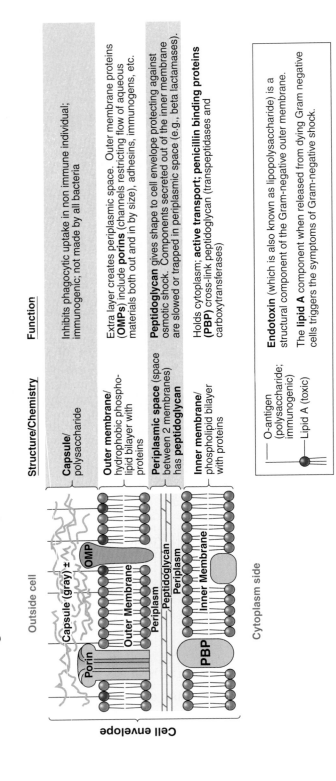

Structure/Chemistry	Function
Capsule/polysaccharide	Inhibits phagocytic uptake in non immune individual; immunogenic; not made by all bacteria
Outer membrane/hydrophobic phospholipid bilayer with proteins	Extra layer creates periplasmic space. Outer membrane proteins (**OMPs**) include **porins** (channels restricting flow of aqueous materials both out and in by size), adhesins, immunogens, etc.
Periplasmic space (space between 2 membranes) has **peptidoglycan**	**Peptidoglycan** gives shape to cell envelope protecting against osmotic shock. Components secreted out of the inner membrane are slowed or trapped in periplasmic space (e.g., beta lactamases).
Inner membrane/phospholipid bilayer with proteins	Holds cytoplasm; **active transport; penicillin binding proteins (PBP)** cross-link peptidoglycan (transpeptidases and carboxytransferases)

O-antigen (polysaccharide; immunogenic)

Lipid A (toxic)

Endotoxin (which is also known as lipopolysaccharide) is a structural component of the Gram-negative outer membrane.

The **lipid A** component when released from dying Gram negative cells triggers the symptoms of Gram-negative shock.

FIGURE 2.2. Gram-negative cell envelope showing structures and describing their chemistry and function. (Updated from Hawley LB. *High-Yield Microbiology and Infectious Diseases.* 2nd ed. Baltimore, MD: Lippincott Williams & Wilkins; 2007.)

3. **Peptidoglycan** (also called **mucopeptide** or **murein**) is unique to prokaryotes. It is found in all bacterial cell walls except *Mycoplasma*.
   a. **Structure:**
      (1) This **complex polymer** consists of a **backbone** composed of alternating *N*-cetylglucosamine and *N*-acetylmuramic acid and a set of identical tetrapeptide **side chains.**
      (2) The tetrapeptide side chains are attached to the *N*-acetylmuramic acid and are frequently linked to adjacent tetrapeptides by identical peptide **cross-bridges** or by direct peptide **bonds.**
      (3) The β-1, 4 glycosidic bond between *N*-acetylmuramic acid and *N*-acetylglucosamine is cleaved by the bacteriolytic enzyme **lysozyme** (found in mucus, saliva, and tears).
      (4) It may contain **diaminopimelic acid,** an amino acid unique to prokaryotic cell walls.
   b. Peptidoglycan is the site of action of certain antibiotics such as **penicillin** and the **cephalosporins.**
   c. In Gram-positive bacteria, it comprises up to 50% of the cell wall. In Gram-negative bacteria, it comprises only 2% to 10% of the cell wall.
4. **Teichoic** and **teichuronic acids** are **water-soluble polymers,** containing a ribitol or glycerol residue linked by phosphodiester bonds.
   a. They are found in **Gram-positive** cell walls or membranes.
      (1) Teichoic acid is found in cell walls and is chemically bonded to peptidoglycan.
      (2) Lipoteichoic acid is found in cell membranes and is chemically bonded to membrane glycolipid, particularly in mesosomes.
   b. **Functions:**
      (1) Contain important bacterial surface antigenic determinants, and lipoteichoic acid helps anchor the wall to the membrane.
      (2) May account for 50% of the dry weight of a Gram-positive cell wall.
5. **Lipoprotein** is found in **Gram-negative** bacteria.
   a. Lipoprotein cross-links the peptidoglycan and outer membrane.
   b. A peptide bond links the lipoprotein to diaminopimelic acid residues of peptidoglycan tetrapeptide side chains; the lipid portion is noncovalently inserted into the outer membrane.
6. The **periplasmic space** is found in **Gram-negative** cells.
   a. It refers to the area between the cell membrane and the outer membrane.
   b. Hydrated peptidoglycan, as well as hydrolytic **enzymes including β-lactamases, specific carrier molecules,** and oligosaccharides are found in the periplasmic space.
7. An **outer membrane** is found in **Gram-negative** cells.
   a. **Structure.** The outer membrane is a phospholipid bilayer in which the phospholipids of the outer portion are replaced by lipopolysaccharides. It contains:
      (1) Embedded proteins, including matrix **porins** (nonspecific pores).
      (2) Some non-pore proteins (phospholipases and proteases).
      (3) Transport proteins for small molecules.
   b. **Functions:**
      (1) Protects cells from harmful enzymes and some antibiotics.
      (2) Prevents leakage of periplasmic proteins.
8. **Lipopolysaccharide** is found in the outer leaflet of the outer membrane of **Gram-negative** cells.
   a. **Structure:**
      (1) Lipopolysaccharide consists of **lipid A,** several long-chain fatty acids attached to phosphorylated glucosamine disaccharide units, and a polysaccharide composed of a core and terminal repeating units.
      (2) It is negatively charged and noncovalently cross-bridged by divalent cations.
   b. **Functions:**
      (1) Also called **endotoxin;** the toxicity is associated with the lipid A.
      (2) Contains major surface antigenic determinants, including **O antigen** found in the polysaccharide component.

table **2.1**	Protein Secretion Systems Associated with Virulence
Secretion System Type	**Bacteria**
Type II (T2SS)	*Vibrio cholerae, Legionella pneumophila,* enterotoxigenic *E. coli,* and *Pseudomonas aeruginosa*
Type III (T3SS)	*Salmonella typhimurium, Shigella,* enterotoxigenic *E. coli,* and *Yersinia enterocolitica*
Type IV (T4SS) (also transport nucleic acids)	*Helicobacter pylori, Pseudomonas aeruginosa, Bordetella pertussis, E. coli,* and *Legionella pneumophila*
Type V (T5SS)	Adhesins—*E. coli, Haemophilus influenzae, Yersinia enterocolitica,* and *Bordetella pertussis;* Toxins—*Helicobacter pylori;* and IgA proteases—*Neisseria gonorrhoeae* and *N. meningitidis, Shigella,* and *Helicobacter pylori*
Type VI (T6SS)	*Vibrio cholerae, Pseudomonas aeruginosa,* and *Francisella tularensis*
Type VII (T7SS)	*Corynebacterium diphtheriae, Nocardia,* and *Staphylococcus aureus*

9. **Protein secretion systems (T1-7SS)** play a major role in bacteria interacting with their environment and helping to determine pathogenicity, particularly in Gram-negative bacteria (Table 2.1).
   a. **Distribution**.
      (1) Gram-negative bacteria have six classes of systems; Gram-positive bacteria have an additional unique class and some of the other six classes.
      (2) Some Gram-negatives contain more than one type of secretion system in a class (*Salmonella typhimurium* has two types of T3SS coded on different pathogenicity islands).
   b. **Structure.** There are some simple systems like T1SS that consist of transporters, outer membrane factors, and membrane fusion proteins, while others (T3SS, T4SS, and T6SS) involve a transmembrane structure **(injectosome)** which consists of more than 25 proteins.
   c. **Functions:**
      (1) Transport proteins or nucleic acids (T4SS) to outside of cell, periplasm, or inside host cells.
      (2) Transported proteins can be surface proteins like adhesins or toxins and effector proteins which modify the host-cell physiology, causing pathological consequences.

J. **External layers.**
   1. **Surface proteins:**
      a. These antiphagocytic proteins are external to the cell wall of some Gram-positive bacteria.
      b. **Functions:** act as **adhesins** facilitating tissue colonization with several species (e.g., *Staphylococcus aureus* [fibronectin-binding proteins] and *Streptococcus pyogenes* [F proteins]).
   2. **Capsule:**
      a. The capsule is a well-defined structure of polysaccharide surrounding a bacterial cell and is external to the cell wall. The one exception to the polysaccharide structure is the poly-D-glutamic acid capsule of *Bacillus anthracis.*
      b. **Functions:** protects the bacteria from phagocytosis and plays a role in bacterial adherence.
   3. **Glycocalyx:**
      a. The glycocalyx refers to a loose network of polysaccharide fibrils that surrounds some bacterial cell walls.
         (1) It is sometimes called a slime layer.
         (2) It is synthesized by surface enzymes.
      b. **Functions:** associated with adhesive properties of the bacterial cell and contains prominent antigenic sites.

K. **Appendages.**
   1. **Flagella** are protein appendages for locomotion and contain prominent antigenic determinants.
      a. They consist of a basal body, hook, and a long filament composed of a polymerized protein called **flagellin.**

    b. Flagella may be located in only one area of a cell **(polar)** or over the entire bacterial cell surface **(peritrichous)**.
  2. **Pili (fimbriae)** are rigid surface appendages composed mainly of a protein called **pilin**.
    a. **Types:**
      (1) **Common pili (adhesins)** are involved in bacterial adherence and Gram-positive cell conjugation.
      (2) **Sex pili** are involved in attachment of donor and recipient bacteria in Gram-negative cell conjugation.
    b. **Functions:**
      (1) Ordinary pili are the colonization antigens or **virulence factors** associated with some bacterial species such as *S. pyogenes* and *Neisseria gonorrhoeae*.
      (2) They also may confer antiphagocytic properties, such as the **M protein** of *S. pyogenes*.

L. Endospores.
  1. **General characteristics.** Endospores are formed as a survival response to certain adverse nutritional conditions, such as depletion of a certain resource. These metabolically **inactive bacterial cells** are highly resistant to desiccation, heat, and various chemicals. They are helpful in identifying some species of bacteria (e.g., *Bacillus* and *Clostridium*).
  2. **Structure:**
    a. Endospores possess a core that contains many cell components, a spore wall, a cortex, a coat, and an exosporium.
    b. The core contains **calcium dipicolinate,** which aids in heat resistance within the core.
  3. **Function:** endospores germinate under favorable nutritional conditions after an activation process that involves damage to the spore coat. They are not reproductive structures.

M. Biofilms are aggregates of bacterial cells that form in soil and marine environments and the surface of **medical implant devices** (e.g., prostheses). They enhance nutrient uptake and often exclude antimicrobials.

II. BACTERIAL GROWTH AND REPLICATION

A. Growth.
  1. **General characteristics: bacterial growth**
    a. Bacterial growth refers to an increase in bacterial cell numbers (multiplication), which results from a programmed increase in the biomass of the bacteria.
    b. It results from bacterial reproduction due to binary fission, which may be characterized by a parameter called **generation time** (the average time required for cell numbers to double).
    c. It may be determined by measuring **cell concentration** (turbidity measurements or cell counting) or **biomass density** (dry weight or protein determinations).
    d. It usually occurs asynchronously (i.e., all cells do not divide at precisely the same moment).
  2. **Cell concentration:**
    a. Cell concentration may be measured by **viable** cell counts involving serial dilutions of sample followed by a determination of colony-forming units on an agar surface.
    b. It may be determined by **particle cell counting** or **turbidimetric density** measurements (includes both viable and nonviable cells).
  3. **Bacterial growth curve** (Fig. 2.3):
    a. The bacterial growth curve involves the inoculation of bacteria from a saturated culture into fresh liquid media. It is unique for a particular nutritional environment.
    b. It is frequently illustrated in a plot of logarithmic number of the number of bacteria versus time; the **generation time** is determined by observing the time necessary for the cells to double in number during the log phase of growth.

  c. The bacterial growth curve consists of **four phases:**
      (1) Lag—metabolite-depleted cells adapt to new environment.
      (2) Exponential or log—cell biomass is synthesized at a constant rate; cells in this stage are generally more susceptible to antibiotics.
      (3) Stationary—cells exhaust essential nutrients or accumulate toxic products.
      (4) Death or decline—cells may die due to toxic products.
 4. **Synchronous growth:**
      a. This type of growth refers to a situation in which all the bacteria in a culture divide at the same moment.

A.   Bacterial Growth and Division

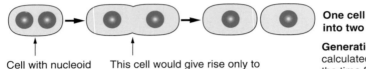

One cell always divides into two cells!

Cell with nucleoid already duplicated

This cell would give rise only to one colony, so a "viable" count = 1. With optical density or cell mass, it would look like 2.

Generation time (always calculated in log phase) is the time for one cell to divide into two.

1→2→4→8→16→32→64→128→etc.

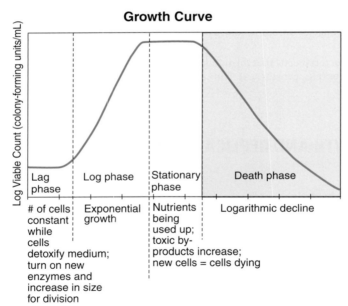

Growth Curve

Typical Problem:

A broth is inoculated to 2×10^2 cells/mL. If the lag phase is 20 minutes and the generation time is 10 minutes, how many cells are there at the end of 60 minutes? (Work problem and then check your work below.)

Log Viable Count (colony-forming units/mL)

Lag phase | Log phase | Stationary phase | Death phase

# of cells constant while cells detoxify medium; turn on new enzymes and increase in size for division | Exponential growth | Nutrients being used up; toxic by-products increase; new cells = cells dying | Logarithmic decline

B.   Answer to Growth Curve Problem

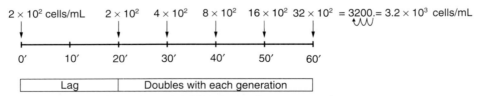

2×10^2 cells/mL 2×10^2 4×10^2 8×10^2 16×10^2 32×10^2 = 3200.= 3.2×10^3 cells/mL

0′   10′   20′   30′   40′   50′   60′

Lag | Doubles with each generation

FIGURE 2.3. Bacterial growth and division. **(A)** Binary fission (which is asexual), growth curve, and typical problem. **(B)** Explanation of growth curve problem. (Updated from Hawley LB. *High-Yield Microbiology and Infectious Diseases*. 2nd ed. Baltimore, MD: Lippincott Williams & Wilkins; 2007.)

    b. It may be achieved by several methods, including thymidine starvation (thymidine-requiring bacteria), alternate cycles of low and optimal incubation temperatures, spore germination, selective filtration of old (large) and young (small) cells, or "trapped cell" filtration.

B. Cultivation.
  1. General characteristics: bacterial cultivation
    a. Bacterial cultivation refers to the propagation of bacteria based on their specific pH, gaseous, and temperature preferences.
    b. It is performed in either liquid (broth) or solid (agar) growth medium and requires an environment that contains:
      (1) A carbon source
      (2) A nitrogen source
      (3) An energy source
      (4) Inorganic salts
      (5) Growth factors
      (6) Electron donors and acceptors
  2. Superoxide dismutase is an enzyme in aerobes and facultative and aerotolerant anaerobes that allows them to grow in the presence of the superoxide free radical (O_2^-).
    a. This enzyme carries out the reaction $2O_2^- + 2H^+ \rightarrow H_2O_2 + O_2$.
    b. This reaction produces hydrogen peroxide (H_2O_2), which is toxic to cells but is destroyed by **catalase** or is oxidized by a peroxidase enzyme.

C. Oxygen requirements.
  1. Obligate aerobes: require oxygen for growth; contain superoxide dismutase, which protects them from the toxic O_2^-.
  2. Obligate anaerobes: are killed by the O_2; grow maximally at a pO_2 concentration of less than 0.5% to 3%.
    a. They lack superoxide dismutase, catalase, and cytochrome-C oxidase (enzymes that destroy toxic products of oxygen metabolism).
    b. Instead of oxygen, they require another substance such as a hydrogen acceptor during the generation of metabolic energy and utilize **fermentation pathways** with distinctive metabolic products.
    c. General characteristics:
      (1) Outnumber aerobes 1000:1 in the gut and 100:1 in the mouth.
      (2) Comprise 99% of the total fecal flora (10^{11}/g of stool in the large bowel).
      (3) Usually cause polymicrobial infections, those involving more than one genus or species.
      (4) Are foul smelling.
    d. They generally are found proximal to mucosal surfaces, but can escape into tissues by:
      (1) Gastrointestinal obstruction or surgery
      (2) Diverticulitis
      (3) Bronchial obstruction
      (4) Tumor growth
      (5) Ulceration of the intestinal tract by chemotherapeutic agents
  3. Facultative anaerobes: grow in the presence or absence of oxygen.
    a. They shift from a fermentative to a respiratory metabolism in the presence of air.
    b. Their energy needs are met by consuming less glucose under a respiratory metabolism than under a fermentative metabolism **(Pasteur effect)**.
    c. Most **pathogenic bacteria** are facultative anaerobes.
  4. Aerotolerant anaerobes: resemble facultative bacteria but have a fermentative metabolism both with and without an oxygen environment.

D. Nutritional requirements.
  1. Heterotrophs require preformed organic compounds (e.g., sugar, amino acids) for growth.
  2. Autotrophs do not require preformed organic compounds for growth because they can synthesize them from inorganic compounds and carbon dioxide.

E. Growth media.
   1. **Minimal essential growth medium:**
      a. This medium contains only the primary precursor compounds essential for growth.
      b. A bacterium grown in this medium must synthesize most of the organic compounds required for its growth.
      c. Generation time is relatively slow.
   2. **Complex growth medium:**
      a. This medium contains most of the organic compound building blocks (e.g., sugars, amino acids, nucleotides) necessary for growth.
      b. Generation time for a bacterium is faster relative to its generation time in minimal essential medium.
      c. Fastidious bacteria are grown in this medium.
   3. **Differential growth medium** (Table 2.2):
      a. This medium contains a combination of nutrients and pH indicators to allow the visual distinction of bacteria that grow on or in it.
      b. Colonies of particular bacterial species have a distinctive color.
   4. **Selective growth medium** (see Table 2.2):
      a. This medium contains compounds that prevent the growth of some bacteria while allowing the growth of other bacteria.
      b. Dyes or sugars, antibiotics, high salt concentration, or pH are used to achieve selectivity.

F. Metabolism.
   1. **General characteristics:**
      a. **Bacterial metabolism** is the sum of **anabolic processes** (synthesis of cellular constituents requiring energy) and **catabolic processes** (breakdown of cellular constituents with concomitant release of waste products and energy-rich compounds).
         (1) Pathogenic bacteria exhibit **heterotrophic** metabolism.
         (2) Metabolism can vary depending on the nutritional environment.
      b. **Bacterial transport systems** involve membrane-associated binding or transport proteins for sugars and amino acids.
         (1) Energy is frequently required to concentrate substrates inside the cell.
         (2) Transport is usually inducible for nutrients that are catabolized; glucose, which is constitutive, is an exception.
         (3) Phosphotransferase systems are frequently used for sugar transport.

t a b l e **2.2**	Representative Differential and Selective Growth Medias	
Media	Bacteria Identified	Identification Mechanism
Blood agar	Hemolytic bacteria (Staphylococcal and Streptococcal species)	Defibrillated blood in nutrient agar base provides identification of α-hemolytic (green zone around colonies) and β-hemolytic (clear zone around colonies).
Hektoen-enteric agar	Enteric Gram-negative rods (E. coli, Klebsiella, **Salmonella**, and **Shigella**)	Contains bile salts, thiosulfate, ferric ammonium citrate, and lactose, and sucrose. Gram-positives are inhibited and lactose/sucrose fermenters and H_2S producers are observed.
MacConkey agar	Enteric Gram-negative rods (E. coli, Klebsiella, Salmonella, Shigella, and Proteus)	Contains bile salts, crystal violet, lactose, and neutral red pH indicator. Bile salts and crystal violet inhibit Gram-positives; only Gram-negatives that ferment lactose give the colonies a color that determines species.
Löwenstein-Jensen graft media	**Mycobacteria**	Is a glycerated egg-potato media (provides fatty acids and proteins) containing malachite green dye, penicillin, and nalidixic acid to inhibit Gram-positive and some Gram-negative organisms.
Thayer-Martin and Martin-Lewis medium	**Neisseria** species	Variants of chocolate agar (blood agar containing gently heat-lysed RBCs to provide nutrients) and antibiotics to inhibit most normal respiratory and genital flora.

2. **Carbohydrate metabolism:**
   a. **Fermentation** is a method of obtaining metabolic energy that is characterized by **substrate phosphorylation.**
      (1) **Adenosine triphosphate (ATP)** formation is not coupled to electron transfer.
      (2) An organic electron acceptor (e.g., pyruvate) is required.
      (3) Specific metabolic end products are synthesized, which may aid in the identification of bacterial species.
   b. **Respiration** refers to the method of obtaining metabolic energy that involves **oxidative phosphorylation.**
      (1) ATP is formed during electron transfer and the reduction of gaseous oxygen in aerobic respiration.
      (2) A cell membrane electron transport chain composed of cytochrome enzymes, lipid cofactors, and coupling factors is used during this process.
3. **Regulation:**
   a. **Regulation of enzyme activity:**
      (1) Enzymes are **allosteric proteins,** susceptible to binding of effector molecules that influence their activity.
      (2) **Feedback inhibition** involves the end product.
      (3) **Substrate-binding enhancement** regulates catalytic activity.
   b. **Regulation of enzyme synthesis** may involve the following mechanisms:
      (1) Allosteric regulatory proteins that activate (**activators**) or inhibit (**repressors**) gene transcription.
      (2) **End-product feedback repression** of biosynthetic pathway enzymes.
      (3) **Substrate induction** of catabolic enzymes.
      (4) **Attenuation control sequences** in enzyme mRNA.
      (5) **Catabolite repression,** which is under positive control of the **catabolite activator protein.**
   c. **Pasteur effect** is caused by oxygen blocking the fermentative capacity of **facultative bacteria.** The energy needs of the bacteria are met by using less glucose during aerobic growth.

G. **Cell wall synthesis** (Fig. 2.4).
   1. Cell wall synthesis involves the cytoplasmic synthesis of peptidoglycan subunits, which are translocated by a membrane lipid carrier and cross-linked to the existing cell wall by enzymes associated with the plasma membrane of Gram-positive bacteria or found in the periplasmic region of Gram-negative bacteria.
   2. In Gram-positive cells, it involves the covalent linkage of teichoic acid to *N*-acetylmuramic acid residues.
   3. In Gram-negative cells, three components (lipoprotein, outer membrane, lipopolysaccharide) are added, whose constituents or subunits are synthesized on or in the cytoplasmic membrane and assembled outside of the cell.

III. BACTERIAL VIRUSES

A. **General characteristics. Bacteriophages** are bacterial viruses that are frequently called **phages.**
   1. These obligate intracellular parasites are host-specific infectious agents for bacteria.
   2. **Bacteriophage virions** are complete (genetic material and capsid) infectious particles.
   3. Major components are protein and RNA or DNA.

B. **Morphologic classes of bacteriophages.**
   1. **Polyhedral phages** are usually composed of an outer polyhedral-shaped protein coat (capsid), which surrounds the nucleic acid.
      a. They may contain a lipid bilayer between two protein capsid layers (PM-2 phage).

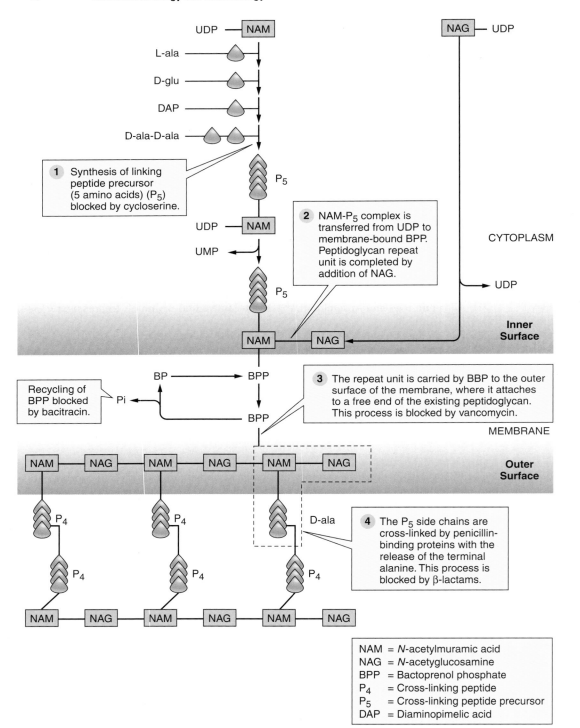

FIGURE 2.4. Synthesis of peptidoglycan.

    b. Their **genetic material** consists of one of the following:
      (1) Circular double-stranded (PM-2) DNA.
      (2) Single-stranded DNA (θX174 and M-12).
      (3) Linear single-stranded RNA (MS2 and Qβ).
      (4) One phage (θ6) that has three pieces of double-stranded RNA.

2. Filamentous phages have a filamentous protein capsid that surrounds a circular single-stranded DNA genome (f1 and M-13).
    a. They infect bacteria through the host's sex pili; thus, they are male-bacteria-specific. (Pili are only present on male bacteria.)
    b. They do not lyse their host cells during the replication process.

3. Complex phages have a protein polyhedral head containing linear double-stranded DNA, a protein tail, and other appendages. They include the T and lambda phages of *Escherichia coli.*

C. Genetic classes of bacteriophages.

1. RNA phages refer to all phages with RNA as their genetic material.
    a. These phages are specific for bacteria with male pili (male specific).
    b. The RNA is single-stranded (except for θ6, see X B-1). It can act as polycistronic mRNA.

2. DNA phages refer to all phages with DNA as their genetic material.
    a. They contain nucleic acid bases that are frequently glycosylated or methylated.
    b. Some of the nucleic acid bases are unusual, such as 5-hydroxymethyl cytosine or 5-hydroxymethyl uracil.
    c. Two classes are recognized: **virulent** or **temperate,** depending on whether their pattern of replication is strictly lytic (virulent) or alternates between lytic and lysogenic (temperate).

D. Bacteriophage replication.

1. General characteristics: Phages replicate by using the biosynthetic machinery of the host cell. During replication, the phage genome is injected into the host cell. (Filamentous phages are the exception.)
    a. The basic sequence of events includes adsorption; penetration; phage-specific transcription, translation, or both; assembly; and release.
    b. It is initiated by the interaction of phage receptors and specific bacterial surface receptor sites.
    c. Two patterns are recognized for DNA phages: **lytic** or **lysogenic.**
    d. For virulent phages, replication is usually complete in 30 to 60 minutes.

2. Lytic replication (also known as productive replication) occurs all of the time when a virulent virus replicates in a permissive host (Fig. 2.5A) and may occur with temperate phages.
    a. Strains of bacteria can be identified based on their lysis by a selected set of phages, a process called **phage typing.**
    b. **One-step growth curve** is the result of an experimental situation in which one cycle of lytic phage replication is monitored.
      (1) It plots the amount of infectious virus produced versus time after infection using a **plaque assay,** an infectious-center assay in which counts are made of focal areas of phage-induced lysis on a lawn of bacteria.
      (2) **Data** obtained from the one-step growth curve includes:
        (a) **Replication time:** average time necessary for a phage to replicate within a specific host cell and be released from that cell.
        (b) **Burst size:** number of infectious phages produced from each infecting phage.
        (c) **Eclipse period:** time from infection to the synthesis of the first intracellular infectious virus.

3. Lysogenic replication occurs only in **temperate phages** (*E. coli* phage lambda) (see Fig. 2.5B).
    a. The synthesis of a phage-specific **repressor protein** inhibits phage-specific transcription, thus limiting phage-specific protein synthesis. If the phage repressor protein is destroyed, the phage can revert to lytic replication.

Lytic Replication of Phage

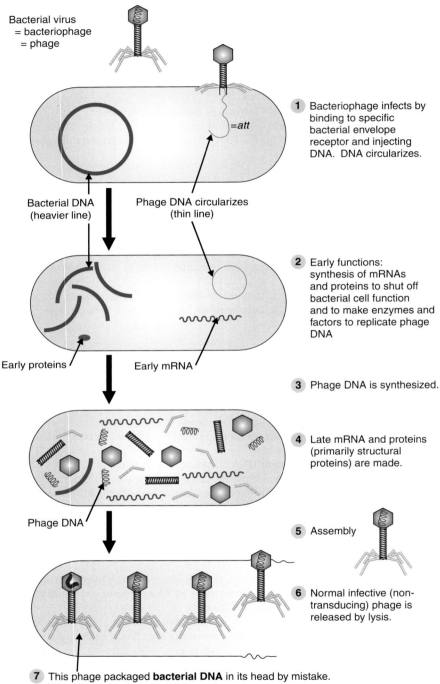

Bacterial virus
  = bacteriophage
  = phage

=att

1 Bacteriophage infects by binding to specific bacterial envelope receptor and injecting DNA. DNA circularizes.

Bacterial DNA
(heavier line)

Phage DNA circularizes
(thin line)

2 Early functions: synthesis of mRNAs and proteins to shut off bacterial cell function and to make enzymes and factors to replicate phage DNA

Early proteins

Early mRNA

3 Phage DNA is synthesized.

4 Late mRNA and proteins (primarily structural proteins) are made.

Phage DNA

5 Assembly

6 Normal infective (non-transducing) phage is released by lysis.

7 This phage packaged **bacterial DNA** in its head by mistake. It is called a **transducing phage.** Because any gene can be incorporated (depending on what bacterial DNA is incorporated), it is called a **generalized transducing phage.**

FIGURE 2.5A. Lytic replication. Note that this productive cycle always occurs in virulent phage and may also occur in temperate phage. (Updated from Hawley LB. *High-Yield Microbiology and Infectious Diseases.* 2nd ed. Baltimore, MD: Lippincott, Williams & Wilkins; 2007.)

Induction/excision of prophage

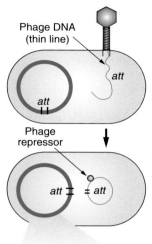

1 The temperate phage Lambda (λ) is shown. Lambda phage binds to specific receptors and injects DNA, which circularizes.

2 If functional repressor protein is made quickly enough, it inhibits transcription of structural proteins and active production of virus, allowing the virus DNA to integrate.

Phage could have gone into lytic life cycle here if the regulatory battles had gone differently.

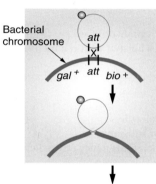

3 Enlarged view of **integration of lambda DNA**: Note that both molecules of DNA have a small area of homology (*att* sites) where the pairing and crossing over occur. This is a classic example of site-specific recombination where the whole molecule is integrated rather than an exchange taking place. Note that *att* site is between the bacterial genes *gal* and *bio*.

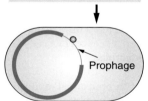

4 This is a **lysogenized cell** (state is called **lysogeny**). When the host bacterial DNA duplicates, so does the phage DNA. As long as the repressor protein continues to be made and is functioning, lysogeny will continue.

5 Prophage integration is somewhat analogous to integration of HIV DNA copy into the human chromosome, where it resides as a provirus.

FIGURE 2.5B. Temperate phage infection: lysogeny. (Updated from Hawley LB. *High-Yield Microbiology and Infectious Diseases*. 2nd ed. Baltimore, MD: Lippincott, Williams & Wilkins; 2007.)

   b. Prophage (phage DNA) is incorporated into specific attachment sites in the host-cell DNA.

      (1) The incorporation of prophage confers immunity to infection by phages of a type similar to the infecting phage.

      (2) The prophage is passed to succeeding generations of the bacteria.

   c. Specialized or restricted transducing phages may be generated.

   d. Lysogenic replication may result in **lysogenic phage conversion,** a change in the phenotype of the bacteria as a result of limited expression of genes within a prophage. This mechanism occurs in the following situations:

      (1) In *Salmonella*, O polysaccharides are changed when lysogenized by the temperate bacteriophage epsilon.

      (2) Conversion of nontoxigenic strains of *Corynebacterium diphtheriae* to toxin-producing strains.

      (3) Conversion of nontoxigenic *Clostridium botulinum* types C and D to toxin-producing strains.

IV. GENETICS

A. Comparison of bacterial and eukaryotic genomes.

   1. Eukaryotic genome:

     a. Structure: The eukaryotic genome:

       (1) Is **diploid** with two homologous copies of each chromosome, except in some fungi.

       (2) Is contained in two or more linear chromosomes located within a membrane-bound nucleus.

       (3) Contains **introns** (DNA sequences not translated into gene products) and redundant genetic information.

     b. Replication:

       (1) Begins at several points along the linear DNA molecule.

       (2) Is regulated by specific gene inducer or repressor substances.

       (3) Involves a specialized structure, the **spindle,** which pulls newly formed chromosomes into separate nuclei during mitosis.

   2. Prokaryotic genome:

     a. Structure: The prokaryotic genome is **haploid** (single, circular chromosome encoding several thousand genes). It may contain extra chromosomal pieces of DNA called **plasmids** and moveable genetic elements called **transposons** and **integrons.**

       (1) Plasmids:

         (a) These DNA pieces replicate independently of chromosomal replication.

         (b) They may exist in an **episome** form that can integrate into the bacterial chromosome and replicate with it.

         (c) Plasmids may carry **antibiotic resistance** genes (e.g., EM-1 β-lactamase gene of *E. coli*), **toxin genes** (e.g., enterotoxins of *E. coli*), and transposons.

       (2) Transposons:

         (a) These **moveable genetic elements** are incapable of independent replication.

         (b) They contain insertion sequences and can transfer genetic information by insertion into bacterial chromosome or plasmids.

         (c) They may contain antibiotic resistance genes like *Neisseria gonorrhoeae*, β-lactamase, or virulence factors like the heat-stable enterotoxin of *E. coli.*

       (3) Integrons:

         (a) These **mobile genetic elements** consist of an integrase gene and a series (cassettes) of antibiotic resistance genes plus insertion sequences (attachment sites) and a promoter region controlling all resistance genes (observed in *Mycobacterium tuberculosis* resistance).

         (b) They are not capable of independent replication.

(4) Pathogenicity islands:
   (a) These **groups of virulence-associated** genes code for unique secretion systems, toxins, adhesins, and regulatory proteins and contain integrase and transposase genes.
   (b) They are associated with tRNA genes on bacterial chromosomes or plasmids.
 b. Replication:
   (1) Replicon is a general term for a double-stranded DNA circle (chromosomes, plasmids) capable of self-replication.
   (2) Replicons replicate bidirectionally (5′ PO_4 to 3′ OH) from a fixed origin.

B. Gene transfer in bacteria.

 1. General characteristics:
   a. Genetic variability in microbes is maintained through **gene transfer** followed by **recombination** of allelic forms of genes.
   b. Transfer is most efficient between cells of the same species.
   c. Gene exchange may also occur as the crossing over of homologous chromosomes or by non-homologous means (e.g., movement of plasmids or transposons, insertion of viral genes).
   d. It can result in the acquisition of new characteristics (e.g., antigens, toxins, antibiotic resistance).
   e. Three mechanisms of gene transfer are recognized: conjugation, transduction, and transformation.
 2. Conjugation: a one-way transfer of genetic material (usually plasmids) from donor to recipient by means of physical contact. In Gram-positive cells, contact occurs between a plasmid-encoded adhesin on the donor cell and receptors on the recipient cell. In Gram-negative cells, contact occurs through sex pili. Gram-negative cell conjugation typically involves one of four types of plasmids:
   a. F (fertility) plasmids, which mediate the creation of a sex pilus necessary for conjugal transfer of the F plasmid to the recipient.
     (1) Cells that contain this plasmid are called **F^+**.
     (2) The F plasmid can integrate into chromosomal DNA, creating **high-frequency recombination (Hfr)** donors from which chromosomal DNA is readily transferred.
   b. R factors, which contain genes for conjugal transfer and genes conferring **drug resistance.**
     (1) Resistance genes are frequently carried on transposons.
     (2) The resistance phenotype is expressed through natural selection.
   c. F′ and R′ plasmids, which are recombinant **fertility** or resistance plasmids in which limited regions of chromosomal DNA can be replicated and transferred by conjugation independently of the chromosome. (Conjugal crosses are shown in Figures 2.6 and 2.7.)
 3. Transduction is the **phage-mediated transfer** of host DNA sequences. It is performed by temperate phages and, under special conditions, by lytic phages. It occurs in two forms:
   a. In **generalized transduction,** by mistake, the phage randomly packages host bacterial DNA inside a bacteriophage coat as was seen back in Figure 2.5A. Thus the transducing particle can transfer any randomly picked up bacterial DNA (Fig. 2.8).
   b. In **specialized transduction,** the lysogenic phage favors the transfer of host DNA segments near the site of prophage integration (Figs. 2.9 and 2.10). Specialized transducing phages contain both viral and host genes.
 4. Transformation is the **direct uptake** and recombination of naked DNA fragments through the cell wall by competent bacteria. Natural occurrence of this process is uncommon (Fig. 2.11).
   a. Surface **competence factors** (DNA receptor enzymes) sometimes mediate transformation. These factors are produced only at a specific point in the bacterial growth cycle.
   b. Bacteria can sometimes be induced into transformation by treatment with calcium chloride and temperature shock.
   c. Transformation is used in recombinant DNA research and commercially to introduce human genes via vectors into bacteria for rapid and large-scale production of human gene products.

Conjugation: F⁺ × F⁻

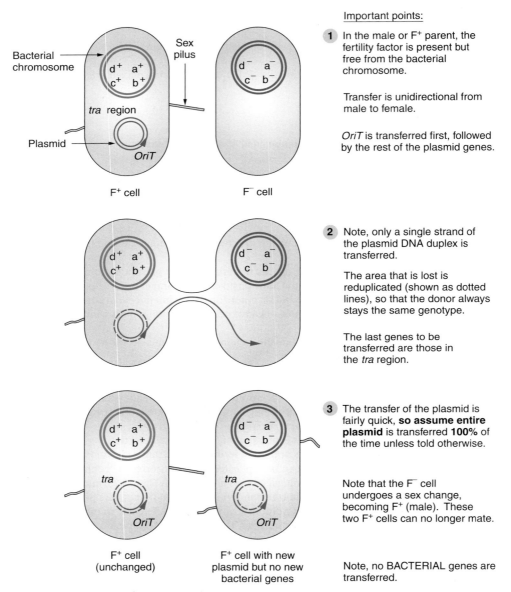

Important points:

1. In the male or F⁺ parent, the fertility factor is present but free from the bacterial chromosome.

   Transfer is unidirectional from male to female.

   OriT is transferred first, followed by the rest of the plasmid genes.

2. Note, only a single strand of the plasmid DNA duplex is transferred.

   The area that is lost is reduplicated (shown as dotted lines), so that the donor always stays the same genotype.

   The last genes to be transferred are those in the *tra* region.

3. The transfer of the plasmid is fairly quick, **so assume entire plasmid is transferred 100%** of the time unless told otherwise.

   Note that the F⁻ cell undergoes a sex change, becoming F⁺ (male). These two F⁺ cells can no longer mate.

   Note, no BACTERIAL genes are transferred.

FIGURE 2.6. Conjugation: F⁺ n F⁻ cross. (Updated from Hawley LB. *High-Yield Microbiology and Infectious Diseases.* 2nd ed. Baltimore, MD: Lippincott Williams & Wilkins; 2007.)

Conjugation: Hfr × F⁻

Important points:

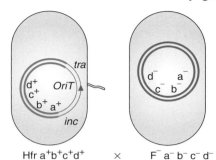

Hfr a⁺b⁺c⁺d⁺   ×   F⁻ a⁻ b⁻ c⁻ d⁻

1 Hfr donor means that the fertility factor (fine red line) is already integrated into the bacterial chromosome (heavier gray line).

In this cross, plasmid genes starting at *OriT* will be transferred first, followed by the bacterial genes in linear order away from the plasmid.

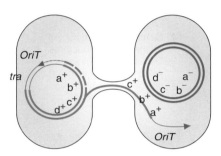

2 Note that as with the F⁺ × F⁻ cross, only a single strand of the DNA duplex is transferred. The area that is transferred is reduplicated (note the rolling model at left), so that the donor always stays the same genotype.

IF the entire chromosome were to be transferred, the last genes to be transferred would be the *tra* region.

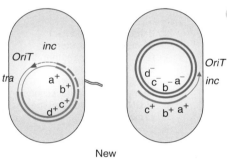

3 It takes approximately 2 hours for a complete transfer to occur. Because the cytoplasmic bridge and DNA are so fine, mating is normally interrupted before the transfer is complete. Assume that mating is interrupted and the recipient gets some new genes but (because it does not get the *tra* operon) does not become Hfr.

New bacterial genes

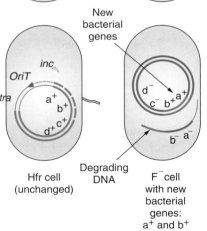

Hfr cell (unchanged)   Degrading DNA   F⁻ cell with new bacterial genes: a⁺ and b⁺

FIGURE 2.7. Conjugation: Hfr × F cross. Newly synthesized DNA is shown as dashed lines. (Updated from Hawley LB. *High-Yield Microbiology and Infectious Diseases.* 2nd ed. Baltimore, MD: Lippincott Williams & Wilkins; 2007.)

Generalized Transduction

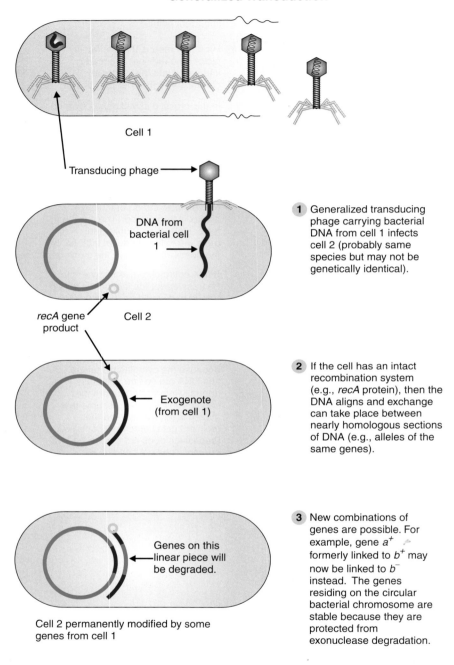

Cell 1

Transducing phage ─────→

DNA from
bacterial cell
1 ────→

recA gene
product

Cell 2

1 Generalized transducing
phage carrying bacterial
DNA from cell 1 infects
cell 2 (probably same
species but may not be
genetically identical).

Exogenote
(from cell 1) ←────

2 If the cell has an intact
recombination system
(e.g., recA protein), then the
DNA aligns and exchange
can take place between
nearly homologous sections
of DNA (e.g., alleles of the
same genes).

Genes on this
←──── linear piece will
be degraded.

Cell 2 permanently modified by some
genes from cell 1

3 New combinations of
genes are possible. For
example, gene a^+
formerly linked to b^+ may
now be linked to b^-
instead. The genes
residing on the circular
bacterial chromosome are
stable because they are
protected from
exonuclease degradation.

In generalized transduction, every bacterial gene has an equal chance
of being incorporated into the phage head and being transferred to the
next bacterial cell that is infected.

FIGURE 2.8. Generalized transduction. (Updated from Hawley LB. *High-Yield Microbiology and Infectious Diseases.* 2nd ed. Baltimore, MD: Lippincott Williams & Wilkins; 2007.)

Production of specialized transducing virus
(Pathway on the right hand side)

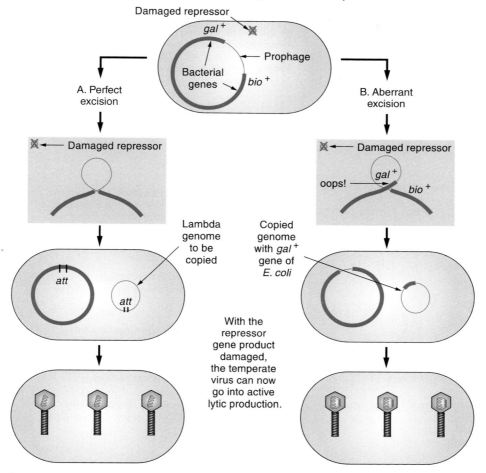

FIGURE 2.9. Transduction: induction/excision of prophage. If the repressor in a lysogenized cell is damaged by ultraviolet light, cold, or alkylating agents, the cell is "induced" into active virus production, which begins with the excision of the prophage DNA. Excision is the reverse of site-specific integration. The normal process of induction/excision of a prophage leading to active temperate phage replication is shown in **(A)**. Aberrant excision leading to production of a specialized transducing phage is shown in **(B)**. (Updated from Hawley LB. *High-Yield Microbiology and Infectious Diseases.* 2nd ed. Baltimore, MD: Lippincott Williams & Wilkins; 2007.)

Specialized Transduction = Restricted Transduction

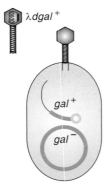

λ.dgal⁺

gal⁺

gal⁻

E. coli gal⁻ cell infected
with a transducing
phage carrying gal⁺

1 Specialized transducing phage created by an
excisional error coming out of lysogeny to lytic
replication of the phage. This defective phage has
some lambda genes and the bacterial gene gal⁺.

2 Transducing gal⁺ phage has now injected its DNA
into a gal⁻ cell.

3 The phage nucleic acid recircularizes in the new cell
and may either undergo reinsertion (the whole circular
molecule) or homologous recombination. Either way
in this cell, some gal⁺ cells may result.

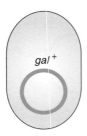

gal⁺

Now gal⁺

Summary of Specialized Transduction
1. Specialized transducing phage are produced by
an excisional error.

2. Only the genes that adjoin the insertion site
(att) of a temperate phage can be integrated
into the phage.

3. Transduced genes may be stabilized by
recombination.

FIGURE 2.10. Specialized or restricted transduction. (Updated from Hawley LB. *High-Yield
Microbiology and Infectious Diseases.* 2nd ed. Baltimore, MD: Lippincott Williams & Wilkins;
2007.)

C. Gene expression.
   1. Transcription is the transfer of DNA-bound protein synthesis instructions to mRNA. A short
     sequence of DNA bases is unwound and complementary ribonucleotide bases are aligned
     onto the DNA template.
     a. In bacteria, it is mediated by **RNA polymerase** and initiated by the binding of **sigma factor,**
       a subunit of RNA polymerase, to the **promoter region** of the DNA molecule.
     b. Transcription occurs in a 5' PO_4 to 3' OH direction.
   2. **Translation** is the assembly of polypeptide chains from the mRNA transcript.
     a. It occurs at the ribosomes.
     b. Amino acids are linked together via tRNAs in accordance with the triplet-encoded mRNA
       transcript.
   3. **Regulation of expression:**
     a. **Operon model:** Expression is regulated **primarily during transcription** and is determined
       partly by the ability of the **DNA promoter region** to bind with sigma factor. Expression is fa-
       cilitated or blocked by regulator proteins binding to operator sequences near the promoter.
       An operator controls a group of genes called an **operon.**
     b. **Negative control** is inhibition of transcription by the binding of a repressor protein.
       (1) *Lac* **operon:**
         (a) This operon controls expression of three structural genes for lactose metabolism
           via a repressor protein.

Gene Transfer: Bacterial Transformation

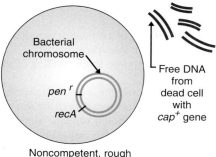

Bacterial chromosome

Free DNA from dead cell with *cap⁺* gene

pen ʳ

recA

Noncompetent, rough (nonencapsulated) *Streptococcus pneumoniae*

1 A bacterium, in this case a *Streptococcus pneumoniae* carrying the gene for capsular formation, has died and released its nucleic acid near a normal, noncompetent, nonvirulent but penicillin-resistant (*penʳ*) *S. pneumoniae*. (It is nonvirulent because it cannot make capsules.)

Most bacteria do not bind and take up DNA, but under certain growth conditions, the ability to do this (called *competency*) occurs. **Competent cells can bind and take up DNA. Competency is required for transformation.**

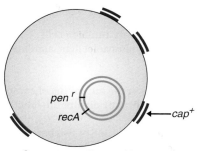

pen ʳ

recA

cap⁺

Competent cell now able to bind DNA

2 The extracellular free DNA binds to the competent cell and is taken up. (Details like single-strand take-up are not important.)

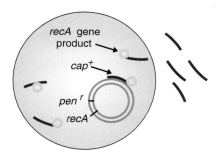

recA gene product

cap⁺

pen ʳ

recA

3 As long as the cell has a functioning recombination system (represented by the circle labeled *recA* gene product), each DNA can find its area of near homology, and **homologous recombination** may mediate the exchange of nearly homologous pieces of DNA.

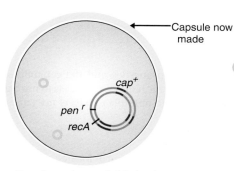

Capsule now made

cap⁺

pen ʳ

recA

Transformed smooth (virulent) *Streptococcus pneumoniae*

4 Stabilization of some genes by homologous recombination has occurred, and the cell has duplicated. The cell is now permanently able to make capsules.

FIGURE 2.11. Gene transfer: bacterial transformation. (Updated from Hawley LB. *High-Yield Microbiology and Infectious Diseases*. 2nd ed. Baltimore, MD: Lippincott Williams & Wilkins; 2007.)

(b) Transcription is induced by the presence of lactose (allolactose), which binds to the repressor protein and frees the *lac* operator.

(2) *Trp* **operon:**
(a) This operon controls **tryptophan synthesis.**
(b) Synthesis of tryptophan is halted by the binding of a repressor protein (tryptophan complex) to the *trp* operator when excess tryptophan is available.

c. Positive control is the initiation of transcription in response to the binding of an activator protein.
(1) Expression of the *ara* operon proceeds only when arabinose binds to a special protein, forming an activator compound necessary for the transcription of the *ara* operon.
(2) Cyclic adenosine monophosphate (cyclic AMP) binding protein, when bound to a specific DNA sequence near the promoter, enhances the expression of many genes associated with fermentation. Cyclic AMP enhances RNA polymerase activity.

D. Mutation.
1. General description: Mutation is an induced or spontaneous heritable alteration of the DNA sequence. It is the means by which variability is introduced into the gene pool, and changes are made in the phenotype.
a. Frequency: occurs approximately once for any gene in every 1 million cells.
b. Causes: may be caused by various mutagens, including ultraviolet light, acridine dyes, base analogs, and nitrous acid.
2. Mutation types:
a. Nucleotide substitutions arise from mutagenic activity or the mispairing of complimentary bases during DNA replication. They often do not significantly disrupt the function of gene products.
b. Frameshift mutations result from the insertion or deletion of one or two base pairs, disrupting the phase of the triplet-encoded DNA message.
c. Deletions are usually large excisions of DNA, dramatically altering the sequence of coded proteins. They may also result in frameshift mutations.
d. Insertions change genes and their products by integration of new DNA via transposons.
3. Results of mutation:
a. Missense mutations result in the substitution of one amino acid for another. They may be without phenotypic effect (silent mutation).
b. Nonsense mutations terminate protein synthesis and result in truncated gene products. They usually result in inactive protein products.
4. Reversions. Function lost to mutation may be regained in two ways:
a. Genotypic (true) reversion: restoration at the site of DNA alteration.
b. Phenotypic (suppression) reversion: restoration of an activity lost to mutation, often by a mutation at a second site (**suppressor mutation**).

V. BACTERIAL PATHOGENESIS

A. General characteristics.
The pathogenesis of a bacterium depends on its virulence properties and the capabilities of the host's defense mechanism. Normal flora may become pathogenic if they gain access to normally sterile body areas or their environmental conditions allow them to multiply to a level not controlled by the host.

B. Virulence factors.
These features may be genetically encoded on the bacterial chromosome or located on plasmids.
1. Structural bacterial components. These virulence factors include:
a. Antiphagocytic surface proteins and capsules
b. Adhesins that promote colonization
c. Endotoxins of Gram-negative bacteria

    d. Immunoglobulin G (IgG) antibody binding surface proteins

    e. Antigenic switching of surface antigens due to phase variation or antigenic variation processes

2. Extracellular gene products. These include:

    a. Degradative enzymes like collagenase and hyaluronidase that facilitate tissue invasion

    b. IgA antibody-degrading proteases

    c. Exotoxins

    d. Protein secretion systems

3. Growth properties include the capacity for intracellular growth and the ability to form biofilms.

C. Toxins.

1. Endotoxins consist of the lipid A component of Gram-negative bacteria. Endotoxins have the following **actions:**

    a. Induce the release of endogenous pyrogens (e.g., interleukin 1 [IL-1], tumor necrosis factor [TNF], prostaglandins, etc.).

    b. Increase vascular permeability.

    c. Initiate complement and blood coagulation cascades.

    d. Cause fever, hypotension, disseminated intracellular coagulation, and shock.

2. Exotoxins are secreted by Gram-positive and Gram-negative bacteria; they may be genetically encoded in the bacterial chromosome, a plasmid, or a phage.

    a. Actions. They have the following five mechanisms of action (see Table 2.3):

        (1) Alter cellular components.

        (2) Act as superantigens that cause inappropriate release of cytokines.

t a b l e   2.3   Examples of Bacterial Exotoxins

Biological Effect	Toxin Name	Organism	Gene Location	Mechanism
Alter Cellular Components	α toxin	*Staphylococcus aureus*	Bacterial chromosome	Forms pore
	Streptolysin 0	*Streptococcus pyogenes*	Bacterial chromosome	Forms pore
	α toxin	*Clostridium perfringens*	Bacterial chromosome and plasmid	Disrupts membranes
	Type III cytotoxin	*Pseudomonas aeruginosa*	Phage	Cytoskeletal changes
	Type III cytotoxin	*Salmonella* species	Bacterial chromosomes	Alters actin cytoskeleton
Superantigens	TSST-1	*Staphylococcus aureus*	Bacterial chromosome	Release of cytokines
	Enterotoxin	*Staphylococcus aureus*	Phage	Release of cytokines
	Erythrogenic toxins A and C	*Streptococcus pyogenes*	Phage	Release of cytokines
Inhibition of Protein Synthesis	Diphtheria toxin	*Corynebacterium diphtheriae*	Phage	ADP ribosylates elongation factor 2
	Exotoxin A	*Pseudomonas aeruginosa*	Bacterial chromosome	ADP ribosylates elongation factor 2
	Shiga toxin	*Shigella dysenteriae*	Plasmid	Inactivates 60S ribosomes
	Vero toxin (also called Shiga-like toxin)	Enterohemorrhagic *E. coli*	Bacterial chromosome or phage	Inactivates 60S ribosomes
Increased Synthesis of cAMP	Cholera toxin	*Vibrio cholerae*	Bacterial chromosome	Turns on stimulatory G protein
	LT toxin ST toxin	Enterotoxigenic *E. coli*	Plasmid	Turns on stimulatory G protein
	Anthrax toxin	*Bacillus anthracis*	Plasmid	Adenylate cyclase activity
	Pertussis toxin	*Bordetella pertussis*	Bacterial chromosome	Turns off inhibitory G protein
Altered Nerve Impulse Transmission	Tetanus toxin	*Clostridium tetani*	Plasmid	Inhibits inhibitory neurotransmitter release
	Botulinum toxin	*Clostridium botulinum*	Phage	Inhibits acetylcholine release

      (3) Inhibit protein synthesis.
      (4) Increase cAMP.
      (5) Alter nerve impulse transmission.
  b. Examples
      (1) Some exotoxins (e.g., Shiga toxin and cholera toxin) have an **A-B subunit structure** in which one or more B subunits are involved in binding and the A subunit possesses the biological activity inside the cell.
      (2) Others are a single polypeptide with:
        (a) Enzymatic activity (e.g., α toxin of *Clostridium perfringens,* which has phospholipase-C activity).
        (b) Other biological activities (e.g., superantigens like toxic shock syndrome toxin 1 [TSST- 1] of *S. aureus*).
  c. Toxoids are chemically altered forms of toxins that may be used as immunization agents. Toxoids induce antibodies that minimize the toxin's biological effects (e.g., diphtheria and tetanus toxins).

VI. HOST DEFENSES TO BACTERIA (SEE CHAPTER 12)

A. Types. Host defenses include:
  1. Nonspecific, antigen-independent mechanisms like anatomic and physiological barriers including skin, lysozyme in tears, stomach acidity, and so on.
  2. Specific antigen-dependent mechanisms involving humoral and cell-mediated immunity.

B. They can become harmful and contribute to the disease process by inducing the formation of auto antibodies (e.g., M proteins of *S. pyogenes* ab-ag complexes can damage the kidneys and lead to acute poststreptococcal glomerulonephritis).

VII. ANTIMICROBIAL CHEMOTHERAPY

A. General characteristics.
  1. Antimicrobial chemotherapy is based on the principle of **selective toxicity,** which implies that a compound is harmful to a microorganism but less damaging to its host.
  2. The **drugs** used in antimicrobial therapy have the following properties (Fig. 2.12):
    a. Are **antimetabolites.**
    b. Inhibit cell wall biosynthesis.
    c. Inhibit protein synthesis.
    d. Inhibit nucleic acid synthesis.
    e. Alter or inhibit cell membrane permeability or **transport.**
  3. Antimicrobial drugs can be either **bacteriostatic** (inhibit growth) or **bactericidal** (kill).
  4. Synergistic combinations of bacteriostatic drugs (e.g., trimethoprim and sulfamethoxazole) are sometimes used in antimicrobial therapy.
  5. Antimicrobial activity can be quantitated and may be modified in certain situations.
    a. A **dilution** or **diffusion** test is used to determine antimicrobial activity, which is quantitated by determining the minimal inhibitory concentration.
    b. Antimicrobial activity may differ in vitro and in vivo.
    c. Drug stability, pH, microbial environment, number of microorganisms present, length of incubation with drug, and metabolic activity of microorganisms can alter antimicrobial actions of certain drugs.
    d. Genetic or **nongenetic drug resistance** may modify the antimicrobial activity of a drug for a specific bacterium.

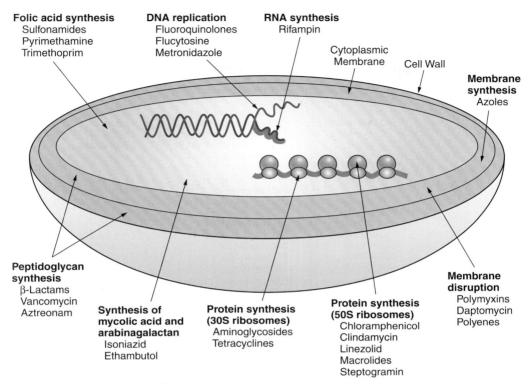

Folic acid synthesis
Sulfonamides
Pyrimethamine
Trimethoprim

DNA replication
Fluoroquinolones
Flucytosine
Metronidazole

RNA synthesis
Rifampin

Cytoplasmic
Membrane   Cell Wall

Membrane synthesis
Azoles

Peptidoglycan synthesis
β-Lactams
Vancomycin
Aztreonam

Synthesis of mycolic acid and arabinagalactan
Isoniazid
Ethambutol

Protein synthesis (30S ribosomes)
Aminoglycosides
Tetracyclines

Protein synthesis (50S ribosomes)
Chloramphenicol
Clindamycin
Linezolid
Macrolides
Steptogramin

Membrane disruption
Polymyxins
Daptomycin
Polyenes

FIGURE 2.12. Sites of antibiotic activity.

B. Mechanisms of action (Table 2.4).

1. **Antimetabolites** are structural analogs of normal metabolites that inhibit the action of specific enzymes.
   a. They include **bacteriostatic** (sulfonamide and trimethoprim) and **bactericidal** (isoniazid) drugs.
   b. Some combinations of individual antimetabolites are bactericidal (e.g., trimethoprim and sulfamethoxazole).
2. **Cell wall synthesis inhibitors** are **bactericidal.**
   a. **General characteristics:**
      (1) **Mechanisms of action:**
         (a) β-lactam drugs inhibit transpeptidation (cross-linking) of peptidoglycan (e.g., penicillins, cephalosporins, and carbapenems).
         (b) Others inhibit the synthesis of peptidoglycan (cycloserine, bacitracin, vancomycin).
      (2) **Location of action:** They may act in the cytoplasm (cycloserine); in the membrane (bacitracin, penicillins, and cephalosporins); or in the cell wall (vancomycin).
      (3) Cell wall synthesis is required for these drugs to be effective.
      (4) Bacteria may take on aberrant shapes or become **spheroplasts** when exposed to these drugs.
   b. **Penicillins** inhibit the transpeptidation enzymes involved in cell wall synthesis. Additionally, they:
      (1) Are active against **Gram-positive bacteria** and **Gram-negative bacteria**.
      (2) React with **penicillin-binding proteins**.
      (3) Have a β-lactam ring structure that is inactivated by β-lactamases (penicillinases), which are genetically coded in some bacterial DNA or some R plasmids.

table **2.4**	Properties of Antibacterial Agents			
Mechanism of Action	**Agent**	**Site of Action**	**Effect**	**Resistance***
Inhibitors of cell wall biosynthesis	Cycloserine	Peptidoglycan tetrapeptide side chain	Bactericidal	2
	Bacitracin	Membrane carrier molecule	Bactericidal	2
	β-Lactams			
	Penicillins	Peptidoglycan cross-linking	Bactericidal	1
	Cephalosporins	Peptidoglycan cross-linking	Bactericidal	1, 2, 3
	Carbapenems	Peptidoglycan cross-linking	Bactericidal	2, 3
	Vancomycin	Translocation of cell wall intermediates	Bactericidal	2, 3
Inhibitors of protein biosynthesis	Aminoglycosides			
	Streptomycin	30S ribosomal subunit	Bactericidal	1, 2, 3
	Kanamycin	30S ribosomal subunit	Bactericidal	1, 2, 3
	Gentamicin	30S ribosomal subunit	Bactericidal	1, 2, 3
	Tetracyclines	30S ribosomal subunit	Bacteriostatic	1, 2, 3, 4
	Spectinomycin	30S ribosomal subunit	Bacteriostatic	1, 2
	Chloramphenicol	50S ribosomal subunit	Bacteriostatic	1, 2, 3
	Erythromycin	50S ribosomal subunit	Bacteriostatic	1, 2, 3, 4
	Clindamycin	50S ribosomal subunit	Bacteriostatic	1, 3
	Linezolid	50S ribosomal subunit	Bacteriostatic	2
Inhibitors of nucleic acid synthesis	Quinolones	DNA gyrase and Topoisomerase IV	Bactericidal	2, 4
	Novobiocin	DNA gyrase and Topoisomerase IV	Bacteriostatic	
	Rifampin	DNA-dependent RNA polymerase	Bactericidal	2
	Metronidazole	Disrupts DNA	Bactericidal	2
Inhibitors of folate metabolism	Sulfonamides	Dihydropteroate synthetase	Bacteriostatic	2, 3, 5
	Dapsone	Dihydropteroate synthetase	Bacteriostatic	2
	Trimethoprim	Dihydrofolate reductase	Bacteriostatic	5
Inhibitor of mycolic acid synthesis	Isoniazid	Mycobacterial mycolic acid biosynthesis	Bactericidal	2
Inhibitor of arabinogalactan synthesis	Ethambutol	Arabinogalactan synthesis	Bacteriostatic	2
Alteration of cytoplasmic membrane	Polymyxins	Bacterial membrane permeability	Bactericidal	
	Colistin	Bacterial membrane permeability	Bactericidal	
	Daptomycin	Depolarization of membrane	Bactericidal	

*1 Drug inactivation
2 Target site mutation
3 ↓ Uptake
4 ↑ Efflux
5 New plasmid-coded enzyme

    c. Cephalosporins have a mechanism of action similar to that of penicillin. They also:

       (1) Are active against both Gram-positive and Gram-negative bacteria.

       (2) Contain a β-lactam ring structure that is inactivated by some β-lactamases.

       (3) Are frequently used to treat patients who are allergic to penicillins.

    d. Carbapenems have a mechanism similar to that of penicillin; they have a β-lactam ring fused to a five-carbon ring and are resistant to β-lactamases.

3. Protein synthesis inhibitors are frequently known as **broad-spectrum antibiotics** and require bacterial growth for their effect.

    a. Aminoglycosides include streptomycin, neomycin, kanamycin, and gentamicin.

       (1) Mechanism of action. These drugs are **bactericidal** for Gram-negative bacteria and **bind to the 30S ribosomal subunit,** irreversibly blocking initiation of translation, or cause mRNA misreading (or both). They are not active against anaerobes or intracellular bacteria.

       (2) Their effective concentration range is narrow before toxicity occurs; toxic effects include renal damage and eighth cranial nerve damage (hearing loss).

       (3) Acetylation may modify their action; they also can be **rendered inactive** by enzymes **contained in R plasmids.**

    b. Tetracyclines include doxycycline, tetracycline, and minocycline.

      (1) Mechanism of action. These drugs are **bacteriostatic, bind to the 30S ribosomal subunit,** and prevent binding of aminoacyl tRNA to the acceptor site. They are transported out of or bound to a plasmid-derived protein in cells containing specific tetracycline R plasmids.

      (2) They may be deposited in teeth and bones, which can cause tooth staining and structural problems in the bones of children.

    c. Chloramphenicol:

      (1) Mechanism of action. This drug is **bacteriostatic** for Gram-positive and Gram-negative bacteria, rickettsia, and chlamydia; it **binds to the 50S ribosomal subunit** and inhibits peptide-bond formation.

      (2) The enzyme chloramphenicol acetyltransferase, which is carried on an R plasmid, inactivates chloramphenicol.

    d. Griseofulvin is a **fungistatic** drug that is active against fungi with chitin in their cell walls. It inhibits protein assembly, which interferes with cell division by blocking microtubule assembly.

    e. Macrolides and **lincomycins** include erythromycin (macrolide) and lincomycin and clindamycin (lincomycins).

      (1) Mechanism of action. These drugs are **bacteriostatic** and **bind to the 23S RNA in the 50S ribosomal subunit,** blocking translocation.

      (2) In bacteria that have a mutation in a 50S ribosomal protein or that contain an R plasmid with genetic information, methylation of 23S RNA occurs, rendering these drugs ineffective by preventing the drug from binding.

4. Nucleic acid synthesis inhibitors:

    a. Mechanism of action. These drugs inhibit DNA (quinolones, derivatives of nalidixic acid) or RNA (rifampin) synthesis. They are generally **bactericidal** and are quite toxic to mammalian cells.

    b. Examples:

      (1) Actinomycin and mitomycin bind to strands of DNA or inhibit replication enzymes.

      (2) Nalidixic acid inhibits DNA gyrase activity.

      (3) Rifampin inhibits DNA-dependent RNA polymerase.

5. Mycolic acid synthesis inhibitor (isoniazid) is a **bactericidal** drug that inhibits mycobacterial mycolic acid biosynthesis.

6. Arabinogalactan synthesis inhibitor (ethambutol) is a **bacteriostatic** drug that inhibits arabinogalactan synthesis in mycobacteria.

7. Cytoplasmic membrane inhibitors:

    a. Mechanism of action. These drugs are **bacteriocidal** and alter the permeability properties of the plasma membrane (polymyxin and polyenes) or inhibit fungal membrane lipid synthesis (azoles: miconazole and ketoconazole).

    b. They are effective against Gram-negative (polymyxin) and sterol-containing mycoplasma and fungal (polyenes: nystatin and amphotericin B) infections; used primarily as topical treatment or with severe infections.

    c. They can react with mammalian cell membranes and are therefore toxic.

C. Drug resistance (Fig. 2.13; see Table 2.4).

    1. Nongenetic mechanisms of drug resistance involve loss of specific target structures, such as the cell wall by L forms of bacteria. It may be caused by metabolic inactivity of microorganisms.

    2. Genetic mechanisms of drug resistance. This form may result from either chromosomal or extrachromosomal resistance.

    a. Chromosomal. A chromosomal mutation alters the structure of the receptor of the drug or the permeability of the drug.

    b. Extrachromosonal:

      (1) A plasmid (R factor or R plasmid) that codes for enzymes is introduced; these enzymes degrade the drug (β-**lactamase**) or modify it (**acetyltransferase**). The plasmid may also code for proteins that pump the drug out of the cell in an energy-dependent fashion.

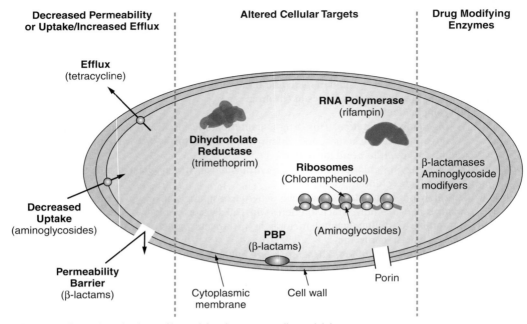

FIGURE 2.13. General mechanisms of bacterial resistance to antibacterial drugs.

(2) The **R factor or R plasmid:**

(a) Contains **insertion sequences** and **transposons.**

(b) Can acquire additional resistance genes by plasmid fusion or from transposons.

(c) Can consist of two components, the **resistance transfer factor (RTF),** which codes for replication and transfer, and the **r or resistance determinant,** which contains genes for replication and resistance.

(d) Can be transmitted from species to species.

(e) Is responsible for the rapid development of multiple drug-resistant bacteria over the past 30 years.

Review Test

Directions: Each of the numbered items or incomplete statements in this section is followed by answers or completions of the statement. Select the ONE lettered answer that is BEST in each case.

1. A bacterial toxin with superantigen activity is produced by

(A) *Clostridium tetani*
(B) *Bordetella pertussis*
(C) *Escherichia coli*
(D) *Staphylococcus aureus*
(E) *Vibrio cholerae*

2. Sugar transport into bacteria is frequently facilitated by

(A) Acetyltransferase
(B) Neuraminidases
(C) Oxidases
(D) Penicillin-binding proteins
(E) Phosphotransferases

3. Thayer-Martin and Martin-Lewis media are used to isolate and identify

(A) *E. coli*
(B) *Mycobacteria*
(C) *Neisseria*
(D) *Salmonella*
(E) *Shigella*

4. β-lactamases confer antibiotic resistance by

(A) Altering antibiotic permeability
(B) Altering penicillin-binding proteins
(C) Altering 70S ribosome structure
(D) Modifying cellular RNA polymerase
(E) Modifying antibiotic structure

5. Polymers of *N*-acetylglucosamine and *N*-acetylmuramic acid are found in which of the following structures?

(A) Teichoic acid
(B) Cell wall
(C) Glycocalyx
(D) Lipopolysaccharide

6. A phage that is not inactivated by proteases is called a

(A) Prophage
(B) Virulent phage
(C) Temperate phage
(D) Filamentous phage

7. Bacteria that synthesize organic compounds from inorganic compounds are

(A) Heterotrophs
(B) Obligate anaerobes
(C) Aerobes
(D) Facultative anaerobes
(E) Autotrophs

8. A bacterial structure involved in adherence is

(A) Capsule
(B) Lipopolysaccharide
(C) Common pili
(D) O-specific side chain
(E) Teichoic acid

9. Aminoglycoside antibiotics are

(A) Bactericidal for Gram-positive bacteria
(B) Inactivated by R-factor phosphotransferases
(C) Mycolic acid synthesis inhibitors
(D) Peptidoglycan synthesis inhibitors
(E) Items that require bacterial growth for the effect

10. A-B subunit structure as it relates to bacterial pathogenesis refers to the structure of

(A) Bacterial exotoxins
(B) Gram-negative bacteria endotoxin
(C) Nucleic acid inhibitor antibiotics
(D) Penicillin-binding proteins
(E) Resistance transfer factors

11. Which of the following displays the Pasteur effect?

(A) Heterotrophs
(B) Obligate anaerobes
(C) Aerobes
(D) Facultative anaerobes
(E) Autotrophs

12. Which of the following toxins acts on synaptosomes?

(A) *E. coli* heat-labile toxin
(B) *Clostridium tetani* exotoxin
(C) *Corynebacterium diphtheriae* exotoxin

(D) *Pseudomonas aeruginosa* exotoxin
(E) *Clostridium perfringens* alpha-toxin

13. Superoxide dismutase-containing bacteria

(A) Need superoxide to grow
(B) Are frequently obligate anaerobes
(C) Grow slowly in the presence of CO_2
(D) Produce hydrogen peroxide from hydrogen ion and the superoxide free radical ($O_2^{\bullet-}$)

14. Lysogenic phage conversion involves

(A) The transformation of a virulent phage to a lysogenic phage
(B) A change in bacterial phenotype due to the presence of a prophage
(C) The conversion of a prophage to a temperate phage
(D) The incorporation of a prophage into the bacterial chromosome

15. Bacteria capable of growth in a high salt concentration are best isolated in which of the following media?

(A) Minimal growth media
(B) Complex growth media
(C) Differential growth media
(D) Selective growth media

16. Bacteria lacking superoxide dismutase are

(A) Heterotrophs
(B) Obligate anaerobes
(C) Aerobes
(D) Facultative anaerobes
(E) Autotrophs

17. The regulation of enzyme activity in bacterial cells can

(A) Be coupled to the binding of effector molecules
(B) Be controlled by a catabolite activator protein (CAP)
(C) Occur via attenuation sequences
(D) Involve inducer molecules

18. The plasma membrane

(A) Contains matrix porins
(B) Includes endotoxin
(C) Contains glycocalyx
(D) Contains the enzymes involved in bacterial oxidative phosphorylation

19. Bacterial antibiotic resistance is frequently conveyed by

(A) A temperate bacteriophage
(B) An R-factor plasmid

(C) A replicon
(D) A lytic bacteriophage
(E) An intron

20. The expression of the *lac* operon

(A) Must be initiated by the binding of an inducer protein
(B) Involves the release of allolactose from a repressor protein
(C) Does not involve the expression of structural genes
(D) Necessitates the finding of RNA polymerase followed by transcription

21. Bacteriophage containing host-cell DNA is involved in which of the following processes?

(A) Transformation
(B) Conjugation
(C) Transduction
(D) Transcription
(E) Recombination

22. The exchange of allelic forms of genes is involved in which of the following processes?

(A) Transformation
(B) Conjugation
(C) Transduction
(D) Transcription
(E) Recombination

23. Which of the following processes creates high-frequency recombination donors?

(A) Transformation
(B) Conjugation
(C) Transduction
(D) Transcription
(E) Recombination
(F) Translation

24. Toxins of enterotoxic Gram-negative bacteria are transferred outside of the cell by

(A) ATP-activated pores
(B) GTP-coupled transporters
(C) PBPs
(D) Pili
(E) Protein secretion systems

25. A mutation which rarely disrupts gene product function is a

(A) Deletion
(B) Frameshift
(C) Insertion
(D) Nonsense
(E) Nucleotide substitution

Answers and Explanations

1. **The answer is D.** *Staphylococcus aureus* produces an enterotoxin and TSST-1 toxins with superantigen activity. *Streptococcus pyogenes* also produces toxins with this activity.

2. **The answer is E.** The transport of sugar into a bacterium frequently involves the transfer of a phosphate group to the sugar molecule.

3. **The answer is C.** These media are variants of chocolate agar and contain antibiotics that inhibit many normal respiratory and genital bacteria but allow the growth of *Neisseria* species.

4. **The answer is E.** β-lactamases cleave the β-lactam ring structure that is important for the antibacterial activity of penicillins, cephalosporins, monobactams, and carbapenems.

5. **The answer is B.** *N*-acetylglucosamine and *N*-acetylmuramic acid are polymerized to form the peptidoglycan backbone of the cell wall.

6. **The answer is A.** A prophage is the intracellular DNA of a phage and is therefore resistant to protease degradation.

7. **The answer is E.** Autotrophic bacteria do not require organic compounds for growth because they synthesize them from inorganic precursors.

8. **The answer is C.** Common pili, adhesins, and the glycocalyx are three bacterial structures that are involved in adherence.

9. **The answer is E.** Bacteria must be actively replicating and synthesizing protein for these compounds, which bind to the 30S ribosomal subunit to have their bactericidal effect.

10. **The answer is A.** Many bacterial exotoxins have an A-B subunit structure in which the B subunit is involved in binding and the A subunit possesses biological activity inside the affected cell.

11. **The answer is D.** Facultative anaerobes shift from a fermentative to a respiratory metabolism in the presence of air because the energy needs of the cell are met by consuming less glucose (Pasteur effect) under respiratory metabolism.

12. **The answer is B.** *Clostridium tetani* exotoxin acts on synaptosomes, thereby causing hyperreflexia of skeletal muscles.

13. **The answer is D.** Superoxide dismutase is found in aerobic and facultative anaerobic bacteria. It protects them from the toxic free radical ($O_2^{\bullet-}$) by combining it with a hydrogen ion to form hydrogen peroxide, which is subsequently degraded by peroxidase.

14. **The answer is B.** Lysogenic phage conversion refers to a change in bacterial phenotype resulting from the presence of a lysogenic prophage of a temperate phage.

15. **The answer is D.** A selective growth medium that contains a high salt concentration would permit bacterial growth.

16. **The answer is B.** Superoxide dismutase, which is present in aerobes and facultative anaerobe organisms, protects them from the toxic $O_2^{\bullet-}$ radical. This enzyme is not present in obligate anaerobes.

17. **The answer is A.** The biochemical activity of an enzyme may be regulated by binding of effector molecules or by biosynthetic pathway end-product feedback inhibition. Enzyme synthesis may be controlled by inducers, attenuation sequences, or catabolite activator protein.

18. **The answer is D.** The plasma membrane contains the enzymes involved in oxidative phosphorylation.

19. **The answer is B.** R-factor (resistance) plasmids contain genes for proteins that degrade antibiotics or alter antibiotic transport, thus conferring antibiotic resistance. They also carry transfer genes, which facilitate their intercellular transfer to other genomes.

20. **The answer is A.** The transcription of the *lac* operon is under negative control. Initiation depends on the binding of allolactose to a repressor protein. This reaction prevents the repressor from binding to the operator region, thus allowing RNA polymerase to bind and transcription to proceed.

21. **The answer is C.** Bacteriophages containing portions of host-cell DNA can introduce this genetic material into new host cells via the process of transduction.

22. **The answer is E.** DNA or genetic recombination is the general term used to describe the exchange of allelic forms of genes in bacteria or eukaryotic cells.

23. **The answer is E.** High-frequency recombination donors, which result from the integration of a fertility (F) factor into chromosomal DNA, are created by recombination.

24. **The answer is E.** Depending on the bacteria, one of four types of protein secretion systems of the Gram-negative bacteria is responsible for transporting exotoxins to the outside of the cell.

25. **The answer is E.** Nucleotide substitution and some missense mutations can be silent and not affect gene product function.

3 Important Bacterial Genera

I. CLINICAL LABORATORY IDENTIFICATION

Taxonomic relationships of the various genera of medically important bacteria are currently determined using molecular techniques and numerical taxonomy. By contrast, clinical identification of pathogens are determined by a variety of methods. New methods are continuously introduced but do not always replace older methods. In this review book, critical identification methods and standard culture media are presented along with the newer methods because many of the older methods will continue to be used by some laboratories and will appear on national examinations.

A. **The identification of the specific causative agent of a bacterial infection is most commonly made by detecting the presence of one or more of the following:**
   1. Bacteria through microscopy or culture
   2. Bacterial components or products such as specific nucleic acid sequences, toxins, enzymes or enzymatic activities, capsules, or antigens
   3. Patient antibodies to a specific organism or its products

B. **Diagnostic tests.** Tests can be performed on the following:
   1. **Clinical specimens.** Some tests (e.g., nucleic acid amplification tests (NAATS) or microscopy) may be performed directly on clinical specimens.
   2. **Isolated pathogen.** Other tests require that the pathogen is isolated by culture and the diagnostic tests then are performed on the isolated pathogen. This is especially true where identification requires running biochemical tests and most often to also be able to do antibiotic susceptibility testing.

C. **Microscopy.**
   1. **Gram stain,** a differential stain, is a key starting point for etiological diagnosis of infection.
      a. On some clinical specimens, it is used to guide initial therapy (e.g., lancet-shaped Gram-positive diplococci in a sputum sample suggesting *S. pneumoniae*).
      b. On clinical specimens with normal flora, it may not be useful (e.g., Gram-negative diplococci are found in normal pharyngeal flora so a Gram stain cannot be used to diagnose gonococcal pharyngitis. However, the finding of Gram-negative diplococci inside polymorphonuclear neutrophils (PMNs) from a urethral discharge is sufficient to start treatment in males.
      c. On the isolated bacterial culture, the source of the isolate, Gram reaction, and oxidase or catalase test results guide the selection of additional identification tests and antibiotic susceptibilities.

Gram-Positive = Purple
Highly coss-linked and thick cell
walls; no outer membrane

Gram-Negative = Red
Thin peptidoglycan with little cross
linkage + phospholipid outer membrane

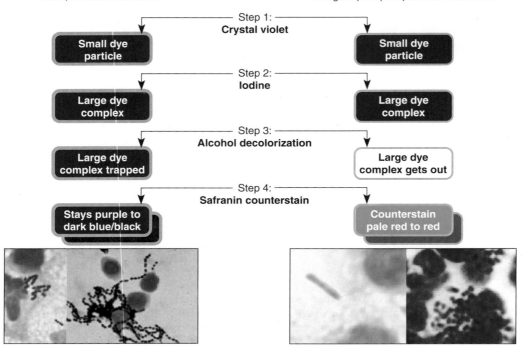

FIGURE 3.1. **The Gram stain**. The photomicrographs at the bottom of the figure show the color variation of Gram-positive cells (left) and Gram-negative cells (right). (In each pair of images, the left image is from the author (LH) and the right graciously provided by Dr. Dilip K. Banerjee from *Microbiology of Infectious Diseases.* London: Gower Medical Publishing, 1986.)

    d. Gram-positive bacteria are purple.

    e. Gram-negative bacteria are red/pink because their cell envelopes lose the large purple dye complex and so the stain pink/red counterstain is shown.

    f. Not reliably showing up on Gram stain: *Mycoplasma, Ureaplasma, Chlamydia, Rickettsia, Anaplasma, Ehrlichia, Coxiella, Legionella,* and spirochetes (especially ***Treponema***).

    g. Review the Gram stain procedure (Fig 3.1) and see the provided examples. On direct clinical specimens (e.g., pus), the background of human cells will stain pale red with red nuclei.

  2. Acid-fast stain (Fig. 3.2). This stain distinguishes **mycobacteria,** all of which are **acid-fast (red),** from all other bacteria, all of which are **not acid-fast (blue).** Additionally:

    a. *Nocardia* are partially acid-fast, sometimes showing some blue rods along with the red ones on the same slide; however, there will always be some red.

    b. Parasitic oocysts of *Cryptosporidium, Cyclospora,* and *Isopora* are acid-fast.

  3. Wet mounts are used for specific specimens such as unspun urine or for motility.

  4. Dark-field microscopy is useful for spirochetes that are too thin to be seen in a Gram stain and to show their motility.

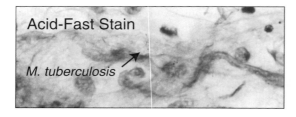

FIGURE 3.2. **Acid-fast stain**. Mycobacteria (acid-fast = red) are shown in this sputum sample. This image has been enlarged greater than is possible with the light or fluorescent microscope, making the images generally easier to read than on the actual microscope. Note how hard it is to see the red acid-fast bacteria. On acid-fast stains, human cells and debris are stained blue. (Image was graciously provided by Dr. David Carter of St. Mary's/Duluth Clinic, Duluth Minnesota.)

FIGURE 3.3. Fluorochrome stain. The auramine binds nonspecifically to the waxy mycobacterial cell well. Because there is no antibody involved in this binding, this is not a specific stain, but it is a sensitive screening test for sputum samples and is easy to read because of the contrast of the bound dye with everything else dark. A positive fluorochrome stain is always confirmed by an acid-fast stain or a mycobacterial fluorescent antibody stain.

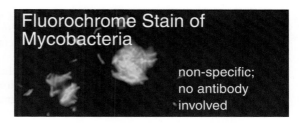

Fluorochrome Stain of Mycobacteria

non-specific; no antibody involved

5. **Fluorescent microscopy** may be used to examine both cultured isolates and directly on clinical specimens.
   a. **Fluorochrome dye methods** (Fig. 3.3) include auramine-rhodamine dyes that bind nonspecifically to waxy cell wall components of both *Mycobacterium* and relatives.
      (1) This stain is more sensitive because it is easier to read than an acid-fast stain. The fluorescent dyes light up the bacteria on the black background without interference from the specimen.
      (2) The fluorochrome dyes are sensitive but not specific like immunofluorescent staining because antibodies are not involved.
   b. **Fluorescent antibody (FA) stains** may be specific to a genus or species depending on the specificity of the primary antibody (Fig. 3.4).
      (1) **Direct fluorescent antibody (DFA)** uses known fluorescent-labeled antibodies that target a specific microbe.
      (2) **Indirect fluorescent antibody (IFA) is a "sandwich technique"** using unlabeled, known antibodies that bind to bacterial antigens on the slide. Then an FA that detects the bound antibody is applied, highlighting any antibody bound to the organism.

D. **Culture** is a complex process that requires that specimens be properly obtained and transported and then grown on appropriate media under the correct conditions. Partial immunity, presence of active white cells (in blood cultures), or partial antibiotic treatment may interfere with growth.
   1. The area from which the specimen is obtained influences the interpretation of results.
      a. If a specimen is obtained from a normally sterile area (e.g., CSF) using aseptic technique, the finding of any microbes in the specimen is significant.

FIGURE 3.4. **Immunofluorescent staining** (also known as fluorescent antibody staining). **(Top)** With **direct fluorescent antibody staining (DFA)**, highly specific (depending on antibody choice) fluorescent staining can be achieved by conjugating fluorescent dye (tagging) to a specific antibody. For example, because *Bordetella pertussis* is often difficult to culture after the characteristic cough has been present for a few days, a nasopharyngeal smear can be made and stained with tagged *B. pertussis* antibody. Thus, the Gram-negative *Bordetella*, which on a Gram stain would be confused with nonpathogenic normal flora, can be positively identified because of the specificity of the antibody–antigen combination. **(Bottom)** With **indirect fluorescent antibody (IFA)**, this test first reacts commercially prepared antibody specific for the agent you are looking for with the fixed patient's specimen. After washing, a fluorescent dye-tagged anti-immunoglobulin is used to detect bound antibody. (Theoretically, if all of the commercially made unlabeled antibodies for the "meat" of this immunofluorescent "sandwich technique" were rabbit antibody, then all tests could use one fluorescent-tagged anti-rabbit antibody to "light" the bound antibody.)

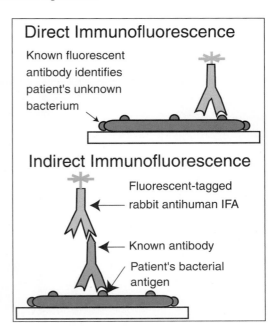

Direct Immunofluorescence

Known fluorescent antibody identifies patient's unknown bacterium

Indirect Immunofluorescence

Fluorescent-tagged rabbit antihuman IFA

Known antibody

Patient's bacterial antigen

   b. If a specimen is obtained from a normally sterile area but passes through tissue with normal flora, specific specimen guidelines are used to evaluate the quality of the specimen and to interpret the results. Examples of these specimens are sputa or urine taken by the clean-catch midstream urine method.

   (1) With "sputum," the finding of many epithelial cells and lack of PMNs suggests that the specimen is saliva rather than material from the lungs.

   (2) With urine, quantitation guidelines suggest whether the patient has an infection or has normal levels of normal flora contaminating the specimen.

   (3) The finding of a specific pathogen that is not part of the normal flora is diagnostic of infection with that agent.

   c. If a specimen is obtained from an area with normal flora such as skin or mucous membranes, interpretation involves isolating pathogens or finding overgrowth of normal flora.

2. The **method** and **transport medium** of the specimen are often critical, especially if it is transported to a reference lab.

   a. Potentially anaerobic specimens such as abscess material must be obtained and transported anaerobically.

   b. Some organisms are sensitive to cold or drying.

3. **Proper culture medium** and **growth conditions** influence growth. A rich medium, often with blood, is commonly used as one isolation medium for most specimens.

   a. **Hemolysis** on blood agar may be used when identifying bacterial species (Fig. 3.5).

   (1) **Alpha-hemolysins** produce **incomplete lysis,** with green pigment surrounding the colony.

   (2) Bacteria producing **no hemolysis** are said to be **gamma-hemolytic** or **nonhemolytic.**

   (3) **Beta-hemolysins** produce **total hemolysis** and break down the hemoglobin creating a clear area around the colony.

   b. **Differential media:** Some specific media (including blood agar) help **differentiate groups of organisms directly on the plate.** Examples are Hektoen and MacConkey agars that distinguish lactose fermenters from nonfermenters (Fig. 3.6).

   c. **Fastidious bacteria** are those with complex nutritional requirements. These bacteria will not grow on standard laboratory agars and require special specific media. The following are **media commonly used to grow fastidious bacteria** (Table 3.1):

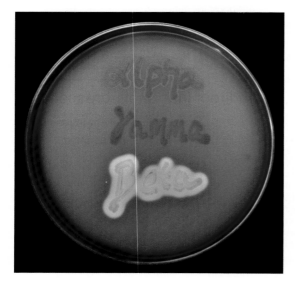

FIGURE 3.5. Hemolysis. Examples of the different types of hemolysis. Plates were inoculated in cursive writing. Note that the growth on these plates does not show up well because transmitted light was used to show the hemolysis. **(Top) Alpha-hemolysis** is partial hemolysis of the red blood cells with a change in the color of hemoglobin resulting in a translucent area with a greenish coloration. **(Middle) Gamma-hemolysis** is no hemolysis. **(Bottom) Beta-hemolysis** is complete lysis of the red blood cells, which results in a transparent area around the colony. (From Engleberg NC, et al. *Schaechter's mechanism of microbial disease.* 5th ed. Baltimore, MD: Wolters Kluwer Health; 2013.)

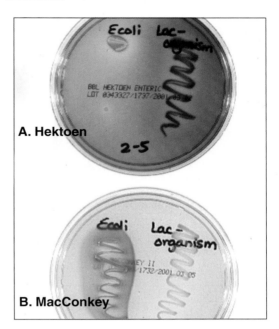

A. Hektoen

B. MacConkey

FIGURE 3.6. Differential media. These media allow the distinction of certain groups from the growth and substrate changes directly on the plate. Thus, on several of the enteric media, Gram-positive bacterial growth is inhibited and Gram-negative bacteria which grow and ferment lactose can be distinguished from those that do not ferment lactose. **(A) Hektoen agar**. Lactose fermentation (here by *Escherichia coli*) produces acid that turns the colonies and medium into colors in the yellow range. **(B) MacConkey medium**. The pale straw color of the medium turns to red when the pH becomes acidic from the lactose fermentation products.

(1) **Chocolate agar (agar made with lysed red blood cells)**
 (a) This medium is used for both ***Haemophilus*** spp. and ***Neisseria*** spp., both of which are nonhemolytic but require nutrients from the lysed RBCs (Fig. 3.7).
 (b) **Thayer-Martin** or **New York City agars** are used to grow *Neisseria* that have been obtained from body areas with competing normal flora (any mucosa). Both are chocolate agars that contain antibiotics to prevent growth of the bacteria and yeasts that are part of the normal mucosal flora. Nucleic acid amplification tests (NAATs) or gene probes may be used instead of cultures for diagnosis of gonorrhea.

(2) **Regan-Lowe** and **Bordet-Gengou agars:**
 (a) These media are used for culture of ***Bordetella pertussis.***
 (b) Rapid, nonculture methods are replacing culture because it is difficult to culture *B. pertussis* either from a vaccinated person or after the early paroxysmal stage of whooping cough.

(3) **Thiosulfate-citrate-bile salts-sucrose.** Thiosulfate-citrate-bile salts-sucrose (TCBS) is an alkaline medium used to grow *Vibrio cholerae*. (Just learn the initials and that TCBS is an alkaline media for *V. cholerae*.)

(4) **(Buffered) charcoal-yeast extract (BCYE) agar** is used to grow ***Legionella.*** It contains needed iron and cysteine plus charcoal.

t a b l e **3.1** Common Bacteriological Media

Common Bacteriological Media	Bacteria
Charcoal-yeast extract agar	*Legionella*
Chocolate agar	*Haemophilus* *Neisseria*
New York City or Thayer-Martin	*Neisseria* from nonsterile specimens
Lowenstein-Jensen Agar or Middlebrook medium	*Mycobacterium*
Regan-Lowe	*Bordetella*
Thiosulfate-citrate-bile salts-sucrose (TCBS), alkaline medium	*Vibrio*

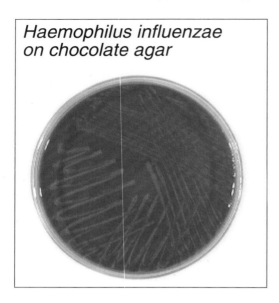

Haemophilus influenzae on chocolate agar

FIGURE 3.7. **Chocolate agar.** Some organisms, such as *Haemophilus influenzae* and pathogenic neisseriae, are nonhemolytic but require complex factors inside blood cells; therefore, they will not grow on blood agar but will grow on chocolate agar, which is made with lysed blood. *Haemophilus influenzae* will also grow on nutrient agar with added hemin and NAD (X and V factors, respectively).

  (5) Lowenstein-Jensen agar:
    (a) Lowenstein-Jensen agar contains egg yolk that provides the necessary lipids for **mycobacteria.**
    (b) It is being replaced with high lipid broth cultures specifically designed for mycobacteria, allowing faster growth and machine detection of growth by quantitative polymerase chain reaction (PCR).

E. **Detection of microbial products.** (Many require isolating the pathogen in culture.)
  1. **Antigen detection** requires specific antibodies and may be done by direct or indirect fluorescent microscopy or by enzyme-linked immunoassay (ELISA).
  2. Tests demonstrating **specific enzymes** or **toxin activities.**
    a. **Nagler test for *Clostridium perfringens* alpha-toxin (a lecithinase):** This test uses a lecithin-containing agar to detect lecithinase activity. One side of the plate has an antibody to the *C. perfringens* alpha-toxin that neutralizes its activity. The test result is positive if there is a visual change around the growth on the side without antitoxin and no change in the media on the side containing the antitoxin since the antitoxin will inactivate the enzyme.
    b. Hemolysin detected on **blood agar** (see I D 3 a).
    c. Growth on media with **one major carbohydrate source.**
      (1) Growth in broths in microtiter plates where there is only one carbohydrate per well.
      (2) MacConkey agar: This agar has peptone and lactose; it supports the growth of all Enterobacteriaceae but only those fermenting the lactose will cause the color change from buff to hot pink red. (It also contains bile salts and crystal violet to inhibit the growth of nonenteric organisms and Gram-positive organisms.) (See Fig. 3.6B.)
    d. Growth in **broths with specific substrates** for detection of specific activities: These tests are the mainstay of commonly used automated identification systems.
    e. **Rapid enzyme tests** detect the presence of the following enzymes:
      (1) Catalase breaks down hydrogen peroxide. This test is used to differentiate the genus *Staphylococcus* (catalase-positive) from *Streptococcus* (catalase-negative). In general, many anaerobes (and some microaerophiles) do not make catalase (Fig. 3.8A).
      (2) Oxidase (cytochrome-C oxidase) is produced by most Gram-negative bacteria but not by members of the Enterobacteriaceae. Oxidase-positive rules the latter out.
      (3) Nitrate reductase reduces nitrate to nitrite. It is used to detect the presence of Enterobacteriaceae in urine (Fig. 3.8B).

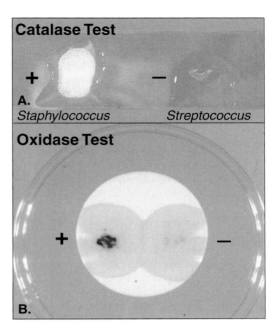

FIGURE 3.8. Important rapid tests used in early identification of some bacteria. (A) Catalase test. Hydrogen peroxide is reacted with a small amount of the bacterial growth. The production of bubbles (oxygen) suggests that the organism contains catalase. The organism on the left side of the slide is positive; the organism (hard to see because there are no bubbles) on the right side is negative. **(B) Oxidase test.** This test detects the presence of cytochrome oxidase and is used largely for Gram-negative bacteria. All Enterobacteriaceae are oxidase-negative. Most others are oxidase-positive.

    (a) *Escherichia coli* and other enterobacteria produce nitrate reductase; this test requires that the bacteria remain in contact with the urine for a sufficient time.

    (b) *Staphylococcus saprophyticus* does not produce nitrate reductase.

  f. Growth under specific conditions can be used to identify certain metabolic features of microbes, such as whether it is an aerobe or anaerobe.

    (1) Suspected *Campylobacter* cultures are grown in incubators at 42°C under microaerophilic conditions.

    (2) Thioglycollate broth is a medium with reducing power that develops an oxygen gradient. The tubes of broth are carefully stab inoculated the full length.

      (a) If an organism grows only at the top of the medium, the isolate is an obligate aerobe.

      (b) If an organism grows throughout the medium but grows more heavily at the top, it is a facultative anaerobe.

  g. Commercial test systems are generally designed to identify a clinical isolate and determine antibiotic susceptibility simultaneously. The general steps used in these systems are as follows:

    (1) Bacterial isolates are grown from the patient specimen.

    (2) Gram stain results (often along with catalase or oxidase tests) are used to select the appropriate identification tests (a series of tests identifying specific enzyme activities such as carbohydrate utilization, urease, etc.). The plates also contain wells with antimicrobials for susceptibility determination.

    (3) Plates are read by machine; results are given as the probability that the isolate is the identified organism and gives minimal inhibitory concentrations for the tested antibiotics.

3. Nucleic acid detection is done with gene probes with or without amplification. Newer techniques may be done directly on clinical specimens as well as cultured growth.

  a. Nucleic Acid Amplification Tests (NAATs) include PCR, reverse transcriptase PCR (RT-PCR), and quantitative (a.k.a. real-time) PCR (utilizing fluorescent dyes on probes to detect and help quantitate amplicons).

  b. Microarrays, which are microchips with hundreds of probes from different bacteria on one slide, expand the ability of NAATs.

  c. Fluorescent in situ hybridization (**FISH**) tests are becoming available for clinical diagnostic use for some organisms or toxins and can be used on tissue sections, specimens such as sputum, or on gels.

F. **Detection of immune response to a specific pathogen.**
1. **Detection of patient antibody** demonstrates current or previous exposure to a pathogen.
   a. Positive titers (levels) are expressed as the highest dilution of the serum still giving a positive test so that a titer written as 1/64 is much higher than a titer of 1/4. Titers may also be written as 1:4. A four-fold increase or greater over a 2-week period is indicative of active infection.
   b. High immunoglobulin M (IgM) titers also suggest recent infection.
   c. High IgG titers with no IgM usually indicate older infection.
2. A positive **skin test** (e.g., tuberculin skin test) in a person who is immunocompetent may demonstrate past or current infection and, unlike serology, cannot differentiate between the two. (Remember that seriously immunocompromised patients may not be able to produce antibody or mount a positive skin test.)
3. **Detection of immune response from whole blood** (QuantiFERON or ELISpot test) has replaced the tuberculin skin test in many situations.

G. **Determination of antimicrobial susceptibility.** Susceptibility testing is done by many methods depending on the organism:
1. **Gene probes** (generally with amplification methods) may be used to determine if an organism carries a specific gene for drug resistance.
2. **Rapid tests** are performed on an isolate mixed with a special substrate such as a chromogenic (colored) β-lactam. If the β-lactam ring is broken by lactamase, it leads to a color change.
3. **Rapid growth detection systems** (such as for *Mycobacterium tuberculosis*) use quantitative PCR to detect growth. These tests are performed in a series of "tubes," some of which contain antimicrobials. Growth can be assessed in the presence or absence of specific antimicrobials (at appropriate levels).

Drug Susceptibility Testing

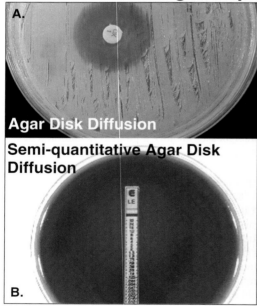
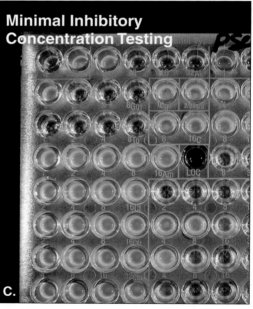

FIGURE 3.9. Drug susceptibility testing. (A) Agar disk diffusion. A disk with a known concentration of dried antibiotic is placed on the surface of an agar plate spread inoculated with the patient's bacterial isolate. After incubation, the diameter of the zone of inhibition determines if the isolate is susceptible intermediate or resistant to that antibiotic. This is a qualitative technique. **(B) E test, a semiquantitative agar disk diffusion.** A sterile plastic "ruler" with a drop of dried antibiotic on the back is placed on a plate inoculated with the patient's bacterial isolate to create a lawn of bacteria. After incubation, the zone of growth inhibition can be correlated with the expected minimal inhibitory concentration from reading the measurements on the ruler. The ruler is different for each antibiotic. **(C) Minimal inhibitory concentration.** Each well has a specific concentration of a single drug and the same approximate number of the patient's bacterial isolate. Drugs are tested in achievable concentration ranges in this test. Growth is measured by a variety of methods.

4. **Minimal inhibitory concentration (MIC)** broth tests are used to determine the minimal concentration in the presence of a particular drug that inhibits the growth of a bacterium.
   a. Commercially prepared microtiter plates with a series of tests to identify an organism (e.g., a Gram-negative isolated from urine) also have a series of wells in which multiple appropriate antibiotics can be tested at a range of concentrations achievable in the body (see Fig. 3.9C). The lowest concentration of each drug that inhibits growth is MIC for that drug. (In other words, the MIC is the level that must be achieved in the site of the infection for the antibiotic to inhibit further growth.)
   b. The killing level or **minimal bacteriocidal concentrations (MBCs)** are usually determined by extrapolation of MICs.
5. **Agar gel diffusion plates (Kirby-Bauer)** use paper disks containing standard concentrations of dehydrated antibiotics (see Fig. 3.9A).
   a. A solid agar medium in a petri dish is spread evenly with a broth of the patient's isolate.
   b. A dispenser drops the appropriate disks containing specific amounts of dried antibiotics on each surface. The disks are tapped to lay flat. The antibiotics hydrate and begin to diffuse out, setting up a concentration gradient.
   c. The plates are incubated, generally overnight, and zones of growth inhibition are then measured and interpreted using charts as to whether the organism is sensitive, has intermediate susceptibility, or is resistant to the drug.
   d. These tests are qualitative, not quantitative.
6. **E-tests** (named for the elliptical zone of inhibition) are also agar diffusion antibiotic susceptibility tests but are made semiquantitative through the incorporation of a small plastic "ruler" with a scale which, through testing hundreds of isolates, correlates the zone of inhibition with quantitative MIC data (see Fig. 3.9B).

II. INTRODUCTION TO MAJOR BACTERIAL GENERA

The following sections include:

A. The major distinguishing characteristics of bacterial genera (and a few families), including important laboratory identifiers and any other important genus information.
B. A list of important species and diseases they cause. For important genera with many species, the characteristics used to distinguish species is included. These characteristics are sometimes presented in tabular form.
   Before continuing, take a quick look at formal and informal nomenclature:
   - Streptococcaceae is a formal family name. (The -aceae is your clue.)
   - Streptococci is a common name, which could refer to the family, species, or any chain of cocci, depending on the context. These are not italicized.
   - *Streptococcus* is a genus name. Note: It is optional to italicize a genus name alone but the formal genus and species binomial should always be italicized. Colloquial (common) names are not italicized. If all of the answer choices to a question on an examination are italicized, they are formal Latin bacterial, fungal, or parasitic names. Formal viral names may now also be italicized. The abbreviation "sp." used after a genus name is singular for any species of that genus. (You will see this on preliminary lab reports.) But "spp." is plural and is used following a genus name to indicate that most species of that genus do something.
   - *Streptococcus pneumoniae* is the proper species name. (The genus name is capitalized, and species name is rarely capitalized even when it is derived from a proper name.)
   - *S. pneumoniae* is the proper abbreviation for the species. *Strep. pneumo.* is colloquial usage; however, it is more precise since "*S.*" could also refer to *Staphylococcus*.
   - Pneumococcus is a nickname for *Strep. pneumoniae*.
   - The term "complex" is used for a series of species so closely related that they do not need to be distinguished in the lab (i.e., *Mycobacterium avium-intracellulare complex* or MAC).

III. GRAM-POSITIVE BACTERIA

A. General characteristics.
1. Gram-positive bacteria have a **highly cross-linked, multilayered (and usually thick) peptidoglycan cell wall** which traps the large Gram crystal violet-iodine complex staining them deep purple.
2. **Teichoic acids** are linked to either the cytoplasmic membrane (the lipoteichoic acids) or to the cell wall peptidoglycan. **Teichoic acids are unique to Gram-positive bacteria** and play roles in **adherence** and **triggering Gram-positive shock** as the cell wall is broken down.
3. A variety of cell surface proteins are present, which are organism specific.
4. Gram-positive bacteria have **no outer membrane** and therefore no hydrophobic barrier to limit access of larger antibiotics to the peptidoglycan.

B. Major genera of Gram-positive bacteria.
1. Genus: ***Staphylococcus.*** Common name: Staphylococci.
   Features:
   a. **Gram-positive cocci** generally in tight grapelike clusters or, in specimens, as singlets, pairs, or short chains as well as clusters.
   b. **Catalase-positive,** breaking down hydrogen peroxide into water and oxygen.
   c. **Facultative anaerobes** producing energy more efficiently aerobically.
   d. **Haloduric** (salt-tolerant).
   e. Speciated medically on the basis of **coagulase and hemolysis.**
   Table 3.2 lists the most important medical species.
2. Genus: ***Streptococcus.*** Common name: Streptococci.
   Features:
   a. **Gram-positive cocci in chains or pairs.** They tend to be oval.
   b. Distinguished from staphylococci on the basis of the catalase test. **Streptococci are catalase-negative, aerotolerant anaerobes** that grow in full oxygen but ferment both in the presence and absence of oxygen.
   c. Subdivided or speciated by three different systems: serology, hemolysin production, and biochemical properties.
      (1) Serology using Lancefield's antibodies to cell wall carbohydrates.
         (a) Streptococci that are positive for these carbohydrates are classified into Lancefield's serogroups (e.g., Group A strep). There are now more than 20 groups.
         (b) Bacteria that have these cell wall carbohydrates produce a pyogenic reaction.
         (c) Some alpha-hemolytic streptococci including *Strep. pneumoniae* and the viridans streptococci lack these cell wall carbohydrates. They are not grouped using Lancefield's antibodies and are not pyogenic.

t a b l e **3.2** Important Streptococcal Species		
Major Species/Epidemiology	**Identifying Characteristics***	**Diseases**
Staphylococcus aureus/ most common in the mucosa of the anterior nares; ↑'s on cutaneous surfaces of HCW, IDU**, diabetics, etc.	Beta-hemolytic Coagulase-positive	Cutaneous infections (impetigo, abscesses, cellulitis) Endocarditis, bacteremia Pneumonia Toxic shock syndrome Food poisoning
Staphylococcus epidermidis/ normal cutaneous flora	Coagulase-negative Nonhemolytic	Opportunist requiring entry (surgical, catheter, shunt, prosthetic devices) causing septicemias, endocarditis, wound infections
Staphylococcus saprophyticus/ urinary mucosa colonization	Coagulase-negative Nonhemolytic	Urinary tract infection, most commonly in newly sexually active young women

*All staphylococci are catalase-positive. **HCW = health care workers; IDU = injection drug users

(2) **Hemolysin testing:** see I D 3 a in this chapter.

(3) **Biochemical tests.** Additional tests used in speciation include the PYR test, CAMP test, growth sensitivity to Optochin, bile lysis, or growth inhibition by bacitracin. You do not need details on these tests.

   d. Streptococci are mainly opportunists but can cause disease in debilitated patients or if they gain entry into the body.

3. Genus: *Enterococcus.*

Features:

   a. Catalase-negative, facultative anaerobes fermenting even in full oxygen; **Streptococcal family**.

   b. Alpha-hemolytic or **nonhemolytic, Gram-positive cocci** in chains that have the **Group D streptococcal cell wall carbohydrate**.

   c. Part of the normal human gastrointestinal (GI) flora.

   d. Tolerant of high concentrations of bile salts and NaCl.

   e. Have a high level of **drug resistance** that continues to increase due to efficient acquisition of plasmid transposon genes for drug resistance.

4. Genus: *Peptostreptococcus.*

Features:

   a. Peptostreptococci are obligate **anaerobic streptococci**.

   b. They are part of the normal flora of the oral, intestinal, and genitourinary tracts.

Table 3.3 lists the most important species distinctions and major diseases of the streptococci and relatives.

5. Genus: *Bacillus.*

Features:

   a. Gram-positive, spore-forming rods that may form chains. Although spores survive for decades in dry environments, they quickly germinate in rich moist conditions (e.g., a macrophage) and transform into metabolically active vegetative cells.

   b. They are **aerobes** (or facultative anaerobes) and grow well in ambient air.

   c. They cause anthrax (*Bacillus anthracis*) and food poisoning (*Bacillus cereus*).

| t a b l e **3.3** | Streptococci, Distinguishing Features Used in Identification, and Common Diseases. All Streptococci Are Gram-Positive, Catalase-Positive Cocci Occurring in Pairs or Chains. |

Major Species	Identifying Characteristics	Diseases
Streptococcus pyogenes Group A	Group A Streptococcal cell wall carbohydrates (Lancefield group) Beta-hemolysis Bacitracin-sensitive	Pharyngitis/scarlet fever Impetigo/cellulitis/fascitis/erysipelas Post-infectious sequelae acute glomerulonephritis rheumatic heart disease
Streptococcus agalactiae Group B (colonizes 15% to 20% of pregnant women)	Group B cell wall carbohydrates Beta-hemolytic Bacitracin resistant	Neonatal septicemia, pneumonia, and meningitis UTIs in pregnant women
Streptococcus pneumoniae	Alpha-hemolytic Sensitive to optochin Lysed by bile No cell wall carbohydrates (no serogroup)	Otitis, sinusitis Lobar pneumonia Meningitis
Viridans streptococci	Normal oral flora Alpha-hemolytic (or nonhemolytic) Not inhibited by optochin Not lysed by bile No cell wall carbohydrates (no serogroup)	Major role in dental caries (*S. mutans*) Role in periodontal disease Endocarditis
Enterococcus faecalis or *Enterococcus faecium*	Group D streptococcal cell wall carbohydrates GI tract flora; drug resistance	Endocarditis Urinary tract infections Septicemia
Peptostreptococcus	Anaerobic streptococci	Opportunists

6. Genus: ***Clostridium.*** Common name: Clostridia.
   Features:
   a. **Anaerobic, Gram-positive, spore-forming rods** that can form chains.
   b. Cause botulism (***Cl. botulinum***) characterized by a flaccid paralysis; gas gangrene and food poisoning (***Cl. perfringens***); and tetanus (***Cl. tetani***), characterized by rigid spasms.

7. Genus: ***Listeria. Listeria monocytogenes*** is the only human pathogen.
   Features:
   a. **Short Gram-positive, non-spore-forming rod** showing weak beta-hemolysis on blood agar.
   b. Motile in broth by tumbling. (They lack forward movement.)
   c. **Facultative intracellular pathogens;** they move from cell to cell by actin polymerization, which may propel the bacterium directly into an adjoining cell without exposure to extracellular milieu.
   d. Grows in the cold and, unlike most non-spore-forming pathogens, survives in the environment. *Listeria monocytogenes* is found in animal feces, rotting vegetation, and occasionally in soft cheeses, deli meats, and cabbage.
   e. Causes mild gastroenteritis, as well as septicemia in pregnant women, leading to potential fetal septicemia or meningitis, and may cause meningitis in immunocompromised patients.

8. Genus: ***Erysipelothrix.***
   Features:
   a. Aerobic **Gram-positive, non-spore-forming rods.**
   b. Found in animals and rotting organic material; entry is through traumatic implantation.
   c. Cause cutaneous erysipeloid primarily in fishmongers, butchers, and veterinarians.

9. Genus: ***Corynebacterium.***
   Features:
   a. Club-shaped, **Gram-positive non-spore-forming bacteria.**
   b. Found in Chinese character-like arrangement of cells.
   c. Aerobic and nonmotile.
   d. Part of **normal flora;** the non-toxin-producing corynebacteria found in the normal microbiota are called **diphtheroids.**
   e. Tox+ ***C. diphtheriae*** causes diphtheria, and ***Corynebacterium jeikeium*** causes infections via catheters and foreign bodies in immunocompromised hosts.

10. Genus: ***Actinomyces.***
    Features:
    a. **Anaerobic, Gram-positive rods** with some branching; nonmotile.
    b. Found in crevices between teeth and gums and female genital tract.
    c. **Not acid-fast.**
       (1) These bacteria are related to mycobacteria.
       (2) They have a similar cell wall but lack the extremely long chain fatty acids found in the mycobacterial cell wall. They have shorter fatty acid chains.
    d. Cause cervicofacial or pelvic infections following trauma that has resulted in necrotic tissue; colonies formed in tissue are sometimes described as "sulfur" granules.

11. Genus: ***Nocardia.***
    Features:
    a. **Gram-positive filamentous bacteria** breaking up into **rods.**
    b. **Aerobic soil organism.**
    c. Often described as **weakly** or **partially acid-fast** as the slide will show some areas where the cells retain some of the carbol-fuchsin (hot pink red color).
    d. Related to mycobacteria—have a cell wall with shorter chain mycolic acids; are somewhat resistant to drying, so they are transmitted in dust.
    e. Cause tuberculosis-like (but not contagious) bronchopulmonary disease in immunocompromised patients.

12. Genus: ***Mycobacterium.*** Mycobacteria are considered Gram-positive even though they do not reliably stain well with the Gram stain. They are presented later with poorly Gram-staining bacteria. (See Section V. following Gram-negative bacteria.)

IV. GRAM-NEGATIVE BACTERIA

A. **General characteristics.**

1. Cell envelope has a **thin (one to three layers) peptidoglycan layer** linked to an **outer membrane;** the peptidoglycan is not highly cross-linked, so on decolorization with alcohol the outer membrane is damaged and Gram-negative cell walls easily lose the large Gram crystal violet/iodine dye complex, thereby becoming colorless until counterstained.

2. **Outer membrane has lipopolysaccharide,** which is released on the death of the cell and has the toxic lipid A component. Entrance of aqueous materials across this outer membrane is through porin channels.

B. **Major genera of Gram-negative bacteria.**

1. Genus: *Neisseria.*
   Features:
   a. **Aerobic, Gram-negative, oxidase-positive diplococci** occurring as pairs with flattened adjoining sides.
   b. All species metabolize glucose.
   c. The two pathogens in this genera are distinguished by maltose fermentation: **meningococcus** ferments **maltose;** gonococcus does not.
   d. Sensitive to cold and drying.
   e. Colonize mucosal surfaces (both nonpathogenic and pathogenic *Neisseria*)
   f. Cause pneumonia, septicemia, and meningitis (***N. meningitidis***) and cervicitis, urethritis, proctitis, and eyesight-threatening conjunctivitis (***N. gonorrhoeae***).

2. Genus: *Moraxella* (*Moraxella catarrhalis*).
   Features:
   a. **Strictly aerobic, oxidase-positive, Gram-negative diplococci.**
   b. Part of **normal oral flora.**
   c. May cause otitis or sinusitis in healthy individuals; bronchitis and bronchopneumonia primarily in patients with chronic obstructive pulmonary disease (COPD).

3. Genus: *Brucella.*
   Features:
   a. Strictly aerobic, **Gram-negative coccobacilli (short rods).**
   b. Fastidious; require special enriched media and 7 to 10 days to grow.
   c. **Facultative intracellular pathogens that infect animals;** humans are infected by direct contact with infected animals; ingestion, inhalation, or implantation of materials contaminated with *Brucella;* or in laboratory accidents. Incidence in the United States is lower than in developing countries as animal disease has been largely eradicated through vaccination and destruction of infected animals.
   d. Cause brucellosis (undulant fever).

4. Genus: *Francisella.*
   Features:
   a. **Strictly aerobic, Gram-negative coccobacilli (short rods).**
   b. **Fastidious;** require cysteine and several days for culture.
   c. Cause tularemia, a **zoonotic** disease seen mainly in rabbits, rodents, and hunters.

5. Genus: *Bordetella.*
   Features:
   a. **Strictly aerobic, Gram-negative coccobacilli (short rods).**
   b. *Bordetella pertussis* is transmitted from person to person; however, humans can acquire kennel cough (*Bordetella bronchiseptica*) from animals.
   c. Very sensitive to drying and inhibitors in normal media; require special media (Bordet-Gengou, charcoal blood agar, Regan-Lowe) to grow.
   d. Causes whooping cough (***Bordetella pertussis***) and a milder version (***Bordetella parapertussis***).

6. Gram-negative, nonfermenting (aerobic) rods: *Pseudomonas, Burkholderia,* and *Acinetobacter:*
  a. Genus: ***Pseudomonas.***
    Features:
    (1) Small, **polar-flagellated, Gram-negative rods** ubiquitous in soil and water.
    (2) **Nonfermentative** and **oxidase-positive (aerobic in infections).**
    (3) Cause pneumonia and septicemia in people with cystic fibrosis and immunocompromised patients (especially those with neutropenia); cellulitis, and septicemia in burn patients; cellulitis in feet where a nail penetrates a tennis shoe; otitis and eye infections.
  b. Genus: ***Burkholderia.***
    Features:
    (1) **Gram-negative opportunists** found in moist environments like *Pseudomonas.*
    (2) Cause infections in people with cystic fibrosis and immunocompromised patients (***Burkholderia cepacia*** complex).
    (3) *Burkholderia pseudomallei* causes melioidosis, an infectious disease endemic in Southeast Asia; it also causes localized infection as well as systemic (e.g., not just pneumonia).

7. Gram-negative, nonmotile, fastidious rods: *Haemophilus, Pasteurella,* and *Legionella:*
  a. Genus: ***Haemophilus.***
    Features:
    (1) **Gram-negative, pleomorphic** rods (elongated forms in culture but very short rods [coccobacilli] in CSF).
    (2) **Fastidious:** *Haemophilus influenzae* requires X (hemin) and V (NAD) factors on nutrient agar but grows well on chocolate agar. They are nonhemolytic, so they do not grow on blood agar.
    (3) Strains without capsules (non-typeable) are part of the normal flora.
    (4) ***Haemophilus influenzae*** **type b** strains cause meningitis or esophagitis in infants and toddlers who have not been vaccinated; some strains cause conjunctivitis and otitis; may cause bronchitis in patients with COPD.
  b. Genus: ***Pasteurella.***
    Features:
    (1) **Gram-negative coccobacilli** (short bacilli) found in the mouths of healthy animals.
    (2) *Pasteurella multocida* may cause cellulitis in humans following untreated animal bites or scratches; *P. pestis* is the causative agent of plague, which is still endemic in the southwest United States.
  c. Genus: ***Coxiella*** (formerly considered a rickettsia) is a Gram-negative rod intracellular organism found in high titers in pregnant animals. It survives drying outside the host and is transmitted by amnionic fluid aerosols or dust from dried parturition materials of infected animals. Taxonomically, *Coxiella* is now considered closer to Legionella (Fig. 3.10).
  d. Genus: ***Legionella.***
    Features:
    (1) **Gram-negative,** short **rod.**
    (2) **Obligate aerobes** and **facultative intracellular organism.**
    (3) Grows in amoeba in streams but survives very long periods in water contaminating water lines (e.g., grocery store vegetable sprayers, dental water lines, etc.) and air-conditioning cooling tanks.
    (4) **Fastidious: Utilizes proteins** rather than carbohydrates as an energy source; charcoal-yeast extract agar (CYE), which has the needed cysteine, is the selective isolation medium.

8. Family: **Enterobacteriaceae.**
  a. General characteristics:
    (1) Gram-negative rods that ferment glucose.
    (2) Facultative anaerobes; oxidase-negative.
    (3) Have **antigens** that may be used in identification: O antigen (cell envelope), H antigen (flagella), K antigen (capsule), Vi antigen (*Salmonella typhi* capsule), and P antigen (pili).

b. Genus: *Escherichia.*
Features:
(1) Ferment lactose as well as glucose.
(2) Major component of **normal colon flora.**
(3) Motile.
(4) May or may not have a capsule, depending on the strain.
(5) Cause urinary tract infections, septicemia, neonatal septicemia and meningitis, several GI tract diseases, and, following bowel perforation, peritonitis.

c. Genus: *Klebsiella.*
Features:
(1) Ferment lactose as well as **glucose.**
(2) Highly motile; found in the human colon and in water.
(3) Produce **copious** amounts of their **polysaccharide capsule.**
(4) Are opportunists; cause ventilator-associated pneumonias.

d. Genus: *Shigella.*
Features:
(1) Do not ferment lactose.
(2) Nonmotile because they lack flagella (so no H antigens).
(3) Do not produce H_2S.
(4) Have **no animal reservoirs,** only human hosts.
(5) Invade M cells of the intestine and then move into adjoining cells via **actin polymerization** (similar to *Listeria*). Shigellae produce shallow ulcerations usually without bloodstream invasion.

e. Genus: *Yersinia.*
Features:
(1) Coccobacilli; show enhanced **bipolar** staining.
(2) Do not ferment lactose.
(3) Lack flagella; no H antigens.
(4) Do not produce H_2S.
(5) Are endemic in rodents in desert southwest of United States; cause plague (*Y. pestis*).

f. Genus: *Proteus.*
Features:
(1) Water organisms; display swarming motility.
(2) Do not ferment lactose.
(3) Produce urease and H_2S.
(4) Cause urinary tract infections and infections in immunocompromised patients.

g. Genus: *Salmonella.*
Features:
(1) Highly motile, nonlactose fermenting Enterobacteriaceae.
(2) Produce H_2S.
(3) Have more than 2000 serotypes; most now classified as *Salmonella enterica* serovar xxxx where the "xxxx" is the former species name. Informally, the former species names are still often used.
(4) Have animal reservoirs except for *Salmonella enterica* serovar typhi (e.g., *S. typhi*), which is strictly a human pathogen.

h. Genus: *Serratia.*
Features:
(1) Slow lactose-fermenting Enterobacteriaceae (Gram-negative, oxidase-negative, glucose-fermenting rod).
(2) Produce a **salmon red pigment.**

Note: END of ENTEROBACTERIACEAE
9. Family: **Vibrionaceae.**
a. General characteristics:
(1) Rods and comma-shaped Gram-negative bacteria with polar flagella.

  (2) Facultative anaerobes, all of which are oxidase-positive.
  (3) Found in water and cause GI and wound infections.
  b. Genus: *Vibrio.*
  Features:
  (1) Curved rods, some requiring salt (halophilic) to grow.
  (2) Cause cholera (mainly O1 and O139 and strains of *Vibrio cholerae*), gastroenteritis (*Vibrio parahaemolyticus*), and cellulitis or hepatitis/septicemia (*Vibrio vulnificus*).
  c. Genus: *Aeromonas.* These ubiquitous Gram-negative rods grow in fresh and salt water (opportunists).

10. Gram-negative spiral-shaped rods: *Campylobacter* and *Helicobacter.*
  a. General characteristics:
  (1) Capnophilic (require elevated CO_2) and **microaerophilic** (grow only in the presence of low oxygen).
  (2) Fastidious (require special media) partially because they **do not metabolize carbohydrates** either oxidatively or by fermentation.
  b. Genus: *Helicobacter.*
  Features:
  (1) Grow at 37°C.
  (2) *Helicobacter pylori* is a chronic colonizer of the human gastric tract with potential to cause ulcers and stomach cancer.
  c. Genus: *Campylobacter.*
  Features:
  (1) Grow at 42°C.
  (2) Cause inflammatory diarrhea (*Campylobacter jejuni*).

11. Gram-negative anaerobes:
  a. General characteristics. These bacteria are prominent colonizers of mucosal surfaces of the oropharynx, female genital tract, and intestines, and thus cause endogenous infections, which are generally polymicrobic.
  b. Genus: *Bacteroides.*
  Features:
  (1) Slender, Gram-negative rods that stain only pale red and have endotoxin with reduced toxicity compared with other Gram-negative bacteria.
  (2) Part of normal GI tract flora.
  (3) Have a **capsule** as their major virulence factor.
  (4) Resistant to bile so they are prominent colonizers of the intestine.
  (5) Although other species of *Bacteroides* are more prevalent in the GI tract, it is usually *Bacteroides fragilis* that is prominent in infections.
  c. Genera: *Prevotella* and *Porphyromonas* are pigmented, **Gram-negative anaerobes** found in oropharyngeal mucosa.
  d. Genus: *Fusobacterium:* **fine needlelike Gram-negative anaerobes** that are part of the normal oral flora.

V. POORLY GRAM-STAINING BACTERIA

Many bacteria do not reliably show up on a Gram stain. These include many of the following groups of bacteria: **spirochetes, rickettsias, chlamydiae, mycoplasmas, mycobacteria,** and members of the genera *Coxiella* and *Legionella.* Most are too thin in diameter for the light microscope to resolve the cylinder of color trapped inside the cell wall. The mycobacterial wall inhibits uptake of the dyes. The legionellae stain Gram-negative as long as the counterstain time is increased. Stains such as silver, Giemsa, or FA stains, which deposit on the surface of the cell, are generally used for these organisms.

A. Spirochetes.
   1. **General characteristics:**
      a. **Flexible, spiral-shaped bacteria with endoflagellum.**
      b. The endoflagellum (also called an axial filament) runs from one end to the other of the bacterium underneath the outer membrane, creating a springing motility.
      c. Not reliably seen by Gram stain (due to its small diameter), but because they have a thin, flexible peptidoglycan layer covered with an outer membrane, they are considered Gram-negative. FA and dark-field microscopy are used to visualize material from lesions.
      d. Classified by their tightness of coiling, cell diameter, and presence of terminal hooks into three genera.
   2. Genus: *Treponema.*
      Features:
      a. **Very thin with tight coiling and no terminal hooks.**
      b. Difficult to culture in the clinical lab, so they are often listed as obligate pathogens. (They are generally extracellular.)
      c. Cause syphilis (*Treponema pallidum*) and related diseases.
   3. Genus: *Leptospira.*
      Features:
      a. Similar to *Treponema* except with **hooks on the ends.**
      b. Cause leptospirosis, a zoonotic disease transmitted by animal urine in water.
   4. **Genus: *Borrelia.***
      Features:
      a. **Larger in diameter and more loosely coiled** than the treponemes or leptospires.
      b. Cause Lyme disease (*Borrelia burgdorferi*) and relapsing fever (other *Borrelia* species).

B. Order: Rickettsiales.
   1. **General characteristics:**
      a. **Obligate intracellular parasites (OIPs).**
      b. Survive only a short time outside of the host cell.
      c. Transmitted by **arthropod vectors** and most are maintained in nonhuman reservoirs.
   2. Genera: *Rickettsia* and *Orientia.*
      Features:
      a. **OIPs** that dissolve the phagosome and **escape into the cytosol of the cell and replicate there.**
      b. Transmitted by arthropod vectors.
      c. **Infect and kill endothelial cells,** causing capillary leakage and vasculitis; cause serious systemic diseases like **Rocky Mountain spotted fever (*Rickettsia rickettsii*)** or scrub typhus (*Orientia tsutsugamushi*).

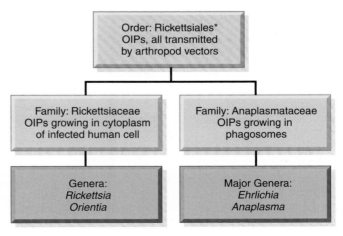

FIGURE 3.10. **Rickettsiales.** Order Rickettsiales are all small bacteria which are obligate intracellular pathogens (OIPs) and divide by binary fission. They require a host for ATP, cofactor A, and NAD. They are poorly Gram staining but have a Gram-negative cell wall structure. They have animal or arthropod hosts; they are spread by arthropod bite and do not survive outside their vectors or hosts. Two major genera—*Coxiella* and *Bartonella*—have been moved out of Rickettsiaceae but are sometimes still listed or referred to as Rickettsiaceae.

* OIPs = Obligate Intracellular Pathogens.

   3. Genera: *Ehrlichia* and *Anaplasma.*
   Features:
   a. Rickettsial OIPs that replicate in vacuoles.
   b. Have animal hosts and tick vectors.
   c. Infect white cells.
   d. Cause human monocytic ehrlichiosis (*Ehrlichia chaffeensis*) and human granulocytic anaplasmosis (*Anaplasma phagocytophilum = Ehrlichia phagocytophila*). Important rickettsias are listed with their reservoirs, vectors, and diseases in Table 3.4.

C. Order: Chlamydiales.
   1. General characteristics:
   a. OIPs unable to generate adenosine triphosphate (ATP).
   b. Have an inner and outer membrane but **no peptidoglycan. Proteins in the outer membrane of the elementary bodies are extensively cross-linked, providing some rigidity.**
   c. Transmitted directly from **person to person** by respiratory droplets or direct mucosal contact, or during the birth process.
   d. Two forms:
   (1) The **infectious form** is the **metabolically inert elementary body.** It has surface ligands that bind to human host cells, triggering the uptake of the chlamydiae.
   (2) In human cell phagosomes, the elementary bodies develop into **reticulate bodies,** which undergo binary fission to produce many more elementary bodies.

t a b l e **3.4**	Important Rickettsial Species			
Group	Disease	Organism	Spread: Vector/ Reservoirs	Clinical Presentation
Anaplasmosis	Primarily NE and north central United States	*Anaplasma phagocytophilum*	*Ixodes* and perhaps other ticks	Human granulocytic anaplasmosis (HGA) = systemic disease from destruction of granulocytes; fever, malaise, myalgias, with thrombocytopenia.
Ehrlichiosis	Primarily in SE and south central United States	*Ehrlichia chaffeensis*	Ticks (*Amblyoma*)	Human monocytic ehrlichiosis (HME) = disease similar to HGA but thrombocytopenia is not as common & monocytes infected.
Typhus	Epidemic (worldwide) or sylvatic typhus (Eastern United States)	***Rickettsia prowazekii***	Human body lice or flying squirrels (FS) (fleas?)/ humans and FS	Trunk rash, progressing to extremities; gangrene, shock, hemorrhages in kidney, heart, brain, and lungs; milder disease in United States from FS
	Endemic	*Rickettsia typhi*	Rat fleas/rats	Trunk rash, progressing to extremities (less severe than epidemic typhus).
Spotted fevers	**Rocky Mountain spotted fever**	*Rickettsia rickettsii*	Dog and wood ticks (*Dermacentor*)/ ticks and dogs are reservoirs	Rash on extremities, progressing to trunk, fulminant vasculitis
	Rickettsialpox	*Rickettsia akari*	Mites/rodents	Rash similar to chickenpox (benign course), adenopathy, eschar at bite site.
Diseases caused by organisms formerly considered rickettsias				
	Q fever	*Coxiella burnetii*	Aerosols of amniotic fluid or dust from dried parturition products	Pneumonitis without rash; atypical pneumonia with hepatitis
	Cat scratch fever	*Bartonella henselae*	Cat scratches	Skin, eye rashes, temporary blindness

    e. Have been demonstrated through molecular techniques to have two different genera (***Chlamydophila*** and ***Chlamydia***); medically, they are often all still called genus *Chlamydia*. The species identification is now done by nucleic acid techniques.

    f. Most commonly diagnosed using fluorescent antibodies on specimens or gene probes.

    g. Cause pneumonia (***Chlamydophila pneumoniae, Chlamydophila psittaci,*** and ***Chlamydia trachomatis***) and sexually transmitted diseases and eye infections (***Chlamydia trachomatis***).

    h. Can be identified by growth in tissue cells, DFA staining, or PCR.

D. Family: Mycoplasmataceae Genera: *Mycoplasma* **and** *Ureaplasma.*
  1. General characteristics:
    a. Smallest extracellular bacteria.
    b. Lack a cell wall; are very flexible and able to pass through filters which are 0.4 microns and which stop most bacteria.
    c. Contain sterols in their cell membrane; however, they cannot synthesize sterols so mycoplasmas acquire sterols from hosts or special media.
    d. Facultative anaerobes except for ***Mycoplasma pneumoniae,*** which is an obligate aerobe.
    e. Spread by direct contact or **fresh respiratory droplets.**
    f. Bind to the exterior of cells and **damage epithelium from the outside.**
    g. Fastidious and slow **to grow** even on special cholesterol-containing medium, so diagnosis is usually clinical or serological with PCR becoming more readily available.
    h. Cold agglutinins (autoantibodies agglutinating red blood cells at 4°C) may be present after 1 to 2 weeks of clinical disease. Titers greater than 1:32 are generally considered positive. Complement fixation is more sensitive.
  2. ***Mycoplasma pneumoniae*** causes respiratory tract infections.
  3. ***Mycoplasma hominis*** and ***Ureaplasma urealyticum*** appear to be involved in genitourinary tract infections.

E. Genus: *Mycobacteria.*
  1. General characteristics:
    a. Poorly Gram staining, thin bacilli.
    b. Have a **waxy cell surface** containing a thin triple layer of peptidoglycan linked to and covered with **long chain fatty acids (mycotic acids).** This waxy cell envelope has the following features:
      (1) Porin proteins allow transport of aqueous materials across the otherwise hydrophobic envelope.
      (2) Confers resistance to drying, allowing respiratory droplet nuclei (the dried remains of respiratory droplets) to spread in air handling systems.
      (3) Allows the survival of nontuberculous mycobacteria in soil.
    c. Aerobic bacteria; when walled off in granulomas, their metabolism slows but they may continue to release antigens that stimulate the continued remodeling of the granuloma wall as long as the immune system remains healthy. If the immune system begins to fail, the granuloma wall thins and may erode, exposing the organism to oxygen and triggering new growth and spread.
  2. ***Mycobacterium tuberculosis*** and ***M. bovis*** (both cause tuberculosis).
  3. ***Mycobacterium kansasii*** or ***M. avium-intracellulare*** (also known as *Mycobacterium avian complex* or **MAC**): grouped as **nontuberculous mycobacteria** or atypical mycobacteria or mycobacteria other than tuberculosis (MOTTS). These opportunists cause respiratory diseases in patients with low CD4+ counts such as acquired immunodeficiency syndrome (AIDS) patients or patients on chemotherapy. They are **not contagious from person to person** and are acquired from showers or dust.
  4. ***Mycobacterium leprae*** causes leprosy.

Review Test

Directions: *Each of the numbered items or incomplete statements in this section is followed by answers or completions of the statement. Select the ONE lettered answer that is BEST in each case.*

1. A 21-year-old male college student who had complained of headache and feeling feverish the night before is brought this morning to the emergency department (ED) when his roommate was unable to rouse him. He had been well until yesterday. Vital signs include fever (39.8°C/103.1°F), tachycardia, and hypotension (BP 70/55). Remarkable on physical examination is petechial rash (purpuric in areas) and nuchal rigidity with positive Kernig and Brudzinski signs. CSF is cloudy with high protein and low glucose. Intracellular, red diplococci are seen on Gram stain. What is the most likely genus?

(A) *Staphylococcus*   **(D)** *Mycobacterium*
(B) *Streptococcus*   **(E)** *Neisseria*
(C) *Chlamydia*

2. A 24-year-old female presents with dysuria, as well as urinary urgency and frequency. A urine dipstick test is positive for both leukocyte esterase and nitrites. What genus or family is noted for the production of nitrites?

(A) *Escherichia*   **(C)** *Streptococcus*
(B) *Staphylococcus*   **(D)** *Vibrio*

3. What rapid test commonly used on Gram-negative rods rules out Enterobacteriaceae if positive?

(A) Catalase   **(D)** Chitinase
(B) Coagulase   **(E)** Urease
(C) Oxidase

4. A patient presents with rapid onset severe respiratory symptoms. Chest radiographs show a hemorrhagic lymphadenitis. The isolation of chains of fairly large, aerobic Gram-positive rods, some of which have started to sporulate from a patient with this presentation, should raise a major concern of which organism? (You should be able to answer this question from the genus alone, although a question might also mention that it was nonmotile.)

(A) *Actinomyces israelii*
(B) *Bacillus anthracis*
(C) *Campylobacter jejuni*

(D) *Clostridium perfringens*
(E) *Haemophilus influenzae*

5. A patient undergoing chemotherapy develops a cough. Acid-fast stain of his sputum shows rods and slightly longer forms, with some branching; they vary in their acid-fast reaction from one area of the slide to the next. The acid-fast stain was performed by an experienced medical technologist and, when redone, showed the same variation. The growth was done aerobically. What is the most likely agent?

(A) *Actinomyces*
(B) *Chlamydophila*
(C) *Mycobacterium avian-intracellulare* (MAI or MAC)
(D) *Nocardia*

6. A female patient with a new genital lesion presents to your sexually transmitted disease clinic. She is homeless, has no health insurance, and is an intravenous drug user. You suspect syphilis. Which of these techniques would be most appropriate to demonstrate treponemes?

(A) Immunological test such as the VDRL
(B) Dark-field microscopy
(C) Acid-fast stain
(D) Gram stain
(E) Electrophoresis

7. The CSF from a 2-week-old infant with meningitis shows rods with tumbling motility. These bacteria are found to be Gram-positive and do not form spores. What is the most likely agent?

(A) *Actinomyces*
(B) *Bacillus*
(C) *Clostridium*
(D) *Corynebacterium*
(E) *Listeria*

8. Both a 53-year-old farmer and his 21-year-old son present in August with fever, myalgia, and malaise, which they came down with within a few hours of each other. The son had been home in southern Minnesota for only 3 weeks to help field train two new hunting dogs. You ask about potential tick bites, and the son did have one on him, which was quite engorged. Platelets and granulocytes are low in each man's blood. You ask one of your experienced techs to do a Giemsa stain on a thick blood smear. He calls, reporting clusters of cells resembling raspberries in granulocytes, even though nothing grows in any of the blood cultures. You realize that the blood cultures you set up will not grow and that you have two patients who have infections with a tick-borne obligate intracellular parasite of granulocytes. What genus does the organism belong to?

(A) *Anaplasma* (formerly *Ehrlichia*)
(B) *Borrelia*
(C) *Chlamydia*
(D) *Haemophilus*
(E) *Mycoplasma*

9. A full-term 6-day-old neonate is brought in with a purulent conjunctivitis which the parents noticed earlier today. On Gram stain of the purulent exudate, no bacteria are seen. Which of the following bacteria is most likely the cause of the conjunctivitis?

(A) *Chlamydia trachomatis*
(B) *Escherichia coli*
(C) *Listeria monocytogenes*
(D) *Neisseria gonorrhoeae*
(E) *Streptococcus pneumoniae*

10. An 83-year-old who still lives in her own home has developed pneumonia following influenza. The Gram stain of her sputa is shown. What is the most likely agent?

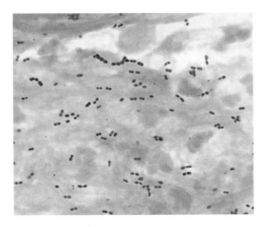

(A) *Chlamydophila pneumoniae*
(B) Influenza virus
(C) *Klebsiella pneumoniae*
(D) *Mycoplasma pneumoniae*
(E) *Staphylococcus aureus*
(F) *Streptococcus pneumoniae*

11. The reagent used to distinguish staphylococci from streptococci is

(A) Hydrogen peroxide
(B) Fibronectin
(C) Fibrinogen
(D) Oxidase

12. A 14-month-old boy is brought in by his parents with fever, fussiness and lethargy, and apparent headache. On examination, the neck is stiff. His parents have not allowed his routine childhood vaccines. Very short Gram-negative rods are seen in the CSF, so antibiotics are immediately started. The organism grows on chocolate agar but not blood agar. No one else in the family is ill. What is the most likely causative agent?

(A) *Escherichia coli*
(B) *Haemophilus influenzae* type b
(C) *Klebsiella pneumoniae*
(D) *Neisseria meningitidis*
(E) *Streptococcus pneumoniae*

13. A healthy 7-year-old boy who has not traveled outside the United States is brought in by his parents in June with signs of meningitis. No bacteria are seen in the Gram stain of the CSF, and no bacterial capsule material is present as determined by a series of latex particle agglutination tests standard to the diagnosis of meningitis. The CSF glucose level is slightly low, protein is near normal, and white cell count is less than 500 cells/microL, mainly lymphocytes. What is the most likely causative agent?

(A) *Chlamydophila pneumoniae*
(B) Enterovirus
(C) *Mycoplasma pneumoniae*
(D) *Mycobacterium tuberculosis*
(E) *Treponema pallidum*

14. In any case, a clue indicating that the causative organism is an obligate intracellular pathogen transmitted by an arthropod bite should lead you to which of the following groups of organisms?

(A) Chlamydiae
(B) Enterobacteriaceae

(C) Rickettsias including *Anaplasma* and *Ehrlichia*

(D) Spirochetes including *Borrelia burgdorferi*

15. What is the main difference between fluorochrome staining (e.g., auramine-rhodamine screening for *Mycobacterium tuberculosis*) and indirect fluorescent antibody (IFA) staining?

(A) Fluorochromes are more specific and used just for *Mycobacterium tuberculosis.*

(B) IFAs are less specific since they use antibody to a different species' antibody (i.e., rabbit antibody to human antibody).

(C) Fluorochrome staining is less sensitive than comparable staining with light microscopy.

(D) IFA's specificity is dependent on the primary antibody used; fluorochromes lack the antibody specificity.

Answers and Explanations

1. **The answer is E.** Gram-negative bacteria should be described as red or pink, so the description fits a Gram-negative diplococcus which is most likely *Neisseria*. *Staph* and *Strep* would be purple, and neither *Chlamydophila* nor *Mycobacterium* will show up on Gram stain.

2. **The answer is A.** Since all choices are in italics, all are genus names and you do not need to look for a family name. Since all Enterobacteriaceae generally produce nitrate reductase, they all eventually produce a positive dipstick nitrite test. *Escherichia* is the only choice belonging to this family. Other members of Enterobacteriaceae that cause urinary tract infections include *Proteus* and *Klebsiella.* Staph and Strep are Gram-positive and *Vibrio* is a genus of Gram-negative, comma-shaped bacteria. A positive nitrite test rules out *Staph. saprophyticus* as the cause of a urinary tract infection.

3. **The answer is C.** Most common Gram-negative rods are oxidase-positive. The major exceptions are members of the Enterobacteriaceae. A catalase test (utilizing hydrogen peroxide) is most commonly used to distinguish Staphylococci (+) from Streptococci (−). (Most aerobes will be catalase-positive and many obligate anaerobes are catalase-negative.) Coagulase is used to distinguish *Staph. aureus* (+) from other medical isolates (coagulase-negative *Staph*). No medically important bacteria have chitinase. There are several medically important urease-positive bacteria, most importantly *Helicobacter pylori, Proteus* sp., and *Ureaplasma urealyticum.*

4. **The answer is B.** *Bacillus* is the correct genus. There are two Gram-positive spore-forming rods. *Bacillus* is aerobic with one species (*Bacillus anthracis*), causing hemorrhagic lymphadenitis and pulmonary edema. The other genus with bacterial endospores, the Clostridia, do not grow aerobically. The other Gram-positive organism listed, *Actinomyces,* often described as a branching bacterium, is also anaerobic. *Campylobacter* and *Haemophilus* are both Gram-negative.

5. **The answer is D.** Either *Nocardia* or MAI is possible from the clinical scenario, but the most likely agent from the acid-fast stain description, the focus of the question, is *Nocardia*. Also, MAI would not grow in 2 days (so some mention of time would be made) and *Actinomyces* would only grow anaerobically, which would also be stated. *Chlamydophila* would not grow except in tissue culture.

6. **The answer is B.** First, notice that the question specifically asks about demonstrating the presence of treponemes and not making the diagnosis of syphilis. (Also, note that the lesions are still present, which suggests that it is too early for serological methods to be reliable.) Then, remember that *Treponema pallidum* is still only cultured by research labs. Because treponemes are so thin in cross-section, they do not reliably show up on a Gram stain; thus, dark-field or FA (not mentioned as a choice) staining would be necessary.

7. **The answer is E.** *Listeria* is the correct answer. Both *Bacillus* and *Clostridium* can be eliminated because they are spore-formers. *Actinomyces* and corynebacteria are both Gram-positive and nonmotile and are not common causative agents of neonatal meningitis. *Listeria* has a tumbling motility when grown in broth, in this case CSF.

8. **The answer is A.** Obligate intracellular bacteria transmitted through arthropods would most likely be the genera: *Rickettsia, Orientia, Anaplasma,* and *Ehrlichia,* with the latter two infecting white cells and *Anaplasma* causing the described disease (Human granulocytic anaplasmosis).

9. **The answer is A.** Neonatal eye infections are most likely to be *Chlamydia trachomatis*, which does not show up on Gram stain. All of the remaining organisms stain well with Gram stain.

10. **The answer is F.** The most common cause of pneumonia in people over 65 years of age has generally been *S. pneumoniae*. Although the other agents also cause pneumonia, *S. pneumoniae* is the only organism that fits the descriptions of Gram-positive cocci in chains. It is also quite common following influenza. If the woman had not been vaccinated for influenza, then she also may not have been vaccinated for pneumococcus.

11. **The answer is A.** The staphylococci are aerobic while the streptococci are aerotolerant anaerobes. Streptococci ferment even in the presence of full oxygen and lack catalase. A standard quick test is the test mixing staphylococci with hydrogen peroxide. The generation of oxygen bubbles indicates that a Gram-positive coccus is a *Staphylococcus* rather than a *Streptococcus*. A coagulase test using serum to see if fibrinogen is clotted is used to distinguish the coagulase-positive staphylococci from coagulase-negative staphylococci. Oxidase is not the reagent but the reactor in the oxidase test.

12. **The answer is B.** Although *Haemophilus influenzae* type b is rarely seen in vaccinated children younger than 2 years of age, it still occurs in unvaccinated children. The description of a chocolate agar-positive organism should suggest either *Neisseria meningitidis* or *H. influenzae* type b. The descriptor as a short rod (from CSF) or pleomorphic rod (from culture) suggests *H. influenzae* type b. Although both *Klebsiella pneumonia* and *Escherichia coli* (a cause of neonatal meningitis) are both Gram-negative rods, neither is likely to cause meningitis in a healthy child, and, like all other Enterobacteriaceae, will grow on blood agar. *Streptococcus* is Gram-positive.

13. **The answer is B.** None of the bacteria listed as choices reliably show up on Gram stain, and none of them is likely to cause meningitis in this scenario. It is much more likely to be an enterovirus. (This one was just to keep you awake!)

14. **The answer is C.** Of the choices, only the chlamydiae and the rickettsia are obligate intracellular organisms. Chlamydiae are spread by direct contact or respiratory droplets, while the rickettsia (the correct answer) are spread commonly by arthropod vectors. Spirochetes like *B. burgdorferi* are not obligate intracellular pathogens and most are also not transmitted by arthropod vectors.

15. **The answer is D.** Fluorochrome dyes, like auramine-rhodamine screening for *Mycobacterium tuberculosis,* lack the specificity of either direct or indirect FA tests because the FA tests use antibodies, making them more specific. The fluorochrome dyes are more sensitive than a comparable acid-fast stain on a bright field light microscope because they light up the microbes on a black background when viewed with the fluorescent microscope. However, the use of antibodies in the IFAs makes them highly specific.

chapter 4

Bacterial Diseases

This chapter describes major bacterial infections by organ system or situation, presenting critical basic details in appropriate detail for medical students.

Seven important species of bacteria are involved in so many different systems that rather than repeating the basic information for each, they are presented in the first section of this chapter under the heading "Major Recurring Species." This clustering also should facilitate learning these species first! These species are: *Chlamydia trachomatis, Escherichia coli, Haemophilus influenzae, Pseudomonas aeruginosa, Staphylococcus aureus, Streptococcus pneumoniae,* and *Streptococcus pyogenes.* Please "bookmark" this section for easy reference.

Antibiotic usage has become increasingly complicated and is beyond the scope of this book. But particularly where antibiotic treatment is straight forward or there is known drug resistance or where treatment involves something in addition to antibiotics, then it may be mentioned. This is done to re-inforce your pharmacology. These drugs are listed as **primary drugs for the treatment for the specific organism** as suggested by *The Sanford Guide to Antimicrobial Therapy* (2012) and *not* the recommended initial therapy for the disease prior to identification of the etiological agent.

I. MAJOR RECURRING SPECIES

A. *Chlamydia trachomatis.*
   Features:
   1. Small, **non-Gram staining,** obligate intracellular pathogen (**OIP**).
   2. Found **only in humans; transmitted as elementary bodies** by **direct contact** (birth, sex, or genitals-to-fingers-to-own eye) or on feet of flies tracking from one eye to next.
   Diseases:
   1. Causes **disease by intracellular replication that elicits** (except in neonates) a **granulomatous response**; if untreated, this leads to damage that depends on body locale (for example, fallopian tube blockage may lead to infertility or ectopic pregnancy).
   2. The **three major serovar groups** each cause a different spectrum of disease; multiple serotypes of each allow reinfection.
      a. *Chl. trachomatis* **serovars D–K** in the United States cause conjunctivitis, genitourinary tract infection, and neonatal pneumonia.
      b. *Chl. trachomatis* **serovars A–C** cause trachoma.
      c. *Chl. trachomatis* **serovars L1, L2, and L3** cause lymphogranuloma venereum.
   3. **Lab ID:** *Chlamydia trachomatis:* NAA tests (nucleic acid amplification tests), which can be done on self-collected vaginal swabs or urines, have replaced cell cultures.
   4. **Treatment:** commonly doxycycline or a macrolide.

B. *Escherichia coli.*

Features:

1. **Motile, lactose-fermenting,** member of the **Enterobacteriaceae** (so oxidase-negative, facultative anaerobe, fermenter of glucose)
2. Colonic **normal flora (NF) (nonpathogenic strains)** of humans and animals. May colonize **lower end of urethra and vagina.** Transmitted during **birth** or via the **fecal-oral** route.

Diseases:

1. *E. coli* causes urinary tract infections (**UTIs**), **neonatal sepsis** and **meningitis,** and **diarrheal diseases.**
2. Disease results when **NF strains enter normally sterile body sites** or **acquire virulence factors, or the host acquires a new virulent strain.**
    a. All strains have endotoxin and constitutively produce common pili that adhere to colon cells.
    b. Like other Enterobacteriaceae, *E. coli* easily receives (or donates) genetic elements from other enterobacteria.
3. **Lab ID:** *Escherichia coli:*
    a. Grows on bile-containing differential media like Hektoen or MacConkey.
    b. Ferments lactose and is identified by a panel of metabolic tests.
4. **Treatment:** treated (except for uncomplicated UTIs) according to drug susceptibility results.

C. *Haemophilus influenzae.*

Features:

1. **Gram-negative, fastidious, pleomorphic rod** (coccobacillary in cerebrospinal fluid).
2. Part of **NF** of the **upper respiratory tract;** NF strains generally do not have a capsule and are called nontypeable; encapsulated virulent strains are stereotyped by the lab; all are transmitted via respiratory droplets by direct contact.

Diseases:

1. Otitis media may be caused by any strain with or without capsule. Virulent strains with type b capsule may cause **meningitis or epiglottitis in unvaccinated children,** generally younger than 5 years of age. *H. influenzae* type d causes exacerbations of chronic bronchitis in patients with chronic obstructive pulmonary disease (COPD).
2. **Lab ID:** *H. influenzae* **is fastidious**—nonhemolytic but **requires protoporphyrin and NAD** and so does not grow on blood agar (BA) but grows on (1) chocolate agar (**chocolate agar positive**) where RBCs are already lysed; (2) near *Staph. aureus* hemolysis on blood agar (satellite colonies); or (3) on nutrient agar with added X (hematin) and V (nicotinamide adenine dinucleotide [NAD]) factors.
3. **Treatment:** treated with cefotaxime or ceftriaxone (for life-threatening infections) or amoxicillin-clavulanate or oral cephalosporins for less serious infections.

D. *Pseudomonas aeruginosa,*

Features:

1. **Gram-negative rod** with polar **flagella**.
2. **Oxidase-positive** (not an Enterobacteriaceae) **aerobe (nonfermentative)**.
3. **Pigments: fluorescein,** a fluorescent pigment, and **pyocyanin, a blue-green pigment.** Blue-green pus is a classic sign of *Ps. aeruginosa* cellulitis in burn patients.
4. **Ubiquitous** and widely distributed in/on **plants, soil,** and **water.** Rapid growth occurs even in distilled or tap water (i.e., sink drains, faucet aerators, cut flowers).

Diseases:

1. Pseudomonas is a frequent cause of **nosocomial infections**, with pneumonias in cystic fibrosis (CF), neutropenic, or ventilated patients; cellulitis in burn patients; plus other infections often involving trauma (e.g., nail penetrating tennis shoe to foot, eye trauma, etc.).
2. **Pathogenesis:**
    a. The **exopolysaccharide layer (slime/capsule) inhibits phagocytic uptake** and **increases adherence** to tracheal epithelium and mucin creating biofilms. It is **up-regulated in CF biofilms. Pili** also aid in adherence.

    b. **Endotoxin** triggers inflammation/shock.

    c. *P. aeruginosa* **exotoxin A** is an **ADP-ribosyl transferase** (similar in activity to diphtheria toxin) that **inactivates EF-2** (elongation factor-2), halting protein synthesis **primarily in the liver**, resulting in liver necrosis.

    d. **Phospholipase-C** damages all membranes, causing tissue necrosis; **elastase and other proteolytic enzymes** damage elastin, immunoglobulins, complement components, and collagen.

  3. Lab ID: often iridescent sheen on colonies; fruity odor.

  4. Treatment: drug resistance; antipseudomonal antibiotics and **susceptibility.**

    a. *Pseudomonas* has a **high inherent resistance** and also acquires resistance (e.g., β-lactamases, decreased carbapenem entrance due to porin loss, DNA gyrase mutations (FQ), and aminoglycoside-inactivating enzymes. **Efflux pump** rids it of antibiotics.

    b. **Antipseudomonal penicillins, dori-, mero-, or imipenems, 3rd generation cephalosporins, tobramycin, or ciprofloxacin;** AP Pen + (tobramycin or ciprofloxacin) in serious disease.

E. *Staphylococcus aureus.*

Features:

  1. Catalase-positive, coagulase-positive, beta-hemolytic, Gram-positive coccus found in **grapelike clusters.**

  2. Colonizes anterior nares' mucosa (~15% of adults are carriers; shed on skin). **Increased cutaneous numbers** are found on **"needle" users.** Transmitted by **direct contact/fomites** (e.g., bedrails.)

Diseases:

  1. Causes **skin/tissue/surgical infections, endocarditis,** infective arthritis, **osteomyelitis,** pneumonias (postinfluenza, very young CF patients, following community-acquired MRSA cellulitis, etc.); **toxic shock syndrome,** scalded skin syndrome, and food poisoning.

  2. Pathogenesis:

    a. **Hemolysins/cytolytic toxins** including the pore-forming exotoxin A.

    b. **Fibrinogen-binding clumping factor** allows *S. aureus* to bind to normal tissue (e.g., heart), thereby facilitating damage by other toxins. This is one of many *S. aureus* MSCRAMMs (microbial surface components recognizing adhesive matrix molecules) playing roles in its ability to adhere to and cause disease in many sites.

    c. **Coagulase binds to prothrombin, triggering fibrin polymerization around** *Staph. aureus,* slowing clearance.

    d. Surface **protein A binds the** antibody **Fc** portion, **reducing opsonization (**as also does the **capsule).**

    e. **Teichoic acids (lipoteichoic** and **cell-wall–bound)** play a role in **adherence;** when the cell wall is breaking up; lipoteichoic acids with peptidoglycan **trigger shock** via the same pathways as endotoxins.

  3. Lab ID: *Staph. aureus:* **positive catalase and coagulase** tests; **beta-hemolytic;** haloduric and ferments mannitol (**mannitol agar positive**), gold colonies.

  4. Treatment: drug resistance; **do susceptibility tests.**

    a. In the 1950s, *Staph. aureus* acquired a **plasmid conferring resistance to many early antibiotics** such as tetracyclines and penicillins; these strains are known in the United States as **methicillin-sensitive Staph. aureus (MSSA).** New β-lactams (methicillin and nafcillin) were developed to treat MSSA.

    b. In the 1980s, some MSSA strains developed new cell wall synthetic enzymes (penicillin-binding proteins or PBP) made by the ***mecA* gene,** which allows these bacteria to build peptidoglycan in the presence of methicillin or nafcillin; these are the **methicillin-resistant Staph. aureus (MRSA).**

    c. Now, there are **vancomycin-intermediate Staph. aureus (VISA)** with thick cell walls that bind fairly high levels of vancomycin and **vancomycin-resistant Staph. aureus (VRSA)** with higher resistance, similar to vancomycin-resistant enterococci (VRE).

F. *Streptococcus pneumoniae* (a.k.a., Pneumococcus).
   Features:
   1. **Catalase-negative, Gram-positive, alpha-hemolytic, lancet-shaped diplococcus.**
   2. **Oropharyngeal mucosal colonizer/opportunist.**
   Diseases:
   1. **Otitis, sinusitis, pinkeye; pneumonia** or **meningitis** in **nonvaccinated young, old, or alcoholics.**
   2. **Pathogenesis:**
      a. Colonizes with the help of **protein adhesins** and an **IgA protease;** reduces numbers of competing NF by production of large amounts of **hydrogen peroxide.**
      b. Thick **polysaccharide capsule** reduces the effectiveness of complement and antibodies, **decreasing phagocytic uptake; there are more than 80 different capsular polysaccharide types.**
      c. Hemolyzes cells through **pneumolysis** and partially reduces hemoglobin to green pigment (**alpha-hemolysis**).
   3. **Lab ID:** *Streptococcus pneumoniae:*
      a. **Alpha-hemolytic, lysed by bile,** and **inhibited by optochin.**
      b. (Has no cell wall carbohydrates so not typeable with Lancefield's antibodies.) **Capsules are typed by the quellung reaction** (apparent capsular swelling when mixed with the matching antibody).
   4. **Treatment: penicillin resistance due to decreased binding to penicillin-binding proteins** mandates testing.
   5. **Prevention:**
      a. A **13-valent polysaccharide-protein conjugate** vaccine (T-cell dependent) for infants.
      b. A **23-valent polysaccharide vaccine** for patients **65 years or older,** asplenics, diabetics, human immunodeficiency virus (HIV) positive, COPD, and so on.

G. *Streptococcus pyogenes* (Group A strep [GAS]).
   Features:
   1. GAS is **beta-hemolytic, Gram-positive, catalase-negative, coccus in chains.**
   2. Also known as **GAS** because it interacts with **Lancefield antibodies for Group A cell wall carbohydrates** (the basis for the rapid antigen test).
   3. **Inhibited by bacitracin** and produces L-pyrrolidone arylamidase (**PYR test positive**).
   4. **Colonizes skin and upper respiratory tract mucosa.** Survives on hard surfaces; spread by **fomites, respiratory droplets,** and **direct contact.**
   Diseases:
   1. GAS causes **pharyngitis, impetigo, erysipelas, cellulitis, necrotizing fasciitis, bacteremia, and streptococcal toxic shock syndrome.** Some strains may cause **rheumatic heart disease (following untreated strep throat),** others **poststreptococcal acute glomerulonephritis (post-pharyngitis or cutaneous infections).**
   2. **Tissue is damaged by enzymes,** including streptolysins and streptokinase A and B, which break down clots, DNase, and hyaluronidase (the spreading factor in necrotizing fasciitis).
      a. **Streptolysin S** is a beta-hemolysin.
      b. **Streptolysin O** is an immunogenic, beta-hemolysin. Antibody to Streptolysin O is a **marker** of recent mucosal infections used in the diagnosis of rheumatic heart disease (**ASO titer**) along with clinical symptoms.
   3. **M proteins** are anchored in *Strep. pyogenes'* cytoplasmic membrane with Class I M proteins extending through the cell wall to the cell surface although Class II M proteins do not.
      a. Strains causing rheumatic heart disease have exposed Class I M proteins, which are responsible for cross-reactivity with human heart antigens.
      b. M-12 strains are associated with glomerulonephritis.
   4. Nonimmunogenic **hyaluronic acid capsule**—inhibits phagocytic uptake until other surface components are opsonized.
   5. *Strep. pyogenes* erythrogenic (SPE) toxins:
      a. SPEs are produced only by **strains of *Strep. pyogenes* carrying a lysogenic phage.**
      b. All SPEs produce a **fine, blanching, "sandpaper" rash** on the arms and upper trunk.

   c. **SPE-A** and **SPE-C are superantigens,** nonspecifically activating large numbers of T cells, triggering proinflammatory cytokines, and ultimately producing shock and multisystem organ failure.
   6. **Lab ID:** *Strep pyogenes* pharyngitis: rapid antigen test and culture if negative; all other infections: culture on blood agar (BA). Isolates are beta-hemolytic, catalase-negative.

SYSTEM-BASED DISEASE

II. EYE INFECTIONS

A. **General aspects of conjunctivitis.**
   1. Bacterial (e.g., *S. pneumo*) conjunctivitis is characterized by a purulent exudate, sticky eyelids, and palpebral papillae. Preauricular lymphadenopathy is usually absent.
   2. Chlamydial (intracellular bacteria) and viral conjunctivitis are generally nonpurulent with preauricular lymphadenopathy and follicles instead of papillae. Because neonates lack a functional lymphoid system at birth, *Chl. trachomatis* (intracellular) conjunctivitis in neonates resembles extracellular bacterial conjunctivitis with purulence.
   3. Etiological diagnosis for some bacterial infections can be made with Gram stain, fluorescent antibody (FA) staining, antigen testing, or NAA tests.

B. **Neonatal conjunctivitis.** Condition acquired during birth. Onset of symptoms and microscopy suggest etiology. Mother may be asymptomatic but she (and her partner) also require treatment.
   1. ***Chl. trachomatis* serovars D–K.**
      Features: (Refer back to this chapter [4] section I A, referenced from now on as: see 4 I A.)
      Disease: Most common neonatal conjunctivitis (~4X more moms infected and routine eye prophylaxis does not prevent).
      a. Onset **3 to 10 days after birth**.
      b. Has **purulent exudate**, sticky eyelids, and **palpebral papillae.**
      c. **Treatment:** treated with *oral* erythromycin; to prevent pneumonitis. (Signs: repetitive staccato cough without wheezing; may lead to asthma.) Treat mother/partner.
   2. ***Neisseria gonorrhoeae:***
      Features:
      a. **Oxidase-positive, Gram-negative diplococcus** with a "paired kidney bean" morphology; **utilizes glucose** but **does not ferment maltose.**
      b. Human oculogenital **mucosal pathogen** is sometimes asymptomatic.
      Disease: hyperpurulent conjunctivitis in neonates
      a. Onset **2 to 4 days after birth**.
      b. Hyperacute and **hyperpurulent** with pus reaccumulating within minutes of lavage.
      c. **Eyesight is rapidly destroyed** from apparent **pressure necrosis** of the corneal surfaces due to the rapid accumulation of pus under the eyelid.
      d. **Prophylaxis** with erythromycin or silver nitrate **prevents!**
      e. **Treatment: Immediate!** Use IV **ceftriaxone *and* lavage** to prevent loss of eyesight. Also treat neonate for ***Chlamydia*** since more common. Treat Mom/partner.
      f. **Lab ID:** rapidly diagnosed by Gram stain; follow-up: culture/susceptibilities.

C. **Bacterial conjunctivitis in children/adults. Acute, mucopurulent with conjunctival injection, eyelid swelling (unilateral to quickly bilateral).**
   1. **Agents/Features: *Staphylococcus* spp., *Strep. pneumoniae*,** and ***H. influenzae*** are the most common bacterial agents in eyes without trauma (see 4 I F, E, C).
   2. ***Ps. aeruginosa*** and ***E. coli* infections** are more commonly associated with trauma (including contact lenses) or from coma (see 4 I D, B).

D. **Adult inclusion conjunctivitis** (a.k.a., TRIC for trachoma inclusion conjunctivitis, not to be confused with trachoma below)/**Chl. trachomatis** most commonly: **serovars D–K** (see 4 I A).

Disease TRIC:

1. Adults; acute follicular conjunctivitis. Starts mucoid.
2. TRIC is often unilateral and is usually in adults; may start from person's own genital infection or another's. Treat orally.

E. **Trachoma/Chlamydia** *trachomatis* **serovars A, B, Ba, C** (see 4 I A).

1. Trachoma initially involves all conjunctival surfaces producing an initial mucopurulent conjunctivitis. Repeated untreated infections lead to chronic follicular keratoconjunctivitis with pannus formation. Ultimately upper palpebral follicles enlarge, leading to distortion of the eyelid and in-turned eyelashes, causing corneal scarring and blindness.
2. **Trachoma** is the leading cause of infectious blindness worldwide, usually in poverty where access to water is limited. Daily face and hand washing reduces transmission. Transmission is by hands or flies "tracking" the chlamydiae from eye to eye.

F. **Keratitis.**

1. Involves deeper levels; is characterized by **eye pain** and associated with eye trauma (e.g., wearing extended-wear contacts for too long, eye surgery, or contaminated eye drops).
2. Also occurs in individuals with coma who do not receive proper eye care.

Agents: Huge variety but **Pseudomonas aeruginosa** commonly occurs with contacts.

G. **Styes (hordeola).**

1. External styes are an inflamed swelling involving an infected eyelash follicle.
2. Commonly caused by mucocutaneous flora: **Staph. aureus** or **Propionibacterium** (a Gram-positive, non–spore-forming, facultative anaerobe of the normal skin flora).
3. Treated with hot packs several times a day until the stye drains and resolves.

III. DENTAL DISEASE

A. **Dental plaque/Viridans streptococci.**

Features:

1. **Alpha-hemolytic streptococci neither inhibited by optochin nor bile soluble.**
2. Normal oral flora. The most common species are *Streptococcus salivarius, Streptococcus mutans, Streptococcus mitis,* and *Streptococcus sanguis.*

Disease: dental plaque:

1. **Strep. mutans (a major player)** secretes dextran and levan capsules which fix the bacteria to teeth dental enamel, facilitating destruction of enamel and dissolution of underlying dentin.
2. If not treated (removal and filling), this invasion ultimately provides access to the tooth root and bloodstream with a high risk of serious infections, including endocarditis.

B. **Oral abscesses and periodontal disease/normal flora.**

1. Caused mainly by anaerobic oral flora including the **viridans streptococci** and many others like the **Gram-negative anaerobic rod Prevotella melaninogenica.**
2. These bacteria are particularly prominent in the gingival spaces. Dental abscesses are often polymicrobic.

Disease: Oral abscesses and periodontal disease:

1. Where oxygenation of tissues is poor from poor oral hygiene.
2. Abscesses generally require drainage to be successfully treated.

IV. EAR AND SINUS INFECTIONS

Otitis and sinusitis are commonly caused by **normal flora (NF).** Since the bacteria do not travel through the bloodstream to reach the middle ear or sinuses, capsules are not a required virulence factor. Pediatric pneumococcal and *Haemophilus* vaccinations have only slightly reduced the incidence of acute otitis media. (Nonencapsulated *H. influenzae* is part of normal oropharyngeal flora.)

Agents:

A. *Strep. pneumoniae* and *H. influenzae.* (See 4 I C and F. Please be sure as you go through this chapter that you repeat the features for each of these agents to yourself; if you are unable to do this, please turn back and re-learn it. These are some of the most tested organisms!)

B. *Moraxella catarrhalis* is a **Gram-negative diplococcus** (microscopically indistinguishable from Neisseria) found in the normal oropharyngeal flora.

C. Less commonly, **Strep. pyogenes** and **Staph. aureus.**
   Disease: Otitis media:
   1. Following viral ear infection, inflammation often causes blockage of sinus or eustachian tube, allowing fluid to accumulate that serves as a lush growth medium for NF whose bacterial growth creates pressure and pain.
   2. Risk factors include toddlers (due to eustachian tube size or position and supine drinking habits) or short eustachian tubes (cleft palate kids and certain ethnic groups); exposure to secondhand smoke; and crowded living conditions.

V. BACTERIAL PHARYNGITIS

A. Streptococcal pharyngitis/*Strep. pyogenes*
   Features: (see 4 I G):
   Disease: Strep throat:
   1. **Fever, headache, and sore throat** with an **intense pharyngeal redness**/edema, creamy-yellow tonsillar exudate, cervical lymphadenopathy, and leukocytosis; with or without nausea or anorexia.
   2. May spread to sinuses or ears; in rare cases, tonsillar abscesses may occur. The extracellular agent causes disease largely through numerous virulence factors such as hemolysins.
   3. **Treatment:** condition commonly treated with penicillin.
   4. **Nonsuppurative sequelae** include acute **rheumatic fever, rheumatic heart disease,** and **acute glomerulonephritis.**

B. Scarlet fever (*scarlatina*)/*Strep. pyogenes.*
   1. Scarlet fever is a **strep throat with the production of one or more of the phage-coded erythrogenic toxins** (SPE-A, B, or C). SPE-A and SPE-C are also superantigens.
   2. Fine, blanching, **sandpaper rash** (largely peripheral) that may **desquamate** and a tongue that becomes raw (**strawberry tongue**).

C. Other organisms that cause pharyngitis: **N. gonorrhoeae,** *Neisseria meningitidis,* or **Mycoplasma pneumoniae** (extracellular, no cell peptidoglycan).

D. Diphtheria (membranous pharyngitis)/*Corynebacterium diphtheriae.*
   1. **Gram-positive, club-shaped rod** often occurring in V- and L-shaped arrangements ("Chinese characters").
   2. **Human respiratory pathogen** colonizing the upper respiratory tract. *Tox*-negative *C. diphtheriae* are normal oral flora.

Disease:
1. **Toxin-mediated** by single **potent exotoxin** which damages the pharyngeal mucosa and circulates in the blood. The toxin is **only produced by strains of _C. diphtheriae_** that are **lysogenized by a bacteriophage carrying the _tox_ gene.** Diphtheria toxin is a **potent ADP-ribosyl transferase** that ADP-ribosylates EF-2, shutting down eukaryotic protein synthesis in the mucosa, heart, and nerves.
2. **Clinical signs: diphtheria:**
   a. Begins as **mild pharyngitis** with only slight fever. The pseudomembrane may not be present initially but grows and spreads up to the **nasopharynx or down to the larynx and trachea,** resulting in a firmly adherent, **dirty gray, pseudomembrane of fibrin, dead cells, and bacteria.**
   b. **The pathogen does not disseminate** beyond the respiratory mucosa; the **toxin circulates** and causes additional signs, such as **hoarseness, stridor, myocarditis,** and, occasionally, more severe **cardiotoxicity** or **paralysis of the soft palate** and more severe **neuropathies due to the circulating diphtheria toxin's** tropism for nerves and heart. Causes **cervical adenitis** and **edema ("bull neck").**
   c. If clinical diagnosis is made, **hospitalize immediately** and treat to prevent asphyxiation and cardiac failure. **Confirm with lab tests.**
3. **Lab ID of _tox_-positive** strains of _C. diphtheriae:_
   a. **Gray/black colonies** on a **tellurite**-containing differential medium.
   b. Demonstrate **production of diphtheria toxin by the isolate,** historically by the **Elek test,** an agar immunodiffusion test. Commonly shown now by NAA tests (some which can be done directly on the clinical isolate.
4. **Treatment:** treated with **antitoxin** and **antibiotics.**
5. **Prevention:** prevented by vaccination with an inactivated form of the diphtheria toxin known as **diphtheria toxoid** and is **part of the DTaP, Td, and Tdap vaccines.**

E. Epiglottitis/*Haemophilus influenzae.* The **_Haemophilus influenzae_ type b** pediatric capsular polysaccharide-protein conjugate vaccine has virtually eliminated pediatric epiglottitis in vaccinated children.

VI. INFECTIONS OF THE RESPIRATORY SYSTEM

Note: Pneumonias are covered in the section following this.

A. Whooping Cough (Pertussis)/*Bordetella pertussis* (*Bp*).
   Features of _Bordetella pertussis_:
   1. **Strict aerobe, Gram-negative coccobacillus.**
   2. **Highly infectious,** human pathogen of **ciliated respiratory epithelium;** transmitted by respiratory droplets from **infected individuals, primarily previously vaccinated individuals whose immunity has waned.** The most severe disease occurs in unvaccinated infants.
   Disease:
   1. *Bp* adheres through its **filamentous hemagglutinin,** its cell-associated **pertussis toxin,** an adherence factor protein called **pertactin,** and the **pili.**
   2. *Bp* does not invade deeper layers but causes submucosa inflammation. As it spreads down the respiratory tract, *Bp* numbers, submucosal inflammation, and lymphadenopathy all increase.
   3. **Additional toxin activities** include:
      a. **Pertussis toxin,** an A/B-component, **ADP-ribosyl transferase** that inhibits the negative regulator of cyclic adenosine monophosphate (cAMP), causing **an increase in cAMP** and inhibiting neutrophil functioning.
      b. A bacterial **adenylate cyclase** that enters host cells and also leads to increased cAMP levels.
      c. A **tracheal cytotoxin** (a peptidoglycan fragment) that kills ciliated respiratory cells.

4. **Clinical symptoms: whooping cough (pertussis):**
   a. **Catarrhal stage** (lasts 1 to 2 weeks): mild upper respiratory tract infection with sneezing, slight cough, low-grade fever, and runny nose.
   b. **Paroxysmal stage** (lasts 1 to 6 weeks): extends to the lower respiratory tract, with the characteristic severe cough (5 to 20 forced hacking coughs per 20 seconds ending in an inspiratory whoop) producing anoxia and vomiting. The cough is so severe to produce eye hemorrhages and possibly the central nervous system (CNS) damage. Epithelial damage predisposes the patient to secondary bacterial pneumonia.
   c. **Convalescent stage:** less severe but persistent cough. The incidence of permanent neurological damage or death is high in unvaccinated infants.
   d. **Pertussis occurs in the vaccinated whose immunity has waned,** which keeps the disease present in the general population. It is less severe and quite common. (**12% to 20% of afebrile adults with coughs lasting more than 2 weeks have pertussis.**)

5. **Lab ID:** Historically diagnosed by posterior nasopharyngeal cultures on Regan-Lowe or Bordet-Gengou medium. Cultures were rarely positive in vaccinated individuals or after paroxysmal cough began in unvaccinated individuals. Now diagnosis is done by **NAA tests** or **DFA** (direct fluorescent antibody) done directly on nasal secretions.

6. **Prevention:** prevented by vaccination or, in an outbreak situation, by antibiotic prophylaxis for unvaccinated individuals.
   a. **DTaP (diphtheria, tetanus, and acellular pertussis)** has **three pertussis components: pertussis toxoid, filamentous hemagglutinin,** and **pertactin.** One dose of the DTaP is given at each of these ages: 2, 4, 6, and 15–18 months and 4–6 years.
   b. **The new booster with pertussis (Tdap: tetanus, diphtheria, acellular pertussis)** is recommended for the adolescent booster at 11 to 12 years and once for all adults. It is also importantly recommended for pregnant women in the third trimester (to boost immunity transferred to their babies) or at delivery (to keep Mom from getting pertussis), as well as to grandparents, family, and caregivers having contact with infants.
   c. **Adult boosters (Td: tetanus, diphtheria) are given every 10 years.**

B. **Mycoplasma bronchitis** leading to **pneumonia ("walking" pneumonia)/Mycoplasma *pneumoniae* (*Mp*). Features:**
   1. **Tiny, non-Gram staining bacterium lacking a rigid cell wall** but has **cholesterol in membrane** and requires cholesterol for growth. *Mp* is extracellular.
   2. Mucosal pathogen most frequently causing **respiratory disease in adolescents and young adults** in outbreaks about every 4 years.
   3. ***Mp* attaches to upper respiratory and bronchial epithelial cells** by the mycoplasmal P1 protein and **releases hydrogen peroxide** and other damaging substances, triggering a largely **monocytic response** and **damaging the respiratory epithelium,** producing a long-lasting, hacking cough. Fusion of the mycoplasma and host membrane deposits **mycoplasma antigens,** which then play a role in autoimmune-like reactions.

Disease:
   1. *Mp* disease starts as **pharyngitis** and spreads, causing **otitis, tracheobronchitis,** and **primary atypical pneumonia** characterized by a gradual onset of fever, throbbing headache, malaise, and severe cough (initially nonproductive).
   2. Over several weeks, interstitial or bronchopneumonic pneumonia develops; radiographic appearances vary but most commonly reveal an infiltrative pattern.
   3. **Lab ID:**
      a. Clinical diagnosis **confirmed by serology or NAA tests.** Previously, cold agglutinins (autoantibodies agglutinating red blood cells at 4°C) present after 1 to 2 weeks of clinical disease were used but are insensitive and not specific. Complement fixation is more sensitive.
      b. **Culture** (rarely done) is **on cholesterol-containing mycoplasma medium,** taking 2 to 3 weeks and producing tiny **"fried egg" appearing colonies.**
   4. **Treatment:** A macrolide, fluoroquinolone, or doxycycline over a prolonged period helps resolve manifestations. Because there is no peptidoglycan, *Mp* is *not* sensitive to β-lactams. Reinfections are common.

VII. PNEUMONIA/PNEUMONITIS

A. **General aspects of pneumonia/pneumonitis.**
 1. Bacterial pneumonias characteristically present with fever, respiratory symptoms including cough (productive or dry), and chest pain.
 2. Some pneumonias (e.g., *Mycoplasma*) are caused by colonization of the upper respiratory tract, which damages the mucociliary elevator, allowing the organism to spread down the respiratory tree. Others (e.g., *S. pneumoniae*) depend on reduction of the cough reflex or inhalation of vomitus for the organism to make it to the alveoli. Tuberculosis, legionellosis, anthrax, some viral pneumonias, most fungal pneumonias, and nocardial pneumonias may be caused by organisms directly inhaled into the lungs.
 3. **Classification.** Pneumonias are classified by many different methods.
    a. Epidemiological categories include community-acquired, nosocomial (more often called health care-associated, with ventilator pneumonias being one of the largest concerns), pneumonias in immunocompromised patients, and aspiration pneumonias.
    b. Radiographically, they are categorized as lobar, bronchopneumonia, interstitial pneumonia, pneumonia with abscess or cavitation, and so forth.
    c. The timing (acute, subacute, or chronic) and age of the patient are other ways to categorize.
    d. Microbiologists and physicians may classify them as "typical" or "atypical."
       (1) **Typical pneumonias** (based on *Strep. pneumoniae*):
          (a) Are **true pneumonias** rather than interstitial pneumonitis.
          (b) Cause a **productive cough**.
          (c) The causative microbe shows up on a **Gram stain** of sputum.
          (d) The causative agents grow out on **blood or chocolate agar**.
          (e) Are caused most commonly by streptococci, staphylococci, haemophili, or neisseriae.
       (2) **Atypical pneumonias: interstitial pneumonitis:**
          (a) Start with a **dry nonproductive cough,** often later becoming more productive.
          (b) Causative agents **do not show up on** standard **Gram stain** of lavage fluids or induced sputum.
          (c) Causative agents **do not grow on blood or chocolate agar**.
          (d) Are caused by mycoplasmas, chlamydiae, or legionellae.
          (e) Resemble viral pneumonias.
 4. **Patient history** should include knowledge of the patient's age; underlying health; symptoms including onset, timing, and severity of current disease; geographic locale of acquisition (travel); and contact with mammals, birds, or dusty environments. **Radiography** along with history not only suggests the most likely groups of agents but will dictate prudent diagnostic workup.
 5. **Lab ID:** Guidelines (beyond the scope of this book) are available for determining in which situations pneumonias are worked up and which are treated empirically. The following items describe for each what is done when etiology is desired.
    a. Gram stain of a culture of sputum sample taken before breakfast is most likely to be useful. The presence of PMNs in sputum suggests the specimen is from the lung. (Some immunocompromised patients may not produce a PMN response.) A large number of epithelial cells suggests the specimen is saliva and not from the lungs. Induced sputa or covered brush biopsy may be used if cough is nonproductive.
    b. Blood cultures are also useful in the diagnosis of pneumonia and, when possible, should be taken before antibiotics are started.
    c. If treatment is listed, it is the treatment after etiology is determined rather than initial treatment.
    d. If initial therapy fails and neither Gram stain, cultures, nor susceptibility testing were performed, the physician does not know if the pneumonia is caused by an unusual organism requiring different therapy or if there is drug resistance.

B. **Typical pneumonias.**

   1. **Pneumococcal pneumonia/*Strep. pneumoniae:***

      Features: (see 4 I F):

      Disease:

      a. Typical pneumonia. At highest risk: unvaccinated infants, the elderly, and immunosuppressed persons including those with splenic dysfunction, chronic alcoholics, and people who have had their ciliated "elevator" damaged by a viral infection, most notably influenza.

      b. Oropharyngeal colonization is aided by **surface protein adhesins** and **IgA protease.**

      c. The lower respiratory tract becomes infected by aspiration after epiglottal reflexes have been slowed due to chilling, anesthesia, morphine use, alcohol use, viral infection, or increased pulmonary edema.

      d. Pneumococcal pneumonia manifests with **abrupt onset, fever, chills, chest pain on inspiration, shortness of breath, and productive cough.**

      e. Lab ID: identified by sputum Gram stain (**Gram-positive, lancet-shaped diplococci**) and culture. *Strep. pneumoniae* is alpha-hemolytic on sheep BA and is lysed by bile; its growth is inhibited by optochin. Capsular typing is by the quellung reaction where binding of specific antibodies results in a refractive change.

      f. Treatment: treated with **ampicillin, amoxicillin, or a macrolide;** however, **penicillin-resistant strains with modified penicillin-binding proteins** that result in lowered penicillin binding are found in about one-third of the strains in the United States. **Fluoroquinolones** are commonly the drug of choice for **resistant strains.**

      g. Prevention:

         (1) Prevented in **infants by a 13-valent pneumococcal conjugate vaccine: 13 different serotypes of** capsular polysaccharides are chemically linked to protein, producing a T-cell dependent immunity in infants.

         (2) Prevented in **adults over 65 years of age by a 23-valent capsular polysaccharide vaccine,** which is also recommended for other risk groups such as asplenics.

   2. **Pneumonia/*Staph. aureus:***

      Features: (see 4 I E):

      Disease:

      a. Causes ventilator or **postinfluenza** pneumonias or pneumonias in people with **CF** (early in life) or **chronic granulomatous disease.**

      b. Oropharyngeal colonization precedes **lower respiratory tract entry,** which is **facilitated by ventilators or defective respiratory protection mechanisms** (as for Pneumococcus); *S. aureus* may also reach the lungs hematogenously following septicemia from endocarditis.

      c. Manifests as **lobar pneumonia** with a **high rate of abscess formation, necrosis, and fatality,** especially following influenza.

      d. Treatment: dependent on susceptibilities (see 4 I E).

   3. **Pneumonia/*Klebsiella pneumoniae:***

      Features:

      a. Gram-negative rod, Enterobacteriaceae, lactose-fermenter with **capsule.**

      b. Found in moist environments and human colon.

      Disease:

      a. Common ventilator-associated pneumonia and is also **associated with alcoholism (pneumococcus is still more common)** and **aspiration.**

      b. Lobar pneumonia with a **high incidence of abscesses** and **thick, bloody (dark red or "currant jelly") sputum.** Because of the abscesses, fatality rates are high even if patients receive treatment.

      c. Treatment: difficult because of abscesses, **drug resistance** (via extended spectrum β-lactamase production), and because patients are debilitated.

      d. Prevention: limit respirators, keep patient upright.

   4. **Pneumonia/*Pseudomonas aeruginosa*** (see 4 I D):

      Features:

      a. Gram-negative, nonfermenting rod, motile.

b. Occurs primarily in **burn, CF,** and **severely neutropenic patients. Exposure is from environmental water or plant sources and respirators.** Once colonized, it is probably impossible to eradicate in the lungs of those with CF.

Disease:

a. Disease is due to difficulty in eradicating the adherent organisms in the biofilms created by **production of copious extracellular alginate slime** (overproduced in CF strains). The production and circulation of **exotoxin A (an ADP-ribosyl transferase inactivating EF-2)** is thought to be responsible for the ultimate liver failure. The lung is also **damaged by directly damaging enzymes** like the **phospholipase, elastase, and proteases, some clipping immunoglobulins. Endotoxin** triggers inflammation and contributes to the systemic symptoms.

b. Treatment: antipseudomonal antibiotics (see 4 I D).

C. Atypical pneumonias.

1. Atypical pneumonia/*Mycoplasma pneumoniae*:

Features and disease: (see bronchitis 4 VI B):

2. Atypical pneumonia/*Chlamydophila pneumoniae* (a.k.a. *Chlamydia pneumoniae*):

Features:

a. *Chlamydophila pneumoniae* is an **OIP**. It is a Gram-nonstaining, pleomorphic rod with no peptidoglycan.

b. Common in humans, often without significant symptoms.

Disease:

a. Caused by **intracellular replication** and **toxic effects of antigens.**

b. Mild disease. Pulmonary symptoms may include bronchitis and atypical pneumonia and possibly inflammation of vascular endothelium associated with atherosclerosis.

c. Treatment: treated with doxycycline, erythromycin, or fluoroquinolone; resistant to all β-lactam drugs.

D. Psittacosis (atypical pneumonia)/*Chlamydophila psittaci.*

Features:

1. OIP, Gram-nonstaining pleomorphic rod with **no peptidoglycan.**

2. Avian pathogen of psittacine birds (**parrots**), **turkeys,** and **chickens** with outbreaks in workers in turkey production facilities (classic zoonosis).

Disease:

1. Intracellular replication and toxic effects of antigens cause psittacosis.

2. Ranges from **subclinical to fatal pneumonia.**

E. *Neonatal pneumonia/Chlamydia trachomatis.*

Features: (see 4 I A):

Disease:

1. This pathogen may be acquired from an infected maternal birth canal, putting the neonate at risk for eye and pulmonary infection.

2. Atypical pneumonia characterized by a staccato cough and treated with systemic erythromycin.

F. Legionnaires' disease (atypical pneumonia)/*Legionella pneumophila* and other legionella species.

Features:

1. Gram-negative, pleomorphic rods (coccobacilli *in vivo*) which are **facultative intracellular pathogens of human macrophages.** They do not stain well with Gram stain in clinical specimens but stain well with silver stain.

2. Legionellae are found in **streams** as facultative intracellular parasites of amoeba; they **contaminate all types of water systems growing in amoeba and surviving in biofilms** including hot water systems, air-conditioning cooling towers in hot weather, grocery store produce sprayers, and many other sources.

Disease:
1. Legionnaires' disease is *not* **contagious from person to person.** It causes **fibrinopurulent pneumonia** primarily in debilitated people; individuals 55 years of age and older who smoke and drink alcohol or immunocompromised patients are at high risk.
2. *L. pneumophila* is endocytosed by **macrophages but survives and grows well in the phagosome by inhibiting phagosome-lysosome fusion.**
3. In healthy individuals, the innate immune system (particularly **tumor necrosis factor-alpha** and **inducing iron sequestration through interferon-gamma**) may limit growth of the bacteria and control infection.
4. **If the immune system is unable to control intracellular replication, bacteria overgrow macrophages.** Infected macrophages produce cytokines and attract blood monocytes and neutrophils into the alveolar spaces, forming microabscesses that may coalesce into **cavities.**
5. **Legionnaires' disease** often presents with **a triad of atypical pneumonia, major confusion,** and **diarrhea.**
6. **Lab ID:** rapid immunoassay for urine antigen and NAA tests have replaced sputa stains (negative by Gram stain but positive by Dieterle silver stain) or DFA stain (low sensitivity partially due to the intracellular nature). Culture on buffered charcoal yeast extract (BCYE) agar, which provides the required cysteine and iron, is sensitive but takes 3 to 5 days.
7. **Treatment and prevention:**
   a. The infection is commonly treated with fluoroquinolones or macrolides because *L. pneumophila* **produces β-lactamases** that inactivate cephalosporins and penicillins.
   b. It can be prevented with careful maintenance of water systems, especially in hospitals.

G. Pulmonary Anthrax/*Bacillus anthracis* (*Ba*).
Features:
1. **Gram-positive, aerobic spore former.**
2. Causes **anthrax,** a disease especially **prevalent in goats, sheep, and cattle** in countries that do not vaccinate their domestic animals. **Spores play an important role in transmission;** they can survive in soil or on the skin of animals for years. Humans are infected by inhalation of spores or traumatic implantation (**cutaneous anthrax**).
Disease:
1. **Pulmonary anthrax starts with inhalation of the spores,** which are small and light enough to enter alveoli, where they are picked up by the residential macrophages.
   a. In the **phagocyte,** the inert **spores survive to germinate** and develop into metabolically active toxin producing vegetative cells which kill the phagocyte, **releasing the vegetative** (and **toxin-producing**) *B. anthracis* **into the bloodstream.**
   b. **Vegetative cells** produce the **polypeptide capsule,** which prevents new phagocytic uptake and allows the bacterium to replicate extracellularly and produce anthrax toxin.
   c. The **tripartite protein exotoxin** consists of **protective antigen** (PA), **lethal factor** (LF), and **edema factor** (EF). PA (the B component) triggers the internalization of both LF and EF. **EF is a calmodulin-activated adenylate cyclase** that leads to the **edema. LF is a metalloproteinase of MAPKK1 & 2 mitogen-activated protein kinases so it interferes with signaling,** ultimately killing the cells.
2. **Clinical symptoms: abrupt onset of high fever, malaise, cough,** myalgias, **marked hemorrhagic necrosis of the lymph nodes,** massive pleural effusions, respiratory distress, and cyanosis.
3. **Lab ID:** diagnosed by visualization of the **large, Gram-positive rods** in blood; confirmed by **aerobic, nonhemolytic, nonmotile cultures on BA.** Faster methods such as **NAA tests and gas chromatography to detect LF** are available from reference labs.
4. **Treatment:** Anthrax is commonly **treated with multiple drugs** including fluoroquinolones with clindamycin (to suppress toxin production) and/or rifampin, but remains fatal in 50%.
5. **Prevention:** strategies include **vaccination of domestic animals** where natural outbreaks have occurred; **gas sterilization of commercial wool, hair, and hides from endemic areas;** and vaccination of at-risk individuals (anthrax lab workers, farmers, animal processors, military personnel).

H. Tuberculosis (TB)/*Mycobacterium tuberculosis* (*Mtb*).

Features:

1. *Mtb* is an **obligate aerobe** that has a highly cross-linked **peptidoglycan–arabinogalactan mycolate cell wall** (~ 60% lipid), so it is **acid-fast (AF), poorly Gram staining,** and **resistant to drying** and many chemicals. It has neither endotoxin nor an outer membrane.

2. *Mtb* is a human pathogen spread from person to person by dried respiratory droplet nuclei that are small enough to be directly inhaled into the lungs. Because of the resistance to drying, these nuclei remain in rooms and can also be spread by the air-handling systems of hospitals. This risk is reduced by placing all suspected TB patients in separately exhausted, negative-pressure rooms. The bacterium is killed by ultraviolet light and can be removed from air by high-efficiency particulate air (HEPA) filters. Patients with untreated HIV infection and TB play a major role in the spread of the organism as they develop high levels of *Mtb* in the lungs.

Disease:

1. **Primary *Mtb* infection:** starts with **inhalation** of the organism into the **alveoli**, usually in the middle area; outcome is dependent on the individuals' immune system.

   a. Initially, *Mtb* is phagocytosed and removed to regional lymph nodes where it replicates and **generally kills the phagocytes.** The organisms are picked up by the lymphocytes and monocytes attracted to the site of infection. Antigen is processed and presented and a T-cell response is triggered, but generally *Mtb* circulates and replicates until an effective cell-mediated and tissue hypersensitivity response occurs. If the infection is not contained, miliary (disseminated) TB results.

   b. *Mtb* stimulates a strong cell-mediated immune response in healthy hosts, which kills many of the organisms or successfully walls them off in granulomas where they may remain viable. **Granulomas** limit the oxygen to the obligate aerobic *Mtb* organisms, slowing their growth within the granuloma. Leakage of antigens from these granulomas maintains an activated immune state.

      (1) Most (90%) individuals with a primary infection will have no immediate clinical symptoms, just a positive tuberculin skin test as a marker of their primary infection and their immune response.

      (2) Immediate disease occurs in individuals who cannot mount a strong cell-mediated immune response.

2. **Reactivational (secondary) tuberculosis:**

   a. This form occurs **most commonly in the lung apices in previously sensitized individuals with a weakened immune response** (e.g., malnutrition, immunotherapy for other diseases). **Failure to maintain the granulomas leads to caseous necrosis, in which the center of the granuloma is liquefied and the lesions coalesce.** Erosion exposes the organism to oxygen and spreads them to other parts of the lung with a resulting pneumonia. Hypersensitivity leads to the **cavitation.**

   b. TB is characterized by chronic **cough** (often with **blood-tinged sputum**), **night sweats, fever, anorexia, and weight loss.**

3. **Lab ID:**

   a. Tentatively diagnosed by **microscopic demonstration of AF bacteria** in sputum, induced sputum, or gastric washings. Sputum samples may be prescreened with **auramine-rhodamine fluorochrome stain;** this stain is a nonspecific interaction with the waxy wall. (No antibody is involved.) It **requires confirmation by an acid-fast stain (AFS).**

   b. Is diagnosed by **culture** in a radiolabeled broth demonstrating the metabolism of ^{14}**C-labeled palmitic acid** with release of $^{14}CO_2$. (These specimens were formerly plated on **Lowenstein-Jensen agar**.) Drug susceptibilities may also be determined in the broth system. Radiometric systems generally are positive in 7 to 14 days. NAA tests are also available including some to identify genes involved in drug resistance.

   c. Demonstration of immune response (previous exposure):

      (1) Whole blood interferon-gamma release assays use *Mtb* antigen not found in nontuberculous mycobacteria including the BCG vaccine strain; therefore, it is better for identifying tuberculosis in Bacille Calmette-Guérin (BCG) vaccinated persons. It still does not distinguish latent from current active infection.

    (2) **Tuberculin skin testing (TST)** with a purified protein derivative (PPD) of *M. tuberculosis* **demonstrates** only that **a primary infection has occurred** and **does not prove current disease. TST** is considered **positive if** the **zone of induration** at 48 hours measures:

        (a) **15 mm or more** if **no known exposure**.

        (b) **10 mm or more** if patient is from a **country with high risk, or drug user.**

        (c) **5 mm or more** if recent known exposure or HIV+.

            Individuals with **known tuberculous** disease **and a negative PPD** test are **anergic** to the antigen (a poor prognostic sign). TST measures delayed type hypersensitivity.

  4. **Treatment:** run susceptibility tests on all cultures.

    a. **Isoniazid** is the drug of choice for (1) all neonates or children <5 years with known exposure but no symptoms; (2) individuals with known *Mtb* exposure, conversion to TST+ but no clinical signs; or (3) anyone asymptomatic but who is TST+ and <35 years of age but has never been treated.

    b. In cases of **uncomplicated pulmonary TB in a previously untreated, healthy, cooperative patient, the treatment is isoniazid, rifampin, pyrazinamide, and ethambutol for 8 weeks followed by 18 weeks of 1X per week isoniazid and rifampin** (unless susceptibility tests indicate drug resistance). Direct observed therapy (DOT) is important to successful treatment.

    c. Multiple drug-resistant strains are emerging and complicating treatment.

  5. **Prevention:** TB is **partially prevented by the BCG vaccine,** an attenuated strain of *Mycobacterium bovis* (the second causative agent of human TB).

I. Atypical mycobacterial pulmonary infection/*Mycobacterium avium-intracellulare* (MAI or MAC for *M. avium* complex).

Features:

  1. Nontuberculous (atypical) mycobacterium are indistinguishable from *Mtb* by AFS or fluorochrome stain.

  2. MAC is an **environmental organism** found in water, soil, birds, and other animals; in humans, it is an **opportunist**. It is **not contagious** from person to person.

Diseases:

  1. **MAC causes active disease only in individuals who are immunocompromised, generally with CD4+ cell counts below 100/mm³ or people with chronic lung disease.** It is an AIDS-defining condition with a poor prognosis.

  2. **MAC causes a chronic bronchopulmonary disease characterized by fever, night sweats, anorexia, weight loss, and diarrhea.** (The gastrointestinal [GI] tract may be the initial site of infection.)

  3. **Lab ID:** diagnosed with **blood cultures** using a variety of procedures, including **radiometric techniques with probes for rapid identification of growth.**

  4. **Treatment:** highly active antiretroviral therapy **(HAART) plus azithromycin** until CD4+ cell counts are **equal to or greater than 100 cells/mm³.**

  5. **Prevention: antibiotic prophylaxis,** which is started when CD4 count <50–100 cells/mm³.

J. Nocardia pulmonary disease/*Nocardia asteroids.*

Features:

  1. **Aerobic,** filamentous **Gram-positive,** and **partially AF** bacterium that fragments into rods. Its cell wall is somewhat waxy so it also withstands drying. It is related to *Corynebacterium, Mycobacterium,* and *Actinomyces.*

  2. Found in the **soil;** transmitted through **inhalation** of dust or traumatic implantation.

Disease:

  1. Pneumonia with cavitation in **immunocompromised individuals with a high rate of metastases** to the brain.

  2. **Lab ID:** often not diagnosed until autopsy, but antemortem diagnosis is made using gastric washings, lung biopsy, and brain biopsy with Gram and AFS and culture.

  3. **Treatment:** treated with **sulfonamides.**

K. **Q Fever/***Coxiella burnetii.***

Features:

1. Small **Gram-negative intracellular rod** replicating in macrophage phagolysosomes; **resistant to lysosomal contents** and **drying.** Undergoes **antigenic phase variation.** (*Coxiella* was formerly considered a rickettsia and obligate intracellular but can be cultured.)
2. Associated with **sheep, cattle, goats, cats, and rabbits. Highest numbers in products of parturition,** which, even after drying, can be spread by **direct contact with animals** or by **contaminated soil transmitted by wind,** infecting people or animals miles away. Small cell variants (stable in environment for years) are rearranged in macrophages to form large cell variants.

Disease:

1. Presents with **influenza-like symptoms with an interstitial pneumonia,** often with **hepatitis.** Chronic forms cause **cardiac problems**.
2. Triggers granuloma formation in lung, bone marrow, heart, liver, and spleen.
3. **Lab ID:** diagnosed by serology or NAA test.
4. **Treatment:** acute treated with doxycycline or fluoroquinolone.

VIII. NERVOUS SYSTEM INFECTIONS: MENINGITIS

A. General aspects of meningitis.

1. **Bacterial meningitis** can be rapidly fatal. Presenting symptoms in **neonates** include **temperature instability and lethargy;** symptoms in **adults are generally fever, stiff neck, severe headache,** and, particularly for meningococcal meningitis, **petechiae.**
2. Treatment must be started quickly (within 30 minutes) without waiting for lab results; if possible, get CSF for culture prior to starting.
3. **Distinction of bacterial meningitis from viral meningitis is based on CSF findings. Bacterial: elevated white cell counts, elevated protein** (presumably from disrupted blood–brain barrier), and **lowered glucose levels** (from the bacterial metabolism). It is also aided by finding of **elevated serum or CSF C-reactive protein.**
4. **Initial etiological diagnosis** generally can be quickly made by **Gram stain of CSF.** (Latex particle agglutination tests are no longer used.)
5. NAA tests are useful, especially if antibiotic treatment was started prior to getting the CSF.

B. Neonatal meningitis/*Streptococcus agalactiae* **(Group B streptococcus [GBS]).**

Features:

1. **Beta-hemolytic, Gram-positive coccus** in chains possessing the **Lancefield Group B cell wall antigens** and a **polysaccharide capsule.**
2. **Epidemiology:**
   a. GBS occurs frequently in vaginal and oral flora in adult women (15% to 40% of women). It is more frequent in younger mothers and those with more sexual partners, suggesting **potential sexual transfer.** Mothers are at risk of UTIs as well as endometritis and amnionitis.
   b. **Colonization of the maternal genital tract predisposes newborns to respiratory infections and septicemia, which may progress to meningitis. Prolonged labor after the rupture of the membranes increases the transmission risk.**

Disease:

1. **GBS**'s polysaccharide capsule inhibits phagocytic uptake.
2. **Early-onset GBS neonatal sepsis** (birth to 7 days) leading to **respiratory distress** and a high fatality rate has been reduced by intrapartum antibiotics.
3. **Much less common late-onset neonatal sepsis** (7 days to 4 months) is characterized by **meningitis,** which **commonly leads to permanent neurologic damage** and has a fatality rate of 15% to 20%.

4. **Treatment and prevention:**
   a. Meningitis is commonly treated with penicillin.
   b. Early-onset GBS infections are **reduced by predelivery testing of pregnant women (35 to 38 weeks) and intrapartum antibiotic** treatment to prevent infection of the neonate.

C. **Neonatal meningitis/***E. coli* (see 4 I B). This disease is caused by birth exposure to **encapsulated (primarily K1) strains of** *E. coli.* It is treated based on susceptibility testing.

D. *Listeria* **neonatal meningitis or meningitis in compromised persons/***Listeria monocytogenes.*
   Features:
   1. Beta-hemolytic, **Gram-positive, facultative intracellular coccobacillus** that has **tumbling motility in broth** at room temperature and is a **psychrophile,** even growing at refrigeration temperatures.
   2. *Listeria* is found in **vertebrate feces** contaminating unpasteurized **dairy products, deli meats, and soft cheeses made from unpasteurized milk, unheated hot dogs (and the package liquid),** and **uncooked cabbage.** Mom is exposed through food: fetus is exposed from placenta infection or exposure to feces at birth.

   Disease:
   1. *Listeria* invades mononuclear phagocytes and epithelial cells. Inside the phagosome, *Listeria* produces **listeriolysin O,** which facilitates its rapid **egress into the rich cytoplasm prior to phagosome–lysosome fusion,** allowing protected **cytoplasmic replication.** *Listeria* is then able to **"reorganize" host cell actin to propel itself directly into adjoining cells,** avoiding the extracellular environment.
   2. In healthy individuals, ingestion of *Listeria* causes **transient diarrhea** with subsequent fecal carriage.
   3. In **pregnant women,** *Listeria* causes **GI disease with septicemia (flulike symptoms) and the possibility of neonatal infection** by:
      a. **Crossing the placenta,** leading to severe disease in the neonate with abscesses and granulomas throughout the body.
      b. **Fecal contamination at birth** may cause septicemia and late onset neonatal meningitis.
   4. In **immunocompromised patients,** particularly in transplant patients, *Listeria* causes **septicemia and meningitis.**
   5. **Lab ID:**
      a. **Often missed in Gram stain of CSF** because of low numbers and intracellular nature (and may be misidentified as streptococci).
      b. Diagnosed by growth on BA where it is **weakly beta-hemolytic with hemolysis enhanced by growth near *Staph. aureus* hemolysis (positive CAMP test).**
      c. Shows **"tumbling motility" in 25°C broth cultures,** having lost its forward "gears." Additional tests done to distinguish from corynebacteria.
   6. **Prevention:** prevented through limiting exposure and pasteurization. Women and immunocompromised patients should avoid raw cabbage and heat all processed meats before eating.

E. **Pneumococcal meningitis/***Streptococcus pneumoniae* (see 4 I F).
   Pneumococcus also causes **septicemia and meningitis in the very young** and is the **dominant cause of bacterial meningitis in older adults.** It is not considered highly contagious as it must colonize the oropharyngeal mucosa, invade the bloodstream, and survive the trip to the blood–brain barrier where it must cross. Vaccination reduces the risk of infection by vaccine strains. For details return to Chapter 4 section B 1.

F. **Meningitis in unvaccinated children under 2 years/***Haemophilus influenzae* **type b.**
   Features:
   1. Gram-negative, fastidious pleomorphic rods; coccobacilli in CSF (see 4 I C).
   2. Prior to *H. influenzae* type b vaccines, an estimated 30,000 cases per year of invasive *H. influenzae* disease occurred in infants and toddlers, including meningitis, osteomyelitis, and

epiglottitis. With vaccination: around 500 cases/year occur in the United States. It has almost eliminated epiglottitis in toddlers, the major affected group. Disease occurs primarily in **un-vaccinated children 3 months to 2 years** of age. Strains that cause childhood meningitis have the **type b polyribitol capsule.** (Strains without capsules are called "nontypeable"; they are part of our normal oropharyngeal flora and do not cause disease.)

Disease:

1. **Rapidly progressive with permanent** CNS deficits (hydrocephalus, mental retardation, paresis, and speech and hearing problems) in a third of the cases.
2. **Lab ID: Gram stain of CSF;** fastidious, growing on **chocolate agar.**
3. **Prevention:** capsular polysaccharide-protein conjugate vaccine at 2, 4, 6 months.

G. **Meningococcal meningitis/*Neisseria meningitidis* (*Nm*).**

Features:

1. **Gram-negative, oxidase-positive, kidney-shaped diplococcus** with a **polysaccharide capsule** and the ability to **use both glucose and maltose.**
2. Human pathogen colonizing upper respiratory membranes. About 10% of healthy people are carriers who have sufficient immunity to block disease but still have mucosal colonization.

Disease:

1. Meningococcal meningitis is **most prevalent in children 6 months to 2 years,** with **a second peak in young adults,** especially those housed together (college students living in residence halls or frequenting college bars and military recruits). Even the previously healthy can die within 24 hours.
2. *Nm* has more than 12 capsular serogroups; **most U.S. infections are caused by the B, C, W-135, and Y serogroups, the B capsule being notoriously nonimmunogenic. Serotype A** strains cause epidemics in **Africa and China.**
3. *Nm* **binds** to nonciliated mucosal cells **with pili.** *Nm* reaches the submucosa by **passing through mucosal cells** into the submucosa. The **capsule, IgA protease,** and **serum resistance allow this extracellular pathogen to survive in the bloodstream.** If it reaches the **blood–brain barrier, pili** and the outer membrane endotoxins (**lipo-oligosaccharides** [LOS]) cause **inflammation, facilitating entry of *N. meningitidis* into the CNS.** It then causes extensive tissue necrosis, hemorrhage, circulatory collapse, intravascular coagulation, and shock. *Nm* overproduces outer membrane (and thus LOS), causing the rapid shock and early petechiae.
4. *N. meningitidis* disease begins as **mild pharyngitis** with occasional slight fever but, in the immunologically naive, organisms disseminate to most tissues (especially the skin, meninges, joints, eyes, and lungs), resulting in a **fulminant meningococcemia, pneumonia,** and **meningitis** that can be fatal in 1 to 5 days.
5. Characterized by **fever, vomiting, headache, and stiff neck.** Pneumonia may be present. A **petechial eruption** develops that progresses from erythematous macules to frank purpura. **Vasculitic purpura** is the hallmark. **Waterhouse-Friderichsen syndrome** is a fulminating meningococcemia with hemorrhage, circulatory failure, and adrenal insufficiency.
6. May leave eighth-nerve deafness, CNS damage (learning disabilities and seizures), and severe skin necrosis that may require skin grafting or amputation.
7. **Lab ID: Gram-negative diplococci** on Gram stain CSF. Culture of CSF and blood on chocolate agar in high CO_2; do antibiotic susceptibility testing.
8. **Treatment:**
   a. Meningococcal meningitis requires **rapid diagnosis, treatment,** and **prompt hospitalization.**
   b. Treated with IV **ceftriaxone,** which passes through the inflamed blood–brain barrier but **may also require rifampin to eradicate oropharyngeal colonization.**
   c. Manage shock and intravascular coagulation.
9. **Prevention:**
   a. **The meningococcal conjugate vaccine** includes capsules from serotypes Y, W-135, C, and A, each conjugated to protein. **However, ~50% U.S. cases are serogroup B, whose capsule is poorly immunogenic.** Routine use is recommended for high-risk children (e.g., those with late complement component deficiency or asplenia) ages 2 to 10 years; all children age 11 to 12 years; and military recruits or college students if not previously vaccinated.

IX. NERVOUS SYSTEM INFECTIONS: NONMENINGITIS CONDITIONS

A. **Central nervous system abscesses.**
   1. Abscesses represent the body **successfully walling off invading organisms,** but they create a space with **limited access to antibiotics and white cells.**
   2. CNS abscesses may **follow trauma, surgery, sinusitis, otitis, or gingival abscesses.**
   3. CNS abscesses are commonly **mixed infections** caused by oropharyngeal flora, including the **Gram-negative anaerobe *Prevotella melaninogenica* and *Fusobacterium nucleatum*.**

B. **Other neurological manifestations of microbes.**
   1. **Guillain-Barré syndrome** associated with previous ***Campylobacter*** GI infections (see 4 XIII H).
   2. **Bell's palsy** associated with **Lyme disease** (see 4 XVIII B).
   3. **Flaccid paralysis** (descending) from **botulinum toxin** (see 4 XIII B).
   4. **Rigid spasm** from tetanus (see 4 XV I 1).

X. CARDIOVASCULAR INFECTIONS: VASCULITIS

Several infections affect the **vascular endothelium.** These infections include the rickettsial diseases of **Rocky Mountain spotted fever** and **typhus**, both discussed later with arthropod-borne infections. Inflammation occurring as a result of ***Chl. pneumoniae*** and possibly other agents like cytomegalovirus replication in the endothelium appears to play a role in atherosclerosis.

XI. CARDIOVASCULAR INFECTIONS: ENDOCARDITIS

A. **General aspects of endocarditis.**
   1. Endocarditis is an inflammation of the **heart endothelium** (endocardium), often involving the valves; it is a direct infection of the endocardium or, in the case of rheumatic heart disease, an immune reaction to untreated streptococcal pharyngitis.
   2. **Endocarditis** is most commonly a **bacterial infection starting from bacteria in the bloodstream** from brushing teeth, untreated cavities, periodontal disease, passing a hard stool, parturition, surgery, prostate exams, IV lines, IV drug use, and so on.
   3. **Clinical symptoms of endocarditis:**
      a. It may present **acutely** with high fever of unknown origin (**FUO**), **new** or increasing **heart murmurs**, and **fatigue.** Acute infections may occur in the healthy or predamaged heart and are most commonly caused by ***Staph. aureus.***
      b. It also may have a **more chronic onset of low-grade fever, with weight loss, night sweats, increasing heart sounds**, and **increasing fatigue**, commonly in someone who already has a **damaged heart.** The infectious agents are more likely to be **opportunists with less virulence** and require help to access the bloodstream (like root canal).
   4. **All endocarditis agents bind to fibronectin.** Fibronectin is found on prosthetic devices, on nonbacterial thrombolytic vegetations, and on the subendothelial matrix exposed by damage to the endothelium but not on the normal cardiac endothelial surface. ***Staph. aureus* also binds fibrinogen,** which is one of the reasons (along with invasiveness and damaging enzymes) that it can attack a healthy heart as well as a damaged heart tissue.
   5. Endocarditis may result in **vegetations**, three-dimensional bacterial growths made up of extracellular bacterial products, platelets, fibrin mesh, but few immune cells. Interior

microbes are less accessible to phagocytic cells and have lowered metabolism and so are tougher to treat with antibiotics. Pieces break off, seeding the bloodstream and creating stroke risk.

6. Major causative agents in native heart with no illicit IV use are streptococci (both viridans and other), enterococci, and staphylococci (both coagulase positive and negative). With IV drug use, it is most commonly *Staph. aureus.*

B. Endocarditis/*Staph. aureus.*
Features:
1. Catalase-positive, coagulase-positive, Gram-positive coccus (see 4 I E).
2. Common cause of endocarditis in IV drug abusers.
Disease:
1. **Causes high fever,** rapidly damaging **endocarditis, usually acute,** in a "normal" or predamaged heart.
2. **Fibrinogen binding aids binding to normal heart.** However, *Staph. aureus* also binds fibronectin.
3. **Coagulase** allows **formation of fibrin clots,** which reduces access of phagocytic cells to clear *Staph. aureus.*
4. *Staph. aureus* **cytolytic toxins such as the** pore-forming **alpha-toxin rapidly damage heart cells.**

C. Endocarditis/viridans streptococci (see 4 III A). These organisms cause subacute endocarditis in individuals with **damaged hearts** who either have **poor oral hygiene or have had recent dental work without prophylactic antibiotics.** Viridans streptococci are not invasive, but they can bind fibronectin, a characteristic of all bacteria causing infective endocarditis.

D. Endocarditis/*Enterococcus faecalis, E. faecium,* and other *Enterococcus* sp. Enterococci (see 3 III B 3) are part of the normal GI flora. Enterococci are a leading cause of nosocomial infections, including endocarditis. They enter the bloodstream via microscopic bowel defects created by **cytotoxic anticancer agents or via medical manipulation of the genitourinary (GU) or GI tract.** Endocarditis is commonly seen in older men with already damaged heart tissue who have recently undergone prostate exams. Antibiotic resistance is common.

E. Endocarditis/*Staphylococcus epidermidis* (plus other coagulase-negative staphylococci).
Features:
1. **Coagulase-negative** and **nonhemolytic staphylococcus.**
2. **Normal skin commensal** with little virulence but may cause infection in individuals with medical devices (e.g., **artificial heart valves** or **knees, pacemakers, IV lines**). The hydrophobicity of both *Staph. epidermidis* and device polymers facilitates their binding; the polysaccharide slime (also known as glycocalyx or extracellular matrix) made by *Staph. epidermidis* serves as a "glue," **creating biofilms** that are difficult to clear without removal of the device.

F. Rheumatic fever (acute disease)/Rheumatic heart disease (chronic damaged heart)/*Strep. pyogenes* (GAS).
Features:
1. Gram-positive, beta-hemolytic, catalase-negative cocci in chains (see 4 I G for GAS).
2. **Follows untreated Group A streptococcal pharyngitis** in genetically predisposed individuals.
Disease:
1. May result from antistreptococcal antibodies cross-reacting with sarcolemma membrane proteins. The resulting antigen-antibody complexes initiate a damaging inflammatory process.
2. Results in a systemic inflammatory process involving the connective tissue, heart, joints, and CNS, which may get worse with each subsequent *Strep. pyogenes* infection.
3. May **damage heart muscle and valves,** with **mitral stenosis** as a lesion hallmark.
4. **Treatment:** treat promptly with penicillin. In persons exposed to children (the major source of the streptococcal infection), continue to prevent recurring infections and increased damage.

XII. CARDIOVASCULAR: MYOCARDITIS

Myocarditis is caused primarily by coxsackie viruses and *Trypanosoma cruzi*. It is also a component of disseminated *Borrelia burgdorferi* (see 4 XVIII B) and diphtheria from the effect of the circulating toxin on the myocardium.

XIII. GASTROINTESTINAL INFECTIONS

A. Gastritis and ulcers/ *Helicobacter pylori* (*Hp*).
   Features:
   1. **Hp is a microaerophilic, Gram-negative, urease-positive, spiral-shaped bacterium with multiple polar flagella** at a single pole.
   2. *Hp* is a complex human colonizer or pathogen with higher rates in developing countries. **Hp** persists in the stomach so the rate of colonization increases with age into middle age. Transmission is fecal or oral or by vomitus. There are genetic predispositions.
   3. Associated with **gastritis, gastric and duodenal ulcers, mucosa-associated lymphoid tissue (MALT) lymphoma, non-Hodgkin lymphoma of the stomach, and gastric adenocarcinoma.** (W.H.O. classifies it as a carcinogen.)
   Disease:
   1. **Colonization and pathogenesis** (Note: Not all strains of *H. pylori* produce high levels of the CagA protein or VacA cytotoxin.):
      a. Produces **urease,** converting urea to ammonia, to facilitate survival during migration to the gastric epithelium.
      b. Penetrates the mucin with the aid of its **mucinase, spiral shape,** and polar **flagellae.**
      c. **Adhesins bind to fucose-containing receptors on gastric mucosa** (Lewis blood group antigens).
      d. Strains with the **CagA pathogenicity island** (a section of DNA coding for the CagA protein and a type VI injection-like secretion system) **inject CagA into epithelial cells** where it ultimately causes **cytoskeletal rearrangement.** Other proteins trigger interleukin 8 (IL-8) production, which also plays a role in the inflammatory response. High CagA producers have a higher association with inflammation and *the subsequent carcinomas.*
      e. Some produce the multifunctional **VacA, a vacuolating cytotoxin** triggering apoptosis. It has a high association with peptic ulcer disease.
   2. **Clinical symptoms:**
      a. **Acute infection** is characterized by epigastric pain, sometimes with nausea, vomiting, anorexia, and belching.
      b. **Chronic superficial gastritis** is caused by hypochlorhydria, which leads to persistent colonization. The immune system appears not to routinely eliminate *H. pylori.*
      c. **Peptic ulcers** are characterized by burning epigastric pain lessened by eating; they are diagnosed by invasive and noninvasive methods.
   3. **Lab ID:**
      a. Invasive tests done on biopsy include:
         (1) **Urease test on biopsy.**
         (2) Histology (silver stain is most sensitive).
         (3) Antigen detection.
         (4) Culture at 37°C is rarely done.
      b. Noninvasive tests include:
         (1) **Urea breath test** in which radioactive carbon-labeled urea is swallowed and urease activity is detected by the radioactive-CO_2 in the breath ($$).
         (2) Demonstration of **serum antibodies**.
         (3) **HpSA:** *Hp* Stool Antigen test FDA approved.

4. **Treatment**: treated most commonly with the combination of a proton-pump inhibitor along with amoxicillin and clarithromycin, but *Hp* resistance to clarithromycin and metronidazole is increasing. Success of treatment is assessed with a fecal antigen test.

B. Botulism/*Clostridium botulinum.*

Features:

1. **Gram-positive, spore-forming, anaerobic rod,** which **requires a low redox potential for growth** in food or tissue.
2. The spores are ubiquitous in **soil** and **dust;** they are highly resistant to heat and drying and can survive decades in a dry environment.
3. Once in a moist, nutritious environment that is not too acidic, the spores germinate and develop into vegetative cells.

Disease:

1. The **vegetative cells** produce a **potent exotoxin** (botulinum neurotoxin), which is **absorbed from the GI tract into the bloodstream,** entering neurons at the myoneuronal junction. Through its endopeptidase activity, it cleaves proteins to **prevent the release of acetylcholine,** producing **flaccid muscle paralysis.**
2. **Food poisoning ("adult" botulism).**
   a. Adult botulism follows **ingestion of the preformed toxin** in contaminated food (improperly canned food, foil-wrapped potatoes, meat pies held in restaurants). Initial **symptoms include double vision, fixed pupils, dry mouth, dizziness, and constipation with bilateral descending paralysis.**
   b. **Treatment:** trivalent equine antitoxin. Recovery may be slow, as nerve endings must regrow.
3. **Infant botulism,** the most common form, occurs in **6-month to 2-year-old infants** after **spore ingestion** (from **dust or honey**). Due to the **immature GI tract flora,** ingested spores germinate and **vegetative cells** grow and **produce botulinum toxin in the GI tract.** This is referred to as a **toxi-infection.**
   a. **Botulinum toxin disseminates** (as described above) causing **a descending flaccid paralysis** resulting in constipation, **weak cry, and loss of eye/head/ limb control, producing a "floppy" baby** and, potentially, diaphragm paralysis with death.
   b. If diagnosed and managed for respiratory arrest, infant botulism is rarely fatal. **Recovery** (prolonged but complete) **is speeded by** one time **use of recombinant human anti-botulinum toxin. Antibiotics are contraindicated!** Prevention is to **avoid honey.**
4. **Lab ID:** diagnosed by symptoms and the presence of the toxin in remaining food, stool, blood, or vomitus and typical electroencephalogram (EEG) results.

C. Vomiting diseases.

1. **Staphylococcal food poisoning/*Staph. aureus:***
   Features:
   a. See 4 I E.
   b. **Spread to food from the nares (sneezing or on hands) or from cutaneous lesions of food preparers;** produces **heat-stable enterotoxins in poorly refrigerated, high-protein foods** (e.g., ham, custard-filled pastries, potato salad).
   Disease:
   a. **Staphylococcal food poisoning** results from the **ingestion of the preformed enterotoxins,** which have a CNS effect with a **rapid onset (1 to 6 hours) of nausea and GI pain.**
   b. It **resolves in less than** 24 hours without treatment.
2. **Food poisoning/*Bacillus cereus:***
   Features:
   a. **Gram-positive, spore-forming aerobe.**
   b. It is found in nature, notably in rice. It germinates and produces toxin in poorly refrigerated **cooked rice (especially fried).**
   Disease:
   a. **Caused by ingestion of toxin; symptoms in 1 to 6 hours.**
   b. Similar to Staphylococcal food poisoning.

D. **Watery (secretory) diarrheas.**
  1. **Cholera/ *Vibrio cholerae* (*Vc*):**
     Features:
     a. **Gram-negative, comma-shaped rod** water organism that is **oxidase-positive.** *V. cholerae* causes cholera; most epidemics are due to biotypes cholerae, El Tor, and O139. The O biotype refers to outer membrane antigens.
     b. Found in and transmitted by water or under the shells of shellfish raised in contaminated water.
     Disease:
     a. Cholera is a toxin-mediated disease with the toxin produced by *Vc* infected with and **lysogenized** by bacteriophage CTX.
        (1) **Cholera toxin** (choleragen) has an A fragment (the active/toxic portion) and a B fragment (binding to cells); it specifically attaches to epithelial cells of microvilli at the brush borders of the **small intestine.**
        (2) The A component is an **ADP-ribosyl transferase triggering an increase in adenylate cyclase to overproduce cAMP, which disrupts the fluid and electrolyte balance, causing hypersecretion of chloride and bicarbonate.**
     b. Following ingestion of contaminated water or food, cholera has an abrupt onset of **intense vomiting and diarrhea** as the key finding. **Copious fluid loss** (15 to 20 L/d) leads to clear stools with flecks of mucus and to rapid metabolic acidosis and hypovolemic shock. It results in remission or death after 2 or 3 days.
     c. **Lab ID:** diagnosed by clinical manifestations, combined with a history of residence in or a recent visit to an endemic area. The organism appears in the stool and can be identified by FA staining.
     d. **Treatment:** treated with **prompt replacement of fluids and electrolytes;** the patient should appear healthier within 1 to 3 hours. Proper therapy reduces the fatality rate from 60% to 1%. Tetracycline should be given to reduce ongoing stool volume and infectivity; if antibiotics are not given, the patient will recover but will shed organisms for as long as 1 year.
     e. **Other *Vibrio* agents:**
        (1) ***Vibrio parahaemolyticus,*** also a marine organism in contaminated shellfish, causes relatively mild gastroenteritis.
        (2) ***Vibrio vulnificus*** contaminates some Gulf of Mexico oyster beds in late summer. It is found in oysters and causes relatively **mild gastroenteritis except in people with liver disease who develop serious septicemia.** It also causes a **serious cellulitis** in cuts from shucking contaminated oysters.
  2. **"Traveler's" diarrhea (a watery diarrhea)/commonly enterotoxigenic *E. coli*:**
     Features:
     a. **Enterotoxigenic *E. coli* (*ETEC*):** (see 4 I B). Gram-negative, oxidase-negative rod that reduces nitrates to nitrites and ferments both glucose and lactose; family Enterobacteriaceae.
     b. Spreads through contaminated food and water and is a **serious cause of diarrhea in children in developing countries as well as travelers.**
     Disease:
     a. **ETEC** adheres to the small intestine via pili and secretes two toxins:
        (1) **LT toxin** is an A-B toxin acting similarly to cholera toxin; it **catalyzes ADP-ribosylation, increasing adenylate cyclase activity. (LT is heat labile.)**
        (2) **ST toxin activates guanylate cyclase,** increasing cyclic guanosine monophosphate (cGMP) and resulting in hypersecretion of fluids and electrolytes. **(ST is heat stable.)**
     b. Produces watery diarrhea for 3 to 5 days.
  3. **Diarrhea with or without ileitis or enteropathogenic *E. coli* (EPEC):**
     Features:
     a. *E. coli* producing **bundle-forming pili** and an **adhesin called intimin.**
     b. Affects mainly infants in **developing countries.**
     Disease:
     a. **Attachment to enterocytes in the small intestines damages the microvilli** (attaching-effacing), causing malabsorption and diarrhea.
     b. Causes a **profuse watery diarrhea for 1 to 3 weeks.**

E. **Hemorrhagic colitis (watery diarrhea to diarrhea with blood** (may be bright red)/**enterohemorrhagic _E. coli_** (EHEC or STEC for Shiga toxin–producing _E. coli_).

Features:
1. **EHEC** is found in **bovine feces.** (The cattle are not sick; they have no receptor.) It is **transmitted by undercooked ground beef** (where contaminated outer surfaces become the interior part of a hamburger), bovine fecal contamination of well water, and so on.
2. The dominant serotype is **O157:H7,** but there are **many other** serotypes. Cattle are the main reservoir.

Disease:
1. **Attaches and effaces (like EPEC** except in **the large intestine),** and secretes a **Shiga-like toxin (a cytotoxin** earlier called verotoxin and now often simply referred to as Shiga toxin**). The toxin nicks the intestinal cell 60S ribosome,** shutting down protein synthesis, **destroying the colonic mucosa,** and causing **bleeding into the intestine.** Pus is normally not present.
2. **Frequently no fever.** Children are more likely to develop **hemolytic uremic syndrome (HUS).** The toxin also damages the kidney. Healthy children may lose kidney function within a few days.
3. **Treatment: NO antibiotics!** The Shiga-like toxin gene is a **prophage gene but the toxin is produced only during lytic replication.** The effect of most antibiotics is to trigger lytic replication, producing more toxin (increasing risk of **HUS**) and more phage, which can infect more _E. coli_ (potentially amplifying the infection).
4. **Prevention:** prevented by thorough cooking of meat, pasteurizing milk and juices, and preventing bovine fecal contamination of wells.

F. **Shigellosis (inflammatory diarrhea or bacillary dysentery)/_Shigella_ spp.**

Features:
1. **Gram-negative, facultative anaerobic, nonmotile rods highly resistant to acid;** therefore, it takes only 100 to 200 shigellae to successfully infect.
2. **Humans are the only reservoirs** (no known animals); organism is not found in soil or water unless contaminated with human fecal material.
3. Shigellae are spread by the **fecal–oral route** through poor sanitation and are readily transmitted from person to person by unrecognized clinical cases and convalescing or healthy carriers via food, fingers, feces, flies, and oral–anal sex.
4. **Classification:** classified into four O antigenic groups:
   a. **_Shigella sonnei_** causes mild disease; the most common cause of shigellosis in the United States.
   b. **_Shigella flexneri_** causes more severe disease; common in the United States.
   c. **_Shigella boydii_** causes more severe disease; rarely found in the United States.
   d. **_Shigella dysenteriae_** causes the most severe disease; rarely found in the United States, unless imported.

Disease:
1. **All strains are invasive in the large intestine and terminal ileum.** Shigellae **traverse the M cells invading from the basal side** of the epithelial cells. In the epithelial cells, they **rearrange cellular actin to "jet propel" themselves into adjoining cells,** producing shallow ulcerations and inflammation with large numbers of PMNs ("excess leukocytes"). Bloodstream invasion is rare because of shallow ulceration.
2. **Only _Sh. dysenteriae_ type 1 secretes** a potent, heat-labile protein exotoxin (**Shiga toxin**), the A subunit of which **nicks the 60S eukaryotic ribosomal subunit,** causing **diarrhea** but also acting as a **neurotoxin.** Like the similar Shiga-like toxin of EHEC strains of _E. coli, Sh. dysenteriae_ type 1 strains also cause HUS; however, because the Shiga toxin gene is chromosomal, **antibiotic treatment does not increase the risk of HUS.**
3. **Clinical symptoms:** characterized by the sudden onset of **abdominal pain and cramps** (may be severe), **diarrhea,** and **fever** after a short incubation period (1 to 4 days). **Stools are liquid and scant;** after the first few bowel movements, they contain **mucus, pus, and occasionally blood.**
4. **Lab ID:** diagnosed from stool culture on differential and selective media. Rapid diagnosis can be made using NAA tests.

5. **Treatment:** generally treated with electrolyte and fluid replacement. Only *Sh. dysenteriae* infections require antibiotic therapy; however, resistance to antibiotics has been developing.

G. **Inflammatory diarrhea/enteroinvasive *E. coli.***

Enteroinvasive *E. coli* (EIEC) causes bloody diarrhea similar to shigellosis by invasion and destruction of colon epithelium; occurs primarily in children in developing countries, rarely the United States.

H. **Inflammatory diarrhea/*Campylobacter jejuni (Cj).***

Features:

1. **Gram-negative, curved rod with polar flagella,** often occurring in "nose-to-nose" pairs with extending polar flagella described as having the appearance of "seagull's wings." It is both **oxidase- and catalase-positive,** is **microaerophilic, and grows at 42°.**
2. *Cj* is found in a wide variety of wild and domestic animals and is transmitted to humans most commonly through contamination from uncooked **poultry.** Outbreaks have been caused by **unpasteurized milk.** *Campylobacter* is the most common bacteria isolated from diarrhea in the United States.

Disease:

1. *Cj* **invades tissue,** causing an inflammatory diarrhea with blood *and* pus.
2. Infections are characterized by **fever, abdominal pain,** and **bloody diarrhea. Diarrhea is a result of prostaglandin production.** It may lead to **extraintestinal** and postinfective complications, including **reactive arthritis** and **Guillain-Barré syndrome.** (About 30% of cases of Guillain-Barré syndrome are due to *Cj.*)
3. **Lab ID:**
   a. Diagnosed by the finding of numerous thin S-shaped **darting microorganisms** in the stool **along with blood and excess neutrophils** (indicating invasion with inflammation).
   b. Immunoassay for stool antigen.
   c. The organism is isolated on special agar (**Campy or Skirrow's agar**) grown at **42°C** (which suppresses most of the growth of other GI tract flora) under **microaerophilic conditions (10% CO_2).**
4. **Treatment:** treated with fluid and electrolytes; the disease is generally self-limiting (lasts less than 1 week). In severe cases, treatment is with azithromycin, erythromycin, or ciprofloxacin, although resistance to ciprofloxacin is increasing.
5. **Prevention:** prevented by sanitation and pasteurization.

I. *Salmonella* **enterocolitis (gastroenteritis)/*Salmonella spp.***

Features:

1. **Gram-negative, motile rods; nonlactose fermenters.**
2. **All from eggs or animals as well as humans except *Sal. typhi* and *Sal. paratyphi,* which have only human hosts.**
3. All serotypes possess **O (outer membrane) antigens used to serogroup;** may possess a **capsular (K) antigen,** or the **virulence (Vi) antigen of *Sal. typhi*** (also a capsular antigen); they are identified further by the presence of different **flagellar (H) antigens.**
4. Important serotypes of *Salmonella enterica* include *Sal. typhi, Sal. paratyphi, Sal. enteritidis, Sal. typhimurium, Sal. schottmuelleri,* and *Sal. choleraesuis.*

Disease:

1. **Mechanisms:**
   a. The endotoxin causes fever, leukopenia, hemorrhage, hypotension, shock, and disseminated intravascular coagulation.
   b. Some may produce an exotoxin (enterotoxin).
   c. They are aided by antiphagocytic activity of the capsule.
   d. They can survive within macrophages by an unknown means.
2. **Enterocolitis** is a **self-limiting illness** manifested by **fever, nausea, vomiting, and diarrhea** and is the most common form of salmonella infection in the United States (approximately 2 million cases per year).
   a. Source is food contaminated by human carriers or ill individuals (particularly food handlers), exotic pets (turtles and snakes), or contaminated animal products (most commonly poultry and poultry products).

  b. Most common causes are *Sal. typhimurium* and *Sal. enteritidis,* which usually require a high infecting dose with an **8- to 48-hour incubation** period.

  c. Disease is usually characterized by the **following pattern:**

   (1) Ingestion of organisms followed by colonization of the ileum and cecum.

   (2) Penetration of epithelial cells in the mucosa and invasion, resulting in acute inflammation and ulceration with the release of prostaglandin. Enterotoxins, resulting in activation of adenylate cyclase and increased cAMP, cause increased fluid secretion in the intestines.

3. Septicemic (extraintestinal) disease is an **acute illness,** most often of nosocomial origin, with abrupt onset and early invasion of the bloodstream.

  a. Clinical symptoms: characterized by a precipitating incident that introduces bacteria (e.g., catheterization, contaminated intravenous fluids, abdominal or pelvic surgery), followed by a **triad of chills, fever, and hypotension.**

  b. Wide dissemination of the organisms may cause local **abscesses, osteomyelitis, and endocarditis. In sickle cell disease patients, *Salmonella* osteomyelitis is a serious and recurring problem.**

  c. Septicemia is caused by *Salmonella* species as well as other Enterobacteriaceae organisms.

  d. Mortality rate is high (30% to 50%) and depends on the degree of preexisting debilitation.

  e. Septicemia is **diagnosed by blood culture** because the organisms do not localize in the bowel and stool cultures are often negative.

4. Enteric fever (typhoid fever) is caused mainly by *Sal. typhi* with **less severe disease (paratyphoid fever)** caused by *Sal. paratyphi,* **both strict human pathogens** (i.e., no animal reservoirs).

  a. Infection occurs through ingestion of food or water contaminated by an unknowing carrier; the organism is **highly infective even with small numbers** of bacteria (e.g., 200).

  b. During the **7- to 14-day incubation** period, the organisms **multiply in the small intestine** and then **enter the intestinal lymphatics.**

  c. Dissemination into the bloodstream (and ultimately to **multiple organs**) causes malaise, headache, and gradual onset of a fever that increases during the day, reaching a plateau of 102–105°F (38.8–40.6°C) each day. **Blood cultures are positive in this first symptomatic phase** but not earlier.

  d. Multiplies in the reticuloendothelial system and lymphoid tissue of the bowel, producing **hyperplasia and necrosis of the lymphoid Peyer's patches.**

  e. A characteristic **rash ("rose spots")** may appear on the trunk in the **second to third weeks**.

  f. Typically, the **disease lasts 3 to 5 weeks**; the **major complications are GI hemorrhage and bowel perforation with peritonitis**.

  g. After recovery, **3% of patients become carriers;** the organism is retained in the **gallbladder** and **biliary passages,** and cholecystectomy may be necessary.

  h. Lab ID: Salmonellae are commonly first isolated in blood or bone marrow, or after 1 to 2 weeks from stool. The specimens are plated onto differential media, selective media, or both.

  i. Treatment: treated with ciprofloxacin; watch for relapse.

J. Diarrhea developing into pseudomembranous colitis (PMC) (also called antibiotic associated diarrhea)/*Clostridium difficile* (less commonly *Staph. aureus*).

Features:

1. *C. difficile* is a Gram-positive, spore-forming, anaerobic rod.

2. Colonizes in 2% to 3% of healthy individuals and 5% to 15% of people who have recently had antibiotics but do not have diarrhea. Hospital environments and personnel may become contaminated with spores.

3. Many strains are resistant to antibiotics relative to other members of the gut flora. Antibiotic treatment kills organisms that normally restrict growth of *C. difficile,* resulting in overgrowth of the latter.

Disease:

1. *C. difficile* produces two toxins: an **enterotoxin (toxin A) that causes fluid accumulation and damages the mucosa of the large bowel** and a **cytotoxin (toxin B) that causes cytoskeletal changes and then kills mucosal cells.**

2. Manifests **first** as **diarrhea** and then develops into **pseudomembranous colitis**, also known as **antibiotic-associated colitis** because it follows antibiotic therapy to treat other bacterial infections.
3. **Treatment:** treated with oral rehydration and metronidazole; discontinue other antibiotics if possible; enteric isolation; avoid antimotility drugs.

K. Abdominal abscesses/*Bacteroides fragilis* (*Bf*).
   Features:
   1. *Bf* **is a Gram-negative, anaerobic rod** that produces some superoxide dismutase and catalase, making it somewhat resistant to short exposure to oxygen.
   2. Is found in the human GI tract and female genital tract, grows rapidly under anaerobic conditions, and is stimulated by bile. It accounts for 1% of gut anaerobes along with other *Bacteroides* species.
   3. It is usually involved in **polymicrobic infections** that involve more than one genus or species; consequently, therapy with several antibiotics may be necessary.
   Disease:
   1. *Bf*'s **capsule** inhibits phagocytosis; collagenase and hyaluronidase aid its spread, but its endotoxin lacks potency and it has no exotoxins.
   2. **Abdominal abscesses** occur after damage to intestinal mucosal barriers; they are **foul smelling.**

XIV. URINARY TRACT INFECTIONS

A. **General aspects of UTIs.**
   1. Host factors that increase the risk of UTIs include obstructions, sexual intercourse, catheters, diaphragms, and voiding impairment.
   2. **Cystitis** is characterized by **painful, frequent urination; hematuria; and urgency;** it is more common in women due to the shorter urethra and its proximity to the anal area.
   3. **Pyelonephritis** is an infection of the kidneys commonly from an ascending UTI; it is characterized by **fever, flank pain, and tenderness and may lead to endotoxic shock.**
   4. UTIs in pregnancy, even those that are asymptomatic, can lead to pyelonephritis, often resulting in premature delivery of the fetus.
   5. **Prostatitis** occurs in older men.

B. **UTI/*E. coli* (see 4 I B).**
   Features:
   1. Lactose-fermenting Enterobacteriaceae (all ferment glucose, are oxidase-negative, and reduce nitrates to nitrites).
   2. The **most common cause of UTIs** occurring after contamination/colonization of the genital area with fecal microbiota.
   Disease:
   1. *E. coli* causes cystitis through **adherence to the lower urinary tract** through mannose-sensitive **fimbriae (pili)** and **inflammation from the endotoxin. Strains causing pyelonephritis have additional adhesins like P-pili which attach to renal cell receptors.**
   2. **Lab ID:** Most strains **reduce nitrate to nitrite;** therefore, urine dipstick tests for nitrites are positive as long as the urine has been in contact with the agent for a sufficient amount of time.
   3. **Treatment: treated according to local susceptibility patterns,** generally with trimethoprim-sulfamethoxazole or ciprofloxacin.
   4. Other Enterobacteriaceae may also cause UTI but are much less common.

C. **UTI/enterococci.**
   Features:
   1. **Gram-positive coccus** of streptococcal heritage.
   2. Opportunists of fecal origin.

Disease:
1. Major cause of UTIs.
2. Cause endocarditis in patients with preexisting heart damage who undergo prostate surgery, · cystoscopy, or urethral dilatation.
3. **Treatment:** relatively **resistant to many antibiotics**; it is inhibited but not killed by penicillin.

D. UTI/*Staphylococcus saprophyticus* (*Ss*).
Features:
1. *Ss* is a **nonhemolytic, coagulase-negative, catalase-positive, Gram-positive staphylococcus.**
2. *Ss* causes **cystitis**, commonly in autumn in **newly sexually active adolescent women** ("honeymoon cystitis"), although *E. coli* is still more common in this population.
Disease:
1. Uncomplicated cystitis.
2. **Lab ID:** is always **nitrite-negative** on urine dipsticks.

E. UTI/*Proteus mirabilis.*
Features:
1. **Lactose-nonfermenting Enterobacteriaceae** known for its **swarming motility.**
2. Primarily an opportunist, **transmitted via catheters.**
Disease:
1. Produces a powerful **urease** that hydrolyzes urea to ammonia and CO_2, **leading to struvite kidney stones**, then to urinary tract obstruction.

F. Acute glomerulonephritis *Streptococcus pyogenes* nephritogenic strains cause an immune complex disease **following either pharyngitis or impetigo** even when treated.

XV. SKIN, MUCOSAL, SOFT TISSUE, AND BONE INFECTIONS

A. General aspects of skin, mucosal, soft tissue, and bone infections.
1. Many of these infections involve *Staph. aureus* and *Strep. pyogenes* (see 4 I E and G).
2. Staphylococci and streptococci are distinguished by the catalase test. (Mnemonic: Staphylococcus is catalase-positive or "cat-pos"; the name "S t **a** p h y l o **c** o c c u s" contains the letters C, A, and T, but streptococcus does not.)

B. Systemic bacterial diseases with rashes or cutaneous lesions include the following diseases:
1. **Scarlet fever/*Strep. pyogenes.*** Clinical symptoms are a **fine sandpaper body rash with pharyngitis** with or without nausea.
2. **Toxic shock syndrome (TSS)/*Staph. aureus.*** Case definition requires the presence of a **diffuse macular rash that desquamates, especially on extremities.** Streptococcal TSS may also have a rash.
3. **Petechial rash with septicemia** with either *Neisseria meningitidis* or *N. gonorrhoeae.*
4. **Secondary syphilis.** Mucocutaneous lesions cover all surfaces **including palms and soles.**
5. **Rocky Mountain spotted fever.** Petechial rash begins on extremities and migrates to the body (**centripetal rash**); **palms and soles have a rash.** (Typhus causes a centrifugal rash.)
6. **Lyme disease. Target-shaped lesions** are found in the primary stage of the disease (see 4 XVIII B).

C. Impetigo. This infection of the epidermis often starts with bug bites or eczematous lesions. It is caused by:
1. *Staph. aureus,* which is characterized by **bullae** (fairly large fluid-filled vesicular lesions).
2. *Strep. pyogenes,* which is characterized by transient vesicular lesions easily rupturing and taking on an **old varnished** appearance, also described as honey crusted.
3. Commonly, **mixed infections** of the two.

D. **Folliculitis.** These infections are most commonly caused by ***Staph. aureus*** with the exception of "**hot tub folliculitis**," which is caused by ***Ps. aeruginosa*** and acquired in a contaminated swimming pool or hot tub.

E. **Furuncles/carbuncles/(***Staph. aureus***).** Commonly called boils; often start with an infected hair follicle. Carbuncles are the larger, coalescing aggregates of boils.

F. **Erysipelas and cellulitis.**
   1. **Erysipelas** is a painful cellulitis involving blockage of the dermal lymphatics so lesions have sharp raised borders. **Cellulitis** is infection of the deeper dermis and subcutaneous fat.
   2. Both are more commonly caused by *Strep. pyogenes* but may be ***Staph. aureus.***
   3. ***Strep. pyogenes*** may cause TSS following invasive disease (e.g., cellulitis) with encapsulated strains of M1 or M3. These strains produce SPE-A or SPE-C toxins (see 4 I G 5). These toxins are superantigens that have direct cardiotoxicity in addition to decreasing normal liver clearance of endotoxin from the body.

G. **Necrotizing fasciitis.** This infection involves the fascia and overlying fat. It is most commonly caused by ***Strep. pyogenes,*** but may involve mixed bowel flora if the infection originates in the abdominal area. The hyaluronidase facilitates spread.

H. **Surgical wounds.** In breeching the integument, surgery raises the risk of infection even when great care is taken. Additionally, it decreases the responsiveness of the immune system for about 2 days. The etiology varies with surgical site and hospital or clinic. Very common organisms include ***Staph. aureus, Staph. epidermidis, Gram-negative*** enteric bacteria, ***Bacteroides fragilis, and clostridia.***

I. **Trauma.** Trauma often introduces soil or plant microbes as well as normal skin, mucosal, or fecal flora into normally sterile tissues. One fairly common toxin-producing organism, *Clostridium tetani,* is often in the soil and, if not properly prevented or treated, can lead to death.
   1. **Tetanus/*C. tetani*:**
      Features:
      a. **Gram-positive, spore-forming anaerobe** with **terminal spores,** resulting in a characteristic "**tennis racquet**" morphologic appearance.
      b. *C. tetani* vegetative cells and spores are ubiquitous in soil and are a major concern during wars and for babies born to unvaccinated mothers. Infection follows trauma where the oxygen supply to the wound is compromised.
      Disease:
      a. Causes disease through **vegetative cell production of tetanus neurotoxin (TeNT; also called tetanospasmin). TeNT *acts* on synaptosomes to obliterate the inhibitory reflex response of nerve fibers, producing uncontrolled spasms.**
      b. Manifests as descending muscle stiffness, **tetanospasms** of **lockjaw,** back arching (**opisthotonus**), and short, frequent spasms of voluntary muscles. Death occurs after several weeks from exhaustion and respiratory failure.
      c. **Treatment of actual tetanus:**
         (1) Hospitalize and start specialized supportive care immediately.
         (2) Antitoxin (tetanus immunoglobulin [TIG]) only neutralizes unbound toxin. It is given around the wound.
         (3) **Metronidazole** should be started: dead tissue should be debrided; and vaccination should be given at a distant site from TIG.
      d. **Prevention:**
         (1) **Routine vaccination** of infants/children with DTaP vaccine containing the tetanus toxoid. Boosters should be given every 10 years (1X Tdap, rest Td).
         (2) **Prevention** (with proper wound care) in **persons with wounds** is as follows:
            (a) **Tetanus-prone wounds in a person with an unknown or incomplete vaccination record: wound care, TIG around wound, vaccination at distant site, and antibiotics.** Tetanus-prone wounds are stellate or avulsion; wounds deeper

than 1 cm; frostbite or burns; wounds contaminated with dirt, saliva, and so on; tissues with a compromised tissue oxygen supply; or wounds older than 6 hours.

(b) **Tetanus-prone wounds in a vaccinated person:** wound care **plus booster vaccine if more than 10 years since last booster.** Antibiotics depend on wound.

(c) If the wound is not tetanus-prone, provide wound care and ensure that the patient is up-to-date on vaccines.

2. **Cutaneous anthrax/*B. anthracis*** (see 4 VII G):
   Disease:
   a. Unlike clostridia, *B. anthracis* can grow in very superficial wounds. However, since near eradication has occurred in animals by vaccination in the United States and gas sterilization of commercial raw wool imports, *B. anthracis* is not common in the environment. People working with imported goat and sheep products and weavers are at highest risk.
   b. **Clinical symptoms:**
      (1) The **early papular lesion** develops into a **vesicular lesion filled with blood or clear fluid** that, due to cell death, develops **central necrosis (black eschar) with an ery-thematous raised margin.**
      (2) Systemic disease is not present in many cases. The fatality rate is 10%.
   c. **Treatment:** ciprofloxacin.

3. **Cellulitis in burn patients/*Ps. aeruginosa* (*Psa*)** (see 4 I D):
   a. *Pseudomonas* is a major problem in burn patients. We are constantly exposed to *Psa* and, at any one time, 10% of us are transiently colonized with *Psa* (different 10% at different times); this colonization increases to 90% in hospitalized patients. GI *Psa* colonization causes loose stools which contaminate perianal skin and spread on the skin, which is a potential source for burn colonization leading to infection. Other sources are environmental associated with water. **Blue-green pus in a burn generally indicates *Pseudomonas* infection.**
   b. In **systemic infection with *Ps. aeruginosa*** (mainly in **neutropenic patients or burn patients**), black skin lesions (**ecthyma gangrenosum**) that resemble anthrax develop. They start as raised and red, tumorlike lesions and then develop necrosis in the middle.

4. **Bites.** Because all animals, including humans, have bacteria in their mouths, **all bites generally require treatment, commonly amoxicillin-clavulinate. Cat bites** (dominant microbe: **Gram-negative *Pasteurella multocida*)** are most likely to become infected.

5. **Puncture wounds.** A nail that passes through the sole of a tennis shoe is most likely to cause *Ps. aeruginosa* cellulitis (probably from the *Ps. aeruginosa* inside the shoe). Some infections will progress to osteomyelitis. Tetanus risk also needs to be evaluated.

J. **Osteomyelitis. Microbiologic diagnosis is essential.**
   1. *Staph. aureus* is the most common causative agent.
   2. In **infants,** the other **agents of neonatal septicemia** (GBS and Gram-negative bacilli) may also be involved.
   3. In people with **thalassemia or sickle cell disease,** osteomyelitis is extremely common and it is **overwhelmingly** caused by *Salmonella.*

K. **Arthritis.**
   1. **Reactive arthritis (Reiter's)** may follow weeks *after* infections with ***Chl. trachomatis, Campylo-bacter, Yersinia enterocolitica, Salmonella* sp., or *Shigella* sp.** It is generally focused on large joints; it may be migratory and associated with cervicitis or urethritis and conjunctivitis. Only anti-inflammatory drugs are needed.
   2. **Septic arthritis** occurs with several diseases and under several conditions; the risk increases anytime there is a septicemia, an artificial joint, or injection into a joint.
      a. **Gonococcal arthritis** occurs primarily as acute disease in undiagnosed/untreated young women at risk of sexually transmitted infections (STIs). It may be mono- or polyarticular.
      b. **Lyme disease** is generally large joints and polyarticular.
      c. **Postarticular injection** infections are commonly caused by *Staph. aureus, Staph. epidermidis,* or *Pseudomonas.*
      d. **Prosthetic joints** are commonly infected by streptococci or *Staph. aureus* or *Staph. epidermidis;* these may be resistant strains.

SITUATIONAL DISEASE

XVI. SEXUALLY TRANSMITTED INFECTIONS (STIs)

(Statistics from 2010 U.S.) All patients with one STI should be tested for other likely STIs. Diagnostic tests may differ for different body sites; common genital sites are listed.

A. **Sexually transmitted infections/*Chl. trachomatis.***
   1. ***Chl. trachomatis* serovars D–K:**
      Features:
      a. **OIP** (see 4 I A).
      b. ***Chl. trachomatis* is the most common <u>bacterial</u> STI** in the United States. (There were 1.3 million cases reported in 2010 with actual new infections estimated to be at 4 million. Reported incidences were *4 times higher than Ng.*)
      Disease:
      a. High incidence of asymptomatic chronic infections, particularly in women where often infection is not obvious (so not treated) until the granulomatous response causes complications. **Reinfection is common** due to the eight serovars. Each new infection increases the risk of infertility. **Chlamydiae** are a major cause of infertility.
      b. **Urethritis in men (milky discharge); urethritis, endometritis, cervicitis, salpingitis, and pelvic inflammatory disease in women; inclusion conjunctivitis in both genders; and conjunctivitis and pneumonia in neonates.** **Reiter's** syndrome is not uncommon several weeks after infections, particularly in males.
      c. **Lab ID:** NAA tests have replaced less sensitive nonamplified tests. Specimens are either first voided urine or urethral discharge for males. Results from self-collected vaginal swabs correlate well with results from physician-collected cervical swabs. DFA available.
      d. **Treatment**: doxycycline or a macrolide.
      e. **Prevention:** Annual screening of all sexually active young people is now recommended. Prevented only by barrier methods.
   2. ***Chl. trachomatis* serovars L1, L2, L3:**
      These strains cause an STI called **lymphogranuloma venereum,** characterized by a suppurative inguinal adenitis progressing to lymphatic obstruction and rectal strictures if the disease is untreated.

B. **Gonorrhea/*Neisseria gonorrhoeae* (*Ng*).**
   Features:
   1. ***Ng* utilizes glucose but does not ferment maltose.**
   2. Most common in 15- to 25-year-olds. Urban incidence > suburban/rural. Incidence per 100,000 is about 100X more common in non-Hispanic Blacks than other groups. More common east of the Mississippi River and south except for Alaska. ***Ng*** is sensitive to drying and cold so it requires intimate contact.
   Disease:
   1. **IgA1 protease** plays a key early role in the colonization of mucosa. **Adherence is through pili** (protein surface fibrils) **and other outer membrane proteins.**
      a. **Pili undergo *phase variation*** (on & off). Nonpiliation greatly reduces virulence.
      b. Pili also exhibit ***antigenic variation* by continuous genetic rearrangement.** There are **10 to 15 incomplete pilin loci (*pilS* for silent) lacking transcriptional promoter elements** and **one complete pilin expression locus (*pilE*)** with all expression elements. Through **homologous recombination, an incomplete gene or pieces of it can be recombined into *pilE*, creating millions of variants. This recombination occurs continuously** and **accounts for the chronicity** of the infections, the lack of protection against subsequent *Ng* infections, and why both partners need to be treated at the same time.

    c. **Outer membrane proteins** add genetic variation. They include outer membrane **porin protein (PI and PIII)** and proteins that determine **clumping (PII) or opacity.** PII-positive strains promote adherence and invasion, leading to septicemia.

2. *Ng* attachment to the microvilli of the nonciliated cells leads to ciliary stasis and death of the ciliated cells as well as internalization of *Ng.* Intracellular gonococci replicate in vacuoles where they are protected from antibodies. Eventually they exit into the subepithelial connective tissue, causing inflammation and possibly gaining entrance into the bloodstream.

3. **Lipooligosaccharide** (LOS is *Ng*'s version of LPS.) triggers TNF-alpha and damage to the mucosa. Strains causing disseminated gonococcal infections have sialylation of the LOS, which provides greater serum resistance.

4. **Clinical symptoms:**
    a. Gonorrhea is a **mucous membrane infection,** the site dependent on gender, sexual practices, and strain virulence. It is **often asymptomatic in women.** Both asymptomatic and symptomatic persons may transmit the disease. Untreated/repeated infections increase the risk of infertility and predispose women to ectopic pregnancy.
    b. **Urethritis** in men is characterized by thick, yellow, purulent exudate containing bacteria and numerous neutrophils; frequent, painful urination; and possibly an erythematous meatus. Complications include **epididymitis** and **prostatitis** in males.
    c. **Endocervicitis or urethritis** in women is characterized by a purulent vaginal discharge; frequent, painful urination; dyspareunia; and abdominal pain. Approximately 50% of cases go undiagnosed. Complications include arthritis, salpingitis, pelvic inflammatory disease, sterility, and ectopic pregnancy.
    d. **Rectal infections** are characterized by painful defecation, discharge, constipation, and proctitis.
    e. **Pharyngitis** ranges from mild to severe with purulent exudate that mimics "strep" throat.
    f. **Disseminated infection** (untreated with bloodstream invasion) presents most commonly as polyarthritis or necrotic skin lesions on an erythematous base.
    g. **Ophthalmia neonatorum** rapidly leads to blindness if not properly treated immediately.

5. **Lab ID:** gonococcal infections are diagnosed with NAA tests, or culture on Thayer-Martin (a chocolate agar with antibiotics to inhibit NF) or New York City agar. Patients with gonorrhea should be treated for *Chl. trachomatis* too.

6. **Treatment and prevention:** most commonly treated with ceftriaxone; test for (and treat if positive) *Chlamydia trachomatis.* Prevent with condom usage.

C. Syphilis/*Treponema pallidum* (*Tp*).
Features:
1. **Spirochete (corkscrew-shaped, motile spiral bacteria** with an endoflagellum [**axial filament**] underneath the outer membrane) which is **too thin to show up on Gram stain** but does have an outer membrane with **endotoxin-like lipids.**
2. Human pathogen that is most prevalent in homosexuals and drug abusers. Infected, drug-abusing women are responsible for most congenital cases; these are totally preventable with early penicillin treatment of the mother.

Disease:
1. **Causes chronic, painless infections** that may last 30 to 40 years if untreated. The number of *Tp* decreases as host defenses are stimulated, causing disappearance of symptoms; subsequently, organisms multiply and symptoms reappear, the mechanism of which is not understood. However, immunosuppressive treponemal components may play a role. The pathogenesis of syphilis varies considerably and is dependent on the person's immune system and the spread.
2. **Primary syphilis:** starts with mucosal implantation of *Tp* by minor trauma. *Tp* replicates locally. Neutrophils and then lymphocytes and plasma cells infiltrate the site and a **painless primary hard chancre** develops that **may heal** without treatment.
3. **Secondary syphilis:** bloodstream invasion leads to infection in almost all tissues and a papular, mucocutaneous rash over all of the body, including the palms and soles. Aggregation near vessels leads to **endarteritis and periarteritis,** resulting in inhibited blood supply and necrosis. The rash self-resolves but may recur.

4. **Latent syphilis:** about two-thirds of the untreated secondary syphilis cases will have persistent treponemes without symptoms.
5. **Tertiary syphilis:** about half of the individuals with latent syphilis will progress to tertiary, which is often characterized by aortitis and CNS problems, which may be fatal.
6. **In utero infection:** has severe manifestations, including abortion, stillbirth, birth defects, or latent infection (most common) with snuffles (rhinitis) followed by a rash and desquamation.
7. **Lab ID:** includes recognition of symptoms.
   a. **Microscopy (for primary):** Since *Tp* cannot be cultured and since antibodies are not reliably present in very early syphilis, **microscopy** of expressed chancre fluids is commonly done. Because the diameter of the cylinder of dye in the Gram-stained treponemes is below the resolution of the light microscope, other methods are used.
      (1) **Darkfield microscopy** of lesion exudate may demonstrate **corkscrew-shaped spiro-chetes** with "springing" motility.
      (2) **Immunofluorescence** may be used with commercially prepared tagged antibodies.
      (3) **Serology.** See below. Negative serology cannot rule out early infection.
   b. **Serology:** Two different antibodies are produced in response to *Tp* infection. Because (1) each has some cross-reactivity and (2) only the treponemal antibodies are positive for life, it is a **positive test for each of the two types of antibodies that is diagnostic** except in tertiary, where the nontreponemal test will often be negative.
      (1) **Nontreponemal (reaginic) antibodies:**
         (a) Triggered by *Tp's damage* to the human cells. The antigens appear to be of **mitochondrial origin and bind *Tp*.** The antibodies triggered cross-react with cow cardiolipin, which is used as an antigen in economical screening tests.
         (b) Tests are **quite sensitive but not very specific** (positive in other diseases). Confirm positive with treponemal antibody test.
         (c) **Nontreponemal antibody tests** are:
            - **VDRL (Venereal Disease Research Laboratory)** test
            - **rapid plasma reagin (RPR)** test
            - **automated reagin test (ART)**
         (d) **Non-treponemal antibody titers may decrease in tertiary syphilis** with or without treatment.
         (e) Titers are useful to monitor successful therapy.
      (2) **Treponemal antibodies.** In screening of asymptomatic individuals, treponemal tests are used to confirm a positive nontreponemal test. For a patient with symptoms, both the screening and the more specific test would be ordered.
         (a) **Treponemal antibody tests are triggered by *Tp*** itself; they are the **first antibody made**.
         (b) Treponemal antibody tests **require treponemal antigens** so they are **more specific** and costly.
         (c) **Treponemal antibody tests** are:
            - **TP-PA test (treponemal particle agglutination test)** where particles have been coated with **treponemal antigens** (replacing FTA-abs test).
            - ***T. pallidum* hemagglutination test (TPHA).**
            - **FTA-abs test** (fluorescent treponemal antibody absorption test) which has been the gold standard but is technically difficult ($$).
         (d) Titers of treponemal antibody tests remain positive even with proper treatment.
      (3) For screening asymptomatic patients, usually just a nontreponemal antibody test is run and a treponemal test is only ordered if the first is positive. For symptomatic patients one of each type would be ordered initially.
8. **Treatment of syphilis:**
   a. Treatment is long-lasting penicillin.
   b. Treatment of secondary syphilis may trigger the **Jarisch-Herxheimer** reaction immediately after antibiotic therapy. This involves intensification of manifestations for 12 hours and indicates that penicillin is effective.
   c. If penicillin is effective, reagin-based serologic tests become negative 6 months after primary syphilis and 12 months after secondary syphilis; beyond the secondary stage, the patient may remain seropositive for years.

D. **Bacterial vaginosis.**
   1. Bacterial vaginosis (BV) involves overgrowth of bacteria common to the NF, most notably ***Gardnerella vaginalis,*** a Gram-variable rod, and **other anaerobes like *Bacteroides. Gardnerella vaginalis*** is present in 20% to 40% of asymptomatic women, but almost 100% of the partners of women with BV, suggesting it is sexually transmitted.
   2. Presents with copious amounts of an unpleasant fishy or musty discharge.
   3. **Lab ID:** diagnosed by the finding of a **pH greater than 4.5, a positive amine "whiff" test** (drop of KOH on discharge will give off an amine odor), and the presence of **clue cells, which are epithelial cells coated with bacteria.**
   4. **Treatment:** treated with metronidazole.

XVII. PREGNANCY, CONGENITAL, AND PERINATAL INFECTIONS

A. **Bacterial infections made worse by pregnancy.** The immune and hormonal changes that occur during pregnancy increase a woman's susceptibility to infection and may worsen or reactivate certain infections.
   1. **UTIs** are more frequent and serious for both mother and fetus. Bladder and ureter atony leads to an increased incidence of cystitis and a greater likelihood of pyelonephritis. Either, but especially the latter, may precipitate premature delivery whenever they occur.
   2. **Listeriosis,** generally a mild enterocolitis, in pregnancy may become invasive and cause septicemia with influenza-like symptoms and may cross the placenta (but does not cause meningitis in the mother).

B. **Neonatal infections.** A fetus is immunologically incompatible with its mother but is not rejected because of the subtle maternal immune defects and because major histocompatibility complex antigens are absent or have low density on placental cells. Placental antigens are covered with blocking antibody. Therefore, the mother is at increased risk of infection. If an organism makes it into the bloodstream, the placenta and ultimately the fetus may be infected. Some infections are transmitted during the birth process.
   1. Some **bacterial infections cross the placenta:**
      a. ***Listeria*** (see 4 VIII D).
      b. ***T. pallidum*** (see 4 XVI C).
   2. Some **bacterial infections may be acquired during the birthing process.** These are from passage in a contaminated birth canal or exposure to feces.
      a. Neonatal ***Chl. trachomatis* D-K** eye infections or pneumonia.
      b. Neonatal ***N. gonorrhoeae*** ophthalmia neonatorum, which can lead to blindness.
      c. **GBS** septicemia and meningitis (see 4 VIII B).
      d. ***E. coli*** septicemia and meningitis (see 4 VIII C).
      e. ***Listeria monocytogenes*** septicemia and meningitis (see 4 VIII D). (Late onset from maternal fecal colonization and exposure of the baby at birth.)

XVIII. ARTHROPOD-BORNE AND ZOONOTIC DISEASES

Arthropod-borne infections are summarized in Table 4.1; **zoonoses** in Table 4.2.

A. **Rocky Mountain spotted fever (RMSF)/*Rickettsia rickettsii* (*Rr*).** (The most important rickettsia has the "double" name.)
   Features:
   1. **Gram-negative, OIP,** with a specific **predilection for endothelial cells of capillaries.**
   2. **Tick transmitted** by bite of ***Dermacentor variabilis*** **(dog tick** nicely named since dogs are so variable!) and ***Dermacentor andersoni*** **(wood tick).**

| t a b l e **4.1** | Important Arthropod-Borne Diseases |

Disease	Organism	Vector	Reservoir Host	Environment/U.S. Geography Hot Spots
Rocky Mountain Spotted Fever	*Rickettsia rickettsii*	*Dermacentor* ticks	Dogs, rodents, and ticks	Highest in SE United States: Tennessee to Oklahoma but all states
Rickettsialpox	*Rickettsia akari*	Mites	Domestic rodents	Rodent-infested low-income housing, New York City
Epidemic typhus	*Rickettsia prowazekii*	Flying squirrel mites/ fleas Human body lice (*Pediculus humanus*)	Flying squirrel Humans	Rural homes in eastern United States War-torn countries
Human monocytic ehrlichiosis	*Ehrlichia chaffeensis*	*Amblyomma* (Lone Star) ticks and others	A wide range of birds & mammals	South central United States
Human granulocytic anaplasmosis	*Anaplasma phagocytophilum*	*Ixodes* ticks	White-footed mice and white-tailed deer	NE and N central United States
Lyme disease	*Borrelia burgdorferi*	*Ixodes* ticks	White-footed mice and white-tailed deer	NE and N central United States
Plague (also respiratory droplet)	*Yersinia pestis*	Fleas	Rodents, lagomorphs, cats	SW United States: Texas to southern California
Tularemia (also a zoonosis)	*Francisella tularensis*	Ticks, fleas, mosqui- toes, trauma, in- gestion, inhalation	Huge variety but mainly rabbits and hares	Northern hemisphere, primarily from 30 to 71 degrees latitude north

Disease:
1. ***Rr* attaches to and invades vascular endothelial cells** by triggering phagocytic-like uptake. *Rr* escapes the phagosome by phospholipase activity and replicates in the cytoplasm where it polymerizes cellular actin to propel progeny out of the cell into the bloodstream or into neighboring endothelial cells, both facilitating spread. Peripheral vascular damage leads to symptoms. Organ damage leads to death in 20% of untreated infections.
2. **RMSF ranges** from mild to **highly fulminant** and fatal from the damage to the vascular en-dothelial cells, resulting in hyperplasia, thrombus formation, inhibited blood supply, and peripheral vasculitis.
3. **RMSF manifests** as **abrupt onset of high fever, chills, headache** (severe, frontal, unremitting), **myalgias with the macular rash, and edema starting on the extremities and spreading to the trunk; a few days later, hemorrhagic rash, stupor, delirium, and shock develop.**
4. **Lab ID:**
   a. **Diagnosis depends heavily on clinical manifestations,** especially rash and abrupt on-set of fever, headache, and chills with recent exposure to ticks. **Treatment is started on suspicion!**
   b. Diagnosis is confirmed by immunofluorescence, enzyme immunoassay, or complement fixation tests.
5. **Treatment started on suspicion with doxycycline. Cell-mediated immunity and repair of the vasculature is important in recovery;** thus, the elderly and those with poor cell-mediated im-munity are more likely to die even with treatment.

B. **Lyme Disease/*Borrelia burgdorferi* (*Bb*).**
   Features:
   1. ***Bb* is a large** (thicker in cross-section and with a looser spiral), **motile spirochete.**
   2. *Bb* is **taxonomically related to *Treponema;*** there are some parallels between syphilis and Lyme disease in terms of spread, stages, and crossing of both the placenta and the blood–brain barrier.
   3. Also related to ***Borrelia recurrentis*** (louse-borne) and the other *Borrelia* species (tick-borne), all notorious for antigenic variation, which explains why these borreliae cause **relapsing fever.** *Bb* shares with them the tendency for **antigenic variation.**

table 4.2	Important Bacterial Zoonoses	
Disease/Type	*Organism* **and Features**	**Reservoir/Transmission**
Anthrax/pulmonary Anthrax/cutaneous	*Bacillus anthracis* Gram-positive, aerobic rod	Hoofed animals & spores in animal skins or soil contaminated by sick animals/inhalation or traumatic implantation
Brucellosis/systemic	*Brucella melitensis, B. abortus, B. suis, B. canis,* Gram-negative rod	Goats, cattle, pigs, dogs (respectively)/contact with animals/ingestion or trauma
Campylobacter/inflammatory diarrhea	*Campylobacter jejuni,* Gram-negative	Food contaminated with bacteria from raw chicken or other animal sources/ingestion
Cat scratch fever/cellulitis with lymphadenopathy	*Bartonella henselae,* Gram-negative pericellular rod	Cats/scratches
Erysipeloid/cellulitis (dark red) in butchers and fish mongers	*Erysipelothrix rhusiopathiae,* Gram-positive rod	Raw meat or fish/trauma
EHEC/bloody diarrhea and HUS	*Escherichia coli* O157 and others with a Shiga-like toxin	Cattle/contaminated hamburger
Leptospirosis	*Leptospira interrogans* Spirochete with hooked ends	Rodent, cattle, dog urine in water/swimming or inhalation
Listeriosis/GI/septicemia	*Listeria monocytogenes,* Gram-positive	Cabbage and deli soft cheeses & meats, unpasteurized milk & cheeses/ingestion
Listeria meningitis	nonspore-forming rod; somewhat resistant to heat; grows in cold	
Pasteurellosis/animal bite	*Pasteurella multocida*	Oral flora of cats, dogs, and other mammals/bite
Plague/bubonic Plague/pneumonic	*Yersinia pestis*/Gram-negative rod nonlactose fermenting (Enterobacteriaceae)	Rodent flea bite or inhalation from a patient with pneumonic plague
Psittacosis	*Chlamydia psittaci*/OIP*	Birds, turkeys, chickens/inhalation
Q fever/pneumonia with or without hepatitis	*Coxiella burnetii,* a Gram-negative rod somewhat resistant to drying	Pregnant domestic animals' amniotic fluid and dried dust contaminated with *Coxiella*
Salmonellosis/diarrhea	Almost all *Salmonellae* except *Sal. typhi* and *Sal. paratyphi*	Wide variety of animals, but commonly from raw chicken/contaminates other food or eating undercooked chicken
Tularemia: ulceroglandular, pneumonic, or gastrointestinal	*Francisella tularensis,* Gram-negative rod	Rabbits primarily; arthropod bite or traumatic implantation or ingestion
Vibrio cellulitis or septicemia (in people with liver disease)	*Vibrio vulnificus,* Gram-negative flagellated vibrio that is oxidase-positive	Raw oysters from contaminated water/traumatic implantation or ingestion

*OIP = obligate intracellular pathogen

4. **Tick transmitted** by bite of deer ticks *Ixodes scapularis* (**NE and N Central United States**) and *Ixodes pacificus* (NW [Pacific] states.)
   a. Life cycle of tick (eggs → larvae → nymphs → adults).
      (1) Larvae and nymphs feed on the **white-footed mouse,** the most important source of *Bb*; nymphs drop on to grass and then on to humans. **Nymphs** or adults **spread disease**.
      (2) Adults feed on **white-tailed deer** but also drop off on vegetation to then infect humans.
      (3) There is evidence that the *Bb* in the tick must be exposed to human blood for 24 hours to change the outer surface proteins from OspA to OspC to become infectious.

Disease:

1. **Lyme disease** starts at the **bite site** but spreads via the **bloodstream** to seed other tissues, especially the **brain, heart, and joints.** It is most common during tick season (early spring through fall hunting).
   a. **Stage 1.** The hallmark is **erythema migrans (EM), an annular lesion with a rashy border and central clearing** that spreads out from the site of the tick bite. Constitutional symptoms are mild, but, just as in syphilis, the organism may disseminate as early as 1 week. EM is missing in 25% of cases.
   b. **Stage 2. Malaise, fatigue, headache, fever, chills, stiff neck, aches, and pains occur for several weeks, leading to more severe neural and cardiac problems,** including meningitis, cranial neuropathy (most commonly **Bell's palsy**), radiculoneuropathy, and some cardiac dysfunction; follows stage 1 by weeks to months.

    c. **Stage 3. Joint problems** occur, especially in large joints, producing oligoarthritis. Intermittent bouts of arthritis may recur for 3 to 7 years. **Neural dysfunction** may lead to dementia and paralysis; it follows stage 1 by months to years.

2. **Lab ID: Lyme disease** is diagnosed by several methods, but the key to diagnosis is recognition of clinical manifestations along with the tick bite. (Tick attachment, particularly, may be missed by patients because *Ixodes* are small (especially the nymphs) and **ticks inject an antihistamine, anesthetic, and anticoagulant** so you keep bleeding for them.)

    a. The diagnosis is confirmed most frequently by **serology. Western blot is recommended which distinguishes IgM and IgG.** But any may be falsely negative in serious infection; they are negative early in infection and may remain negative if the patient is promptly treated with antibiotics.

    b. The organism can be cultured on special media from skin biopsy and may be seen in biopsy of EM with Giemsa stain.

    c. **Lyme urine antigen capture tests** are used primarily to follow treatment.

    d. **NAA tests** are used to test joint fluid and CSF for the presence of an organism's DNA.

3. **Treatment:** Lyme disease is treated depending on the stage of infection. Primary is treated with doxycycline or amoxicillin.

4. **Prevention:** Lyme disease risk can be reduced by limiting exposure (long pants tucked in) and performing nightly tick checks in the endemic areas. In endemic areas with a partially (or more) deer tick removed, use one dose of oral doxycycline.

C. **Plague/*Yersinia pestis* (*Yp*).**
Features:
1. *Yp* is a pleomorphic **Gram-negative rod** that is a **facultative intracellular pathogen.** It is a **nonlactose-fermenting** Enterobacteriaceae that grows slowly on blood or MacConkey agars. It has **bipolar staining** on Giemsa or Wayson's stains.

2. Endemic in the desert SW United States in wild rodents and lagomorphs (e.g., rabbits); it is **spread to humans by infected rodent flea bite.** Cats that bring infected rodents home play a role. **Pneumonic cases are highly contagious from person to person.**

Disease:
1. **Pathogenesis:**

    a. *Yp* produces a **coagulase** that coagulates the blood in the flea midgut, providing a fibrin clot in which *Yp* replicates. The starved fleas feed, regurgitating high numbers of *Yp* into the host, thereby spreading the agent.

    b. Once **in the human** it is **phagocytosed by PMNs and monocytes and taken to lymph nodes;** however, the **intracellular *Yp* are able to kill the monocytes due to V and W surface components.**

    c. The higher human temperature triggers production of the antiphagocytic **FI capsular protein**; when the new encapsulated *Yp* are released after killing the infected monocytes, the new cells **replicate rapidly extracellularly in the lymph nodes, causing inflamed swellings called buboes.**

    d. *Yp* invades the bloodstream (spread facilitated by the *Yp* plasminogen activator) and the **envelope endotoxin** plays a major role in the peripheral vascular collapse and disseminated intravascular coagulopathy seen in plague. **Thrombi formed in the pulmonary vasculature lead to the highly contagious pneumonic plague.**

2. **Bubonic plague** is characterized by **fever** and exquisitely painful **buboes.**

3. **Septicemic plague** results from bacteria bypassing lymph nodes and multiplying in blood, **presenting as fever without a buboe.**

4. **Pneumonic plague** occurs either from bacteria seeding the lungs in bubonic plague or with respiratory exposure to *Yp*. This form is a rapidly necrotic pneumonia, with death occurring within days. It is highly contagious.

5. **Lab ID:** Diagnosis is hazardous and requires expertise. (The lab should be warned.) Bubo aspirate, sputum, and blood is stained with **Wayson's stain** or **Giemsa** stain (bipolar staining) and **fluorescent antibodies** to confirm.

6. **Treatment:** treated with gentamicin, streptomycin, or doxycycline. If untreated (or delays due to lack of recognition in nonendemic areas), death rate is as high as 75% for pneumonic plague.

D. **Human granulocytic anaplasmosis (HGA)/***Anaplasma phagocytophilum*

Features:

1. **OIP of granulocytes** belonging to the **rickettsias.**
2. **Endemic to the northern United States** in the same areas as Lyme disease and is **tick-borne** by *Ixodes scapularis* and possibly other ticks. Reservoir hosts are deer, rodents, and other wild mammals.

Disease:

1. **Infection starts with a tick bite. When *Anaplasma*** enters the bloodstream, it infects **granulocytes** by inducing phagocytosis. It **replicates in phagosomes**.
2. **Clinical symptoms** include **fever, myalgia, headache, malaise, leukopenia,** and **thrombocytopenia,** but **rarely rash.** There have been some fatalities. (It appears similar to Rocky Mountain spotted fever but without the rash.)
3. **Lab ID:** diagnosed by clinical symptoms and the findings of **mulberry-like clusters of cells (morulae)** in the phagosomes of granulocytes.
4. **Treatment**: treated with doxycycline, which penetrates human cells.

E. **Human monocytic ehrlichiosis (HME)/***Ehrlichia chaffeensis or E. ewingii.*

Features:

1. **OIP of monocytes** belonging to the **rickettsias.**
2. Endemic in the **southern United States;** moves north in **white-tailed deer** and is transmitted by the *Amblyomma* **ticks (Lone Star tick).**

Disease:

1. As for *Anaplasma,* **except it infects monocytes** and causes human monocytic ehrlichiosis.
2. HME is similar to HGA except that the thrombocytopenia may not be as severe. The organisms are also not as likely to be seen in the cells.

F. **Tularemia/***Francisella tularensis* (*Ft*).

Features:

1. **Gram-negative bacterium** causing **tularemia** (also called deer fly fever or rabbit fever). It is a **facultative parasite of fixed macrophages.**
2. *Ft* is found around the world in the **northern hemisphere infecting hundreds of wild animals (mainly rabbits, hares, squirrels, voles);** some domestic animals and wild birds, and over 100 arthropods. It is also found in mud and water (surviving in cold, including frozen meat). **Arkansas, Missouri, Oklahoma, and South Dakota are rural "hot spots,"** and disease acquisition is often associated with **hunting, especially rabbits.**

Disease:

1. Infection starts at the site of entry, which may be skin (infected blood into cuts or insect bites), leading to **ulcer glandular tularemia;** inhalation of blood or respiratory secretions from a sick animal (**pneumonic tularemia**); blood in the eye (**oculoglandular tularemia**); or ingestion of undercooked meat or contaminated meat (**typhoidal tularemia**).
2. Characterized by macrophage infiltration, **granulomas,** and **necrosis of infected tissues. Regional lymph nodes become infected and suppurate.** Spread to the lungs, liver, and spleen is common.
3. Manifests as **abrupt onset of fever, headache, and regional (painful) adenopathy;** back pain, anorexia, chills, sweats, and prostration follow. The fatality rate is 1%.
4. **Lab ID:** diagnosed by **immunofluorescent stain of biopsy.**

XIX. BACTERIAL VACCINES

Prevention has been a major means to reduce many infections. Bacterial vaccines with their immunogens are presented in Table 4.3. Vaccines are listed by the preferred age of administration or special use, certain occupations, or for U.S. travelers to other countries. **Bacterial pathogens** are summarized in Table 4.4.

table **4.3**   Bacterial Vaccines

Vaccine and Type*	Contents
Pediatric Vaccines	
Diphtheria, Tetanus, acellular Pertussis (DTaP) (all inactivated toxins or components)	Diphtheria toxoid Tetanus toxoid Pertussis toxoid and filamentous hemagglutinin plus one other purified *Bordetella pertussis* component, inactivated pertactin or fimbriae
Haemophilus influenzae type b (conjugate PS-protein vaccine)	Type b polysaccharide (polyribitol) capsule chemically complexed to protein
Pneumococcal conjugate vaccine	13 capsular polysaccharides from the most common pediatric strains of *Streptococcus pneumoniae* complexed to protein
Special Risk Groups: Children and Adults	
Meningococcal polysaccharide: conjugate vaccine (polysaccharide and protein)	Polysaccharides of four capsule (Y, W-135, C, A) types of *N. meningitidis* for those who have late complement component deficiencies or who are asplenic or at risk of becoming asplenic
Vaccines for 11- to 12-Year-Olds	
Tetanus and diphtheria toxoids and acellular pertussis vaccine (Tdap) [Also give 1x to adults.]	
Meningococcal polysaccharide conjugate vaccine (MCV4) (polysaccharide and protein)	Same as above but to all not previously vaccinated; recommended for college freshmen not vaccinated
Adult Vaccines**	
Tetanus-diphtheria absorbed (inactivated proteins) (Td)	Toxoids of tetanus and diphtheria (every 10 years)
Pneumococcal polysaccharide	23-serotypes of capsular polysaccharides for those over 65 years plus many other groups
Anthrax vaccine (only special groups)	Cell-free filtrate of an attenuated strain of *Bacillus anthracis* which makes the protective antigen but not the lethal factor nor edema factor (so $PA^+LF^-EF^-$)

*Live attenuated vaccines are generally contraindicated in immunocompromised or pregnant women.
**There are many special situations of underlying medical conditions which are not presented here.

table **4.4**   Properties of Bacterial Pathogens*

Bacterium	Distinguishing Characteristics	Diseases
Actinomyces	Anaerobe, branching rod, Gr+ "Sulfur" granule (microcolonies) Contiguous growth through anatomic barriers Cervicofacial, thoracic, and abdominal lesions	Actinomycosis
Anaplasma phagocytophilum	*Ixodes* tick-transmitted zoonosis OIP of granulocytes; Gr- Belong to family Rickettsiaceae	Human granulocytic anaplasmosis
Bacillus anthracis	Potent tripartite exotoxin: protective antigen, lethal factor, and edema factor Polypeptide capsule inhibits phagocytosis Spore transmission, Gr+ rod	Cutaneous or pulmonary anthrax
Bacteroides fragilis	Non–spore-forming pleomorphic anaerobe, Gr- Mixed infections Capsule Possesses a β-lactamase Wound débridement important	Intra-abdominal abscesses, gastrointestinal, and cellulitis
Bartonella henselae *Bartonella quintana*	Small Gr- bacterium	Cat scratch disease or bacillary angiomatosis (BA). Trench Fever or BA
Bordetella pertussis	Gr- rod extracellular; attaches via pili; paroxysmal cough due to toxin Toxoid part of DTaP vaccine	Whooping cough
Borrelia burgdorferi	*Ixodes* transmission Corkscrew-shaped motile spirochete, Gr nonstaining (ns)/-	Lyme disease

(*continued*)

t a b l e **4.4**	Properties of Bacterial Pathogens* (continued)	
Bacterium	**Distinguishing Characteristics**	**Diseases**
Campylobacter jejuni	Comma-shaped rod; Gr- Animal hosts frequent cause of diarrhea Invasive Neutrophils and blood in stool	Inflammatory diarrhea
Chlamydophila pneumoniae	OIP Elementary (infectious) and reticulate body Divides by binary fission	Atypical pneumonia
Chlamydia psittaci	OIP, zoonotic (birds, chickens, parrots)	Atypical pneumonia nonbreaking Sudden onset
Chlamydia trachomatis	As for Chl. pneumoniae 8 serovars	Sexually transmitted infection (D–K): inclusion conjunctivitis PID, reactive arthritis neonatal eye, pneumonia Lymphogranuloma venereum (L1, L2, L3) Trachoma (A–C)
Clostridium botulinum	Spore-forming anaerobe, Gr+ Exotoxin acting at myoneural junction Suppresses acetylcholine release by peripheral nerves Produces flaccid muscle paralysis Caused by ingestion of preformed toxin or by ingestion of spores by infants	Botulism
Clostridium difficile	Spore-forming anaerobe, Gr+ Part of normal gastrointestinal flora Activated by antibiotic disruption of other flora Secrete an enterotoxin and cytotoxin	Gastroenteritis Pseudomembranous colitis
Clostridium perfringens	Spore-forming anaerobe Spores introduced by severe trauma Possesses an alpha-toxin (lecithinase)	Gas gangrene Soft tissue cellulitis Food poisoning
Corynebacterium diphtheriae	Gr+ rod Phage-coded A/B exotoxin inhibits EF-2 Toxoid part of DTaP, Tdap, and Td vaccines	Pharyngeal diphtheria Cutaneous diphtheria
Coxiella burnetii	Intracellular bacterium, Gr- Dust/parturition materials transmitted Absence of rash	Q fever Pneumonitis with or without hepatitis
Ehrlichia	Amblyomma tick-transmitted zoonosis OIP of monocytes Belong to family Rickettsiaceae	Human monocytic ehrlichiosis
Enterococcus	Formerly group D streptococci, Gr+ Most are alpha- or gamma-hemolytic Antibiotic resistance is a problem β-lactamase producer Nosocomial opportunist	Urinary tract infection (UTI) Endocarditis following genitourinary (GU) manipulations
Escherichia coli	All strains possess endotoxin Nonpathogenic part of normal microbiota of colon Enterotoxigenic: heat-labile toxin stimulates adenylate cyclase similar to cholera toxin; heat-stable toxin activates guanylate cyclase Enteropathogenic: adherence to enterocytes → infantile diarrhea Enterohemorrhagic: Shiga-like verotoxin → bloody diarrhea (serotype O157) Enteroinvasive: similar to Shigella	UTIs, neonatal meningitis, sepsis Gastroenteritis Bloody diarrhea without invasion; HUS Inflammatory diarrhea
Fusobacterium nucleatum	Polymorphic, slender filaments Oral anaerobe, Gr- Synergizes with Borrelia vincentii	Vincent's angina Brain abscess Head, neck, chest infections
Haemophilus influenzae	Gr- pleomorphic rod Antiphagocytic polysaccharide capsule Pyrogenic IgAase Grow on chocolate agar or with X and V factors Epiglottis requires a tracheotomy Vaccine is polysaccharide capsule linked to protein	Meningitis: type b in 3-mo- to 6-yr-old unvaccinated "kids" Chronic bronchitis: type d in COPD Epiglottitis in unvaccinated toddlers

| t a b l e **4.4** | Properties of Bacterial Pathogens* (*continued*) | |

Bacterium	Distinguishing Characteristics	Diseases
Helicobacter pylori	Spiral rod, polar, flagella tuft, Gr- Produces a potent urease and vacuolating cytotoxin Treat with omeprazole, amoxicillin, and clarithromycin	Gastric and peptic ulcers Increases risk for gastric adenocarcinoma
Legionella pneumophila	Aquaphile with inhalation transmission Association with amoeba in streams Possesses a cytotoxin and endotoxin β-lactamase producery Stains with Dieterle silver stain; not standard Gram stain Requires cysteine and iron for growth; intracellular parasite	Legionnaires' disease (pneumonia often with diarrhea and severe headache).
Listeria monocytogenes	Animal reservoirs; cold growth Infects monocytes (monocytosis) Hemolysin destroys vesicular membranes	Gastroenteritis; septicemia Granulomas, abscesses Meningitis (newborns; trans- plant patients)
Moraxella catarrhalis	Gram-negative diplococcus; normal oral flora	Otitis, chronic bronchitis (COPD)
Mycobacterium avium-intracellulare	Group of acid-fast organisms; non-Gram staining Opportunist (AIDS; chemotherapy) noncontagious; drug resistance	Pulmonary disease
Mycobacterium tuberculosis	Cell wall: peptidoglycan-arabinogalactan, mycolic acids, and so on, make all mycobacteria acid-fast and resistant to drying Cord factor (trehalose dimycolate) induces granuloma formation Purified protein derivative in skin test Multiple drug resistance Bacille Calmette-Guérin vaccine (attenuated)	Tuberculosis
Mycoplasma pneumoniae	Lacks a cell wall Smallest extracellular bacterium; not an L-form Mucosal tissue tropism Requires cholesterol but cannot make it.	Primary atypical pneumonia
Neisseria gonorrhoeae	Intracellular Gram-negative diplococcus Produces an IgAase and a penicillinase (plasmid) Purulent exudate Requires chocolate agar (Thayer-Martin) Oxidase-positive	Urethritis, cervicitis, proctitis Pelvic inflammatory disease Conjunctivitis in newborns Septicemia, arthritis
Neisseria meningitidis	Antiphagocytic capsule, Gram-negative diplococcus Endotoxin (lipooligosaccharide) IgAase Vasculitic purpura Headache and stiff neck are common	Meningococcemia Waterhouse-Friderichsen syndrome
Nocardia	Aerobic soil bacterium Inhalation transmission or traumatic implantation	Pulmonary infections in compromised patients; cellulitis
Prevotella melaninogenica	Anaerobic black colonies on agar Found in mouth, gastrointestinal, and GU tracts Putrid sputum Débride and drain lesion Formerly in genus Bacteroides	Oral, dental, and lung abscesses Female GU infections
Proteus mirabilis	Highly motile Produces urease	Pneumonia, nosocomial infections
Pseudomonas aeruginosa	Glycocalyx slime layer, Gr- Pyocyanin (blue-green pigment) Endotoxin (lipopolysaccharide) Exotoxin A (ADP-ribosyl transferase)	Burn infections/septic shock Pneumonia and septic shock in neutropenic & CF punc- ture wounds, ear, eye
Rickettsia rickettsii	*Dermacentor* tick transmission; OIP (bacterium); invades vascular endothelium	Rocky Mountain spotted fever
Salmonella	Animal reservoirs except *Sal. typhi, Sal. paratyphi* Gram-negative rods; many serotypes Intracellular multiplication (facultative) Can invade bloodstream Endotoxin lipopolysaccharide Enterotoxin	Enterocolitis Septicemia Enteric fever (typhoid) Osteomyelitis in sickle cell disease

(*continued*)

t a b l e **4.4**	Properties of Bacterial Pathogens* (*continued*)	
Bacterium	**Distinguishing Characteristics**	**Diseases**
Shigella	Gr- ; no known animal reservoir Pathogenic in small numbers Perpetuation by human carriers All have endotoxin and are invasive *Sh. dysenteriae* has Shiga toxin Stools can contain mucus, pus, and blood Bloodstream invasion is rare	Shigellosis (inflammatory diarrhea) with shallow ulcers
Staphylococcus aureus	Grape-like cluster morphology, Gr+ Antibiotic resistance Catalase- and coagulase-positive Enterotoxin Short incubation period for food poisoning (2 to 6 hrs)	Local abscesses, impetigo, food poisoning Endocarditis especially IVDA Osteomyelitis Sepsis (MSSA, MRSA)
Staphylococcus epidermidis	Gram-positive cocci, normal skin flora Instrument contamination Adherence through polysaccharide slime	Endocarditis (artificial valve) infections catheter, prosthetic devices
Staphylococcus saprophyticus	Gram-positive, catalase-positive coci Coagulase-negative	Urinary tract infections
Streptococcus agalactiae	Group B Streptococci, Gr+ cocci in chairs Can be part of normal vaginal and oral flora Capsule Inhibits complement	Neonatal sepsis (early and late onset) Neonatal meningitis
Streptococcus pneumoniae	Alpha-hemolytic diplococcus Large antiphagocytic capsule Quellung reaction Sensitive to bile and optochin Vaccines: adult: 23 capsular serotypes; meningitis in infants and elderly Pediatric: 13-valent capsule-protein Anticapsular antibody is protective	Pneumonia Otitis media Septicemia Chronic bronchitis (COPD)
Streptococcus pyogenes	Group A M protein (more than 80 types); anti-phagocytic Beta-hemolytic Sensitive to bacitracin Erythrogenic exotoxins	Pharyngitis Scarlet fever Rheumatic fever and heart disease Acute glomerulonephritis Impetigo Cellulitis–erysipelas
Treponema pallidum	Spirochete not seen in Gram stains Unable to be routinely cultured Immunosuppressive Darkfield microscopy examination Serologic tests	Syphilis, 1°, 2°, 3°
Vibrio cholerae	Comma-shaped morphology, Gr- A/B enterotoxin overproduces cAMP Vomiting and rice-water diarrhea Oral rehydration solution or IV	Cholera
Viridans streptococci	Noninvasive opportunist in normal oral flora, Gr+ Alpha-hemolytic Differentiate from *S. pneumoniae* because the viridans strep are bile insoluble and not inhibited by optochin	Endocarditis Dental caries
Yersinia pestis	Zoonotic disease (rats and fleas), SW United States Intracellular multiplication Fever, conjunctivitis, regional buboes, pneumonia	Bubonic plague Pneumonic plague Yersiniosis

*Abbreviations: Gr+ or Gr- or nsGR = Gram-positive, Gram-negative, or Gram-nonstaining; AIDS, acquired immunodeficiency syndrome; cAMP, cyclic adenosine monophosphate; DTaP, diphtheria and tetanus toxoids and pertussis; EF-2, elongation factor 2; HUS, hemolytic uremic syndrome; PID, pelvic inflammatory disease

Review Test

Directions: *Each of the numbered items or incomplete statements in this section is followed by answers or completions of the statement. Select the ONE lettered answer that is BEST in each case.*

1. A 36-year-old man presents with focal central nervous system signs. Imaging shows a brain abscess. The dominant organism is an anaerobe normally found as part of the oral flora. Which of the following best fits that description?

(A) *Nocardia*
(B) *Actinomyces*
(C) *Mycobacterium*
(D) *Pseudomonas aeruginosa*

2. A 23-year-old man who has recently started working on a sheep farm in Nova Scotia develops pneumonia shortly after helping with lambing. His cough produces little sputum, and a saline-induced sputum sample shows no predominant organism either with Gram stain or with acid-fast stain. It is established that he acquired the pneumonia from parturition products from the sheep. Which agent is most likely to be the cause of his pneumonia?

(A) *Rickettsia akari*
(B) *Rickettsia typhi*
(C) *Rickettsia rickettsii*
(D) *Coxiella burnetii*
(E) *Anaplasma phagocytophilum*

3. A 3-year-old girl presents with difficulty breathing and will not lie down to be examined. You suspect acute bacterial epiglottitis and examine the child's epiglottis, which is highly inflamed. Which vaccine are you most likely to find that the child is missing?

(A) Diphtheria
(B) *Neisseria meningitidis*
(C) Polio
(D) *Streptococcus pneumoniae* (conjugate vaccine)
(E) *Haemophilus influenzae*

4. A 22-year-old man with cystic fibrosis presents with fever and increasing dyspnea.

A Gram-negative organism is found in unusually high numbers in the pulmonary mucus. Which virulence factor is most important in colonization and maintenance of the organism in the lungs?

(A) Exotoxin A
(B) Pyocyanin (blue-green pigment)
(C) Polysaccharide slime
(D) Endotoxin

5. From the above case, exotoxin A of the causative agent most closely resembles the action of which other microbial toxin?

(A) Heat-labile toxin (LT) of *Escherichia coli*
(B) Shiga toxin
(C) Diphtheria toxin
(D) *Vibrio cholerae* toxin
(E) Verotoxin

6. A 36-year-old man who immigrated to the United States 15 years ago and lived in a crowded resettlement camp before coming to the United States presents with a cough that has been bothering him for several weeks. He has also lost 10 pounds. A gamma interferon release blood test is positive. Which of the following factors is known to be most important in triggering the granulomatous reaction to wall off and contain the infection?

(A) Cord factor
(B) Mycolic acid
(C) Purified protein derivative (PPD)
(D) Sulfatides
(E) Wax D

7. A 75-year-old patient develops diarrhea 5 days after starting antibiotic treatment for a serious staphylococcal infection. What is the most likely causative agent?

(A) *Clostridium perfringens*
(B) *Clostridium difficile*
(C) *Pseudomonas aeruginosa*
(D) *Shigella sonnei*

8. A 23-year-old woman presents with mild gastroenteritis a few days after having a variety of sushi at a party. There is no blood or pus in the stool. Which causative agent is most likely to have caused this illness?

(A) *Vibrio cholerae*
(B) *Vibrio parahaemolyticus*
(C) *Salmonella typhi*
(D) *Shigella sonnei*

9. *Yersinia pestis* may be transferred by

(A) *Dermacentor* tick bite
(B) Human body louse bite
(C) *Ixodes* tick bite
(D) Respiratory droplets

10. A patient who had surgery to put in a pacemaker and who states he felt fine for the first 2 months now presents 3 months postoperatively with complaints of malaise and increasing fatigue. He is running a low-grade fever, tires easily, and has worsening heart murmurs. Which of the following staphylococcal organisms causes subacute bacterial endocarditis that generally occurs 2 months or more after heart surgery?

(A) *Staphylococcus aureus*
(B) *Staphylococcus epidermidis*
(C) *Staphylococcus haemolyticus*
(D) *Staphylococcus saprophyticus*

11. A previously healthy 6-month-old boy presents with upper body weakness. He cannot hold his eyes open, pupils do not react, and he cannot hold his head up. What is the proper treatment?

(A) Send him home on amoxicillin and clindamycin (to stop the toxin production quickly)
(B) Give him a dose of equine anti-botulinum immunoglobulin
(C) Offer monitored supportive care with antibiotics and human anti-botulinum immunoglobulin
(D) Offer monitored supportive care with human anti-botulinum immunoglobulin
(E) Offer monitored supportive care with no antibiotics and no antitoxin

12. A 78-year-old man presents with a high fever, cough producing a blood-tinged sputum, and difficulty breathing. Sputum shows an organism consistent with *Streptococcus pneumoniae*. What is the most important virulence factor?

(A) Endotoxin
(B) A phospholipase allowing *Streptococcus pneumoniae* to escape the phagosome quickly
(C) Polypeptide capsule
(D) Polysaccharide capsule

13. Which of the following organisms grows in 40% bile?

(A) *Enterococcus faecalis*
(B) *Streptococcus pneumoniae*
(C) Group B streptococci
(D) Viridans streptococci

14. A 45-year-old man who recently returned from Africa has been febrile for several days and now presents with abdominal pain. His blood cultures grow out *Salmonella typhi*. What was the most likely source of his infection?

(A) Raw chicken
(B) Undercooked hamburger
(C) Contact with baby goats on a farm and then eating without washing hands
(D) A food preparer with bad personal hygiene
(E) Undercooked pork

15. A 4-day-old infant girl now showing signs of sepsis is brought to the emergency department. She was preterm (33 weeks) and born at home to her 16-year-old mom after 22 hours of labor following the rupture of the membranes. A friend helped the mother deliver the baby. What is the best description for the agent most likely causing the sepsis if it was acquired during labor but prior to delivery? All organisms in the answer choices are Gram-positive, catalase-negative cocci found in pairs or short chains.

(A) Nonhemolytic organisms found as part of the normal fecal flora; resistant to bile and optochin; carries a high level of drug resistance
(B) Alpha-hemolytic diplococci sensitive to both bile and optochin
(C) Beta-hemolytic cocci in chains and carrying Lancefield's Group B antigen
(D) Alpha-hemolytic cocci in chains; resistant to bile and optochin

16. A 62-year-old woman presents with signs of a gastric ulcer. She does not regularly take nonsteroidal anti-inflammatory agents. Which characteristic appears to play a central role in the organism's ability to survive transit of the lumen to colonize the stomach?

(A) Phospholipase-C production
(B) Urease production
(C) Microaerophilic lifestyle
(D) O antigens

17. A 54-year-old man develops a pyogenic infection along the suture line after knee surgery. The laboratory gives a preliminary report of a beta-hemolytic, catalase-positive, coagulase-positive, Gram-positive coccus. The most likely causative agent is

(A) *Moraxella catarrhalis*
(B) *Staphylococcus aureus*
(C) *Staphylococcus epidermidis*
(D) *Streptococcus agalactiae*
(E) *Streptococcus pyogenes*

Answers and Explanations

1. **The answer is B.** Only *Actinomyces* is anaerobic; the rest are aerobic. (And, of those mentioned, only *Actinomyces* is part of the normal oral flora. Nocardia can, however, cause brain abscesses as well, but it is acquired from the environment.)

2. **The answer is D.** *Coxiella burnetii* is a rickettsia-like organism that can be spread via amniotic fluid, aerosols, or dust particles. It withstands drying and thus can be transmitted at least 10 miles by the wind.

3. **The answer is E.** Epiglottitis is a medical emergency requiring hospitalization. It can be fatal in 24 hours. Pediatric cases were almost always caused by *H. influenzae* type b and have been dramatically reduced by the conjugate vaccine.

4. **The answer is C.** *Staphylococcus aureus* and *Pseudomonas aeruginosa* are two primary pulmonary colonizers that cause pneumonia in patients with cystic fibrosis. (*Staphylococcus* is usually only in young CF patients.) Of the two, *Pseudomonas* is Gram-negative. Its slime material (alginate) produces the resistance to phagocytic killing and poor penetration of antibiotics to the site, which, in conjunction with the antibiotic resistance of *Pseudomonas,* make these serious infections.

5. **The answer is C.** Both *Pseudomonas* exotoxin A and diphtheria toxin inhibit protein synthesis through the inhibition of elongation factor (EF-2). Incorrect choices include: Shiga toxin, which is a cytotoxin, enterotoxin, and neurotoxin. *Vibrio cholerae* enterotoxin and *E. coli* labile toxin (LT) both result in increased cyclic adenosine monophosphate (cAMP).

6. **The answer is A.** *Mtb*'s cord factor helps trigger the Th1 response, which helps contain the infection.

7. **The answer is B.** *Clostridium difficile* has been shown to be the major causative agent of pseudomembranous colitis, which causes diarrhea that most commonly starts after 3 to 4 days of antibiotic administration.

8. **The answer is B.** *Vibrio cholerae* causes classic cholera, which is not generally mild or self-limited; *Vibrio parahaemolyticus,* in contrast, causes a relatively mild gastroenteritis. It is also found in raw fish. *Sal. typhi* is the causative agent of typhoid. Shigellae infections are always invasive and generally will have a little pus in the stool.

9. **The answer is D.** Most transmission in the United States is from an infected flea bite (a choice not given in the question). The other route of transmission is through respiratory droplets from patients who have developed pneumonic emboli and pneumonia.

10. **The answer is B.** *Staphylococcus epidermidis* is ubiquitous as part of the normal flora. Organisms are introduced into the host during invasive procedures. *Staph. aureus* is more likely to be acute, with high fever and damage developing more quickly.

11. **The answer is D.** *Clostridium botulinum* found in household dust or honey was ingested by the baby and the spores germinated in her GI tract because her normal flora was not sufficient to suppress the germination. It is the vegetative cells that produce the botulinum toxin. Antibiotics disrupt normal flora, prolonging the disease, but administration of human antitoxin can dramatically reduce the length of the hospital stay.

12. **The answer is D.** The Gram-positive organism *Streptococcus pneumoniae* contains no endotoxin. It is not phagocytosed in the immunologically naive, eliminating choice B. It is the capsule that is considered the most important virulence factor.

13. **The answer is A.** Enterococci can be differentiated by their reactivity with group D antiserum, bacitracin resistance, and growth in 40% bile or pH 9.6.

14. **The answer is D.** *Sal. typhi* has only human hosts.

15. **The answer is C.** If the mother is young and has had multiple sexual partners, she is more likely to be colonized with Group B streptococci. If the labor is prolonged after rupture of the membranes, the baby is more likely to be infected. And, since she delivered before her due date and had her baby at home, she was not screened for Group B streptococci and did not receive intrapartum antibiotics to prevent infection of the baby. The other descriptions belong to: (A) *Enterococcus*, (B) *Strep. pneumoniae*, and (D) Viridans strep.

16. **The answer is B.** A major survival and virulence factor of *Helicobacter pylori* is urease, which neutralizes stomach acid to allow the organism to survive to reach the tissue.

17. **The answer is B.** Of the answer choices, only streptococci and staphylococci are Gram-positive. The streptococci are catalase-negative and staphylococci are catalase-positive. Of the two staphylococci, *Staphylococcus aureus* is the beta-hemolytic, coagulase-positive organism.

chapter 5 Viruses

I. NATURE OF HUMAN VIRUSES

A. **Virus particles** are called **virions.**
1. Virions are composed of either RNA or DNA that is encased in a protein coat called a **capsid.**
2. They are either naked or enveloped, depending on whether the capsid is surrounded by a lipoprotein **envelope.**
3. Virions replicate only in living cells and therefore are **obligate intracellular parasites.**
4. They cannot be observed with a light microscope.

B. **Viral genome.**
1. Viral genome may be single stranded or double stranded, linear or circular, and segmented or nonsegmented.
2. Its characteristics are used as one criterion for viral classification.
3. Viral-specific enzymes, other proteins within the virion, or both may be associated with the genome.

C. **Viral capsid.**
1. Capsid is composed of structural units called **capsomers,** which are aggregates of **viral-specific polypeptides.**
2. They are classified as **helical, icosahedral** (a 20-sided polygon), or **complex**; used as a criterion for viral classification.
3. Serves four functions:
   a. Protects the viral genome.
   b. Is the site of receptors necessary for naked viruses to initiate infection.
   c. Stimulates antibody production.
   d. Is the site of antigenic determinants important in some serologic tests.

D. **Viral nucleocapsid** refers to the capsid and enclosed viral genome and is identical to the virion in naked viruses.

E. **Viral envelope.**
1. The viral envelope surrounds the nucleocapsid of enveloped viruses and is composed of **viral-specific glycoproteins** and **host-cell-derived lipids** and **lipoproteins.**
2. It contains molecules that are necessary for enveloped viruses to initiate infection, act as a stimulus for antibody production, and serve as antigens in serologic tests; it also forms the basis of ether sensitivity of a virus.

F. Viroporins.
   1. They are **small, hydrophobic virus-encoded proteins** that oligomerize at host-cell membranes where they are involved in enveloped virus budding and non-enveloped virus cellular lysis (see III Viral Replication and Genetics).
   2. They **form hydrophilic pores** which disrupt physiological properties of the host cell, thereby contributing to viral pathogenicity.

II. VIRAL CLASSIFICATION

Classification is based on chemical and physical properties of virions. Viruses are classified into **major families,** which are further subdivided by physiochemical and serologic characteristics into **genera.**

A. **DNA viruses.**
   1. Contain double-stranded DNA (except for parvoviruses).
   2. Are naked viruses (except for herpesviruses, poxviruses, and hepadnaviruses).
   3. Have icosahedral capsids and replicate in the nucleus (except for poxviruses).

B. **RNA viruses.**
   1. Contain single-stranded RNA (except for reoviruses, rotaviruses, coltiviruses, orthoreoviruses, and orbiviruses).
   2. Are enveloped (except for caliciviruses, picornaviruses, and reoviruses).
   3. Have helical capsids (except for picornaviruses, reoviruses, and togaviruses).
   4. Are classified positive, negative, or ambisense, depending on the ability of virion RNA to act as messenger RNA (mRNA).
   5. Replicate in the cytoplasm (except for orthomyxoviruses and retroviruses, which have both a cytoplasmic and a nuclear phase).

III. VIRAL REPLICATION AND GENETICS

A. **General characteristics of viral replication.** Replication occurs only in living cells. It may lead to the death of the host cell (**virulent viruses**) or may occur without apparent damage to the host cell (**moderate viruses**). Replication involves many host-cell enzymes and functions, including attachment, penetration, uncoating of the viral genome, synthesis of early proteins involved in genome replication, synthesis of late proteins (structural components of the virion), assembly, and release (Fig. 5.1).
   1. **Attachment** involves the interaction of **viral attachment proteins (VAPs)** and specific host-cell receptor sites. It plays an important role in viral pathogenesis, determining **viral cell tropism** it may be inhibited by antibodies (neutralizing antibodies) against viral receptors or cellular receptor sites.
   2. **Penetration** can occur by a cellular mechanism called **receptor-mediated endocytosis,** which is referred to as **viropexis** when viruses are involved. The virus envelope may fuse with the plasma membrane of the host cell.
   3. **Uncoating** refers to the separation of the capsid from the viral genome. It results in the loss of virion infectivity.
   4. **Budding** is the process by which enveloped viruses obtain their envelope; it confers infectivity to enveloped viruses. Budding is preceded by the insertion of virus-specific glycoproteins into the membranes of the host cell. It occurs most frequently at the plasma membrane, but also occurs at other membranes.

B. **Replication in DNA viruses.**
   1. **Transcription** occurs in the host-cell nucleus (except for poxviruses) and is regulated by host-cell DNA-dependent RNA polymerases (except for virion-associated RNA polymerase of

Steps in Generalized Viral Infection

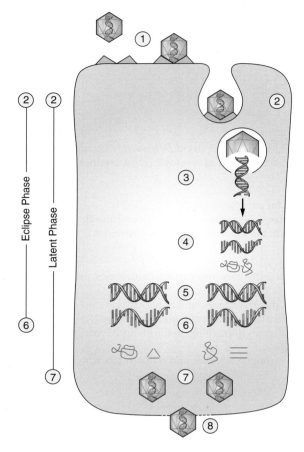

1. Attachment—Specific viral outer proteins (or glycoproteins on envelope viruses) bind to chemical groups on cell membrane.

2. Virus uptake by pinocytosis (as shown) or by fusion of the viral envelope with the cytoplasmic membrane

3. Uncoating (nucleic acid released)

4. Early mRNA and protein (to shut off host synthesis and to make any needed enzymes)

5. Duplication of nucleic acid

6. Late mRNA and protein

7. Assembly and intracellular virus accumulation

8. Release by lysis or by budding out of cell membrane (if enveloped)

Stages 2–6 Eclipse Phase—no internal or external virus
Stages 2–7 Latent Phase—no external virus

FIGURE 5.1. Viral replication: overview of a generalized infection. The eclipse phase is the time from uptake of the virus to just before the assembly of the first intracellular virus (stages 2 to 6). The latent phase is the time from the initial infection to just prior to the first release of the extracellular virus (stages 2 to 7). (Modified from Hawley LB. *High-yield microbiology and infectious diseases.* 2nd ed. Baltimore, MD: Lippincott Williams & Wilkins; 2006:20–4.)

poxviruses). It occurs in a specific temporal pattern, such as immediate early, delayed early, and late mRNA transcription. It may be followed by **posttranscriptional processing** of primary mRNA transcripts (late adenovirus transcripts).

2. Translation occurs on cytoplasmic polysomes and is followed by transport of newly synthesized proteins to the nucleus (except for poxviruses).

3. Genome replication occurs after the synthesis of the early proteins. It is semiconservative and is performed by a DNA-dependent DNA polymerase, which may be supplied by the host cell (adenoviruses) or may be virus specific (herpesviruses).

4. Assembly takes place in the nucleus (except for poxviruses). It is frequently an inefficient process that leads to accumulation of viral proteins that may participate in the formation of **inclusion bodies** (focal accumulations of virions or viral gene products).

C. Replication in RNA viruses.

1. The viral genome may be single stranded or double stranded and segmented or nonsegmented.

a. It may have **messenger (positive-sense) polarity** if it is single stranded and able to act as mRNA (picornaviruses and retroviruses).

    b. It may have **antimessenger (negative-sense) polarity** if it is single stranded and complementary to mRNA (orthomyxoviruses and paramyxoviruses).

    c. It is **ambisense** if it is single stranded with portions of messenger polarity and antimessenger polarity (arenaviruses).

2. Transcription involves a viral-specified RNA-dependent RNA polymerase for all viruses, except retroviruses, which use a host-cell, DNA-dependent RNA polymerase. Negative-sense viruses use a virion-associated enzyme (**transcriptase**).

3. Translation occurs on cytoplasmic polysomes. It may result in the synthesis of a large polyprotein that is subsequently cleaved (in **posttranslational processing**) into individual viral polypeptides (picornaviruses and retroviruses).

4. Genome replication occurs in the cytoplasm (except for orthomyxoviruses and retroviruses) and is performed by a viral-specific **replicase enzyme** (except for retroviruses). A replicative intermediate RNA structure is required for all single-stranded RNA genomes. **RNA viruses have a higher mutation rate than DNA viruses.**

D. Genetics.

1. Phenotypic mixing results when surface antigens from two related viruses enclose the genome of one of the viruses.

2. Phenotypic masking (transcapsidation) occurs when pairs or related viruses infect the same cell. It results when the genome of one virus is surrounded by the capsid or capsid and envelope of the other virus.

3. Complementation can occur when two mutants of the same virus or, less frequently, two mutants of different large DNA viruses infect the same cell. It results when one mutant virus supplies an enzyme or factor that the other mutant lacks.

4. Genetic reassortment can occur when two strains of a segmented RNA virus infect a cell. It results in a stable change in the viral genome (Fig. 5.2).

5. Viral vectors can be constructed with recombinant DNA technology and allow gene transfer into cells. They have been used as an approach to treat diseases, particularly monogenic disorders and some cancers, and are being studied as agents to immunize against other infectious agents.

IV. VIRAL PATHOGENESIS

A. General characteristics. Viral pathogenesis is the process of disease production following infection. It may lead to **clinical** or **subclinical** (asymptomatic) disease. Several viral and host factors are involved.

1. Viral entry into a host:

    a. Viruses enter the host most often through the mucosa of the respiratory tract but may also enter through the mucosa of the gastrointestinal or genitourinary tract.

    b. Entry can be accomplished by direct virus injection into the bloodstream via a needle or an insect bite.

2. Asymptomatic viral disease may also be called **subclinical infection** because no clinical symptoms are evident. It occurs with most viral infections and can stimulate humoral and cellular immunity.

3. Clinical viral disease results from direct or indirect viral effects (e.g., viral-induced cytolysis, immunologic attack on infected cells), which lead to physiologic changes in infected tissues. It is associated with a particular **target organ** for a specific virus.

    a. Disease does not always follow infection and therefore is not an accurate index of viral infection; it occurs much less often than inapparent infection.

    b. It frequently depends on the size of the viral inoculum.

B. Viral aspects of pathogenesis.

1. Viral attachment proteins (VAPs) interact with cellular receptor sites to initiate infection.

    a. VAPs may react with specific antibodies (neutralizing antibodies) and become incapable of interaction with cellular receptor sites.

    b. pH, enzymes, and other host biochemical factors can inactivate VAPs.

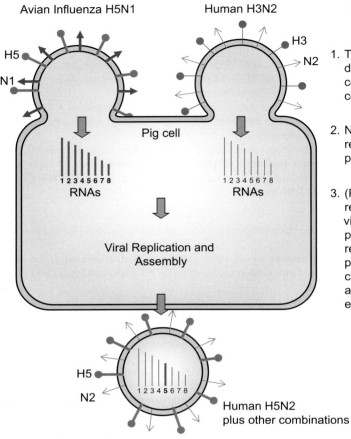

Avian Influenza H5N1   Human H3N2

Genetic Reassortment = Genetic shift

1. Two influenza A viruses from different animals co-infect one cell. Each of the 8 RNAs carries code for a gene product.

2. NOT SHOWN: Each virus replicates all RNAs and all proteins.

3. (Remember two viruses have replicated in one cell.) In the viral assembly, the viral RNAs package randomly (genetic reassortment) which may produce a new virus which now can infect humans (e.g., H5N2) and to which there is no pre-existing immunity.

FIGURE 5.2. Major antigenic changes, called genetic shift or gene reassortment, occur when a single cell is coinfected with two different strains of the same segmented virus. (Modified from Hawley LB. *High-Yield Microbiology and Infectious Diseases.* 2nd ed. Baltimore, MD: Lippincott Williams & Wilkins; 2007.)

2. **Viral virulence** refers to the ability of a particular viral strain to cause disease. It is a composite of all the factors that allow a virus to overcome host defense mechanisms and damage its target organ.
   a. Virulence is genetically determined.
   b. It is decreased with **attenuated strains** of virus.

C. **Cellular aspects of pathogenesis.**
   1. **Cellular receptor sites** interact with VAPs to initiate infection. They help determine **cell tropism** of viruses. Presence or absence of particular sites may be determined by the differentiation stage of a cell.
   2. **Cell tropism** refers to the propensity of a virus to infect and replicate in a cell. Tropism is largely determined by the interaction of virus attachment proteins and cellular receptor sites and the cell's ability to provide other components (e.g., substrates and enzymes) essential for viral replication.
   3. **Target organ** is the organ responsible for the major clinical signs of a viral infection and is largely determined by viral virulence and cell tropism.
   4. **Cellular responses to viral infection** result in clinical disease. These responses may be inapparent or may include:
      a. Cytopathic effects
      b. Cytolysis
      c. Inclusion body formation

table **5.1** Viral Inclusion Bodies

Virus	Inclusion Site	Staining Properties	Inclusion Name
Adenovirus	Nucleus	B	—
Cytomegalovirus	Nucleus	B	Owl's eye
Herpes simplex virus	Nucleus	A	Cowdry type A
Measles virus	Both	A	—
Poxvirus	Cytoplasm	A	Guarnieri bodies (smallpox) Molluscum bodies (molluscum contagiosum)
Rabies virus	Cytoplasm	A	Negri body
Reovirus	Cytoplasm	A	—
Rubella virus	Cytoplasm	A	—

A, acidophilic; B, basophilic

    d. Chromosomal aberrations

    e. Transformation

    f. Interferon (IFN) synthesis

5. Cytopathogenic effects include inhibition of host-cell macromolecular biosynthesis, alterations of the plasma membrane and lysosomes, and development of **inclusion bodies** (Table 5.1).

    a. Infectious virus progeny may not be produced.

    b. Effects may aid in identification of certain viruses (e.g., polykaryocyte formation by measles virus).

D. Types of infections.

1. Inapparent infections occur when too few cells are infected to cause clinical symptoms; they are synonymous with **subclinical disease** (Fig. 5.3).

    a. Sufficient antibody stimulation can cause immunity from further infections.

    b. They frequently occur when the virus inoculum is small.

2. Acute infections occur when clinical manifestations of disease are observed for a short time (days to weeks) after a short incubation period.

    a. Recovery is associated with elimination of the virus from the body.

    b. Acute infections are classified as **localized** or **disseminated,** depending on whether the virus has traveled from its site of implantation to its target organ.

    c. Persistent or **latent** infections may follow acute infection.

3. Persistent infections are associated with the continuing presence of the infectious virus in the body for an extended, perhaps lifelong, period.

    a. Clinical symptoms may or may not be present.

    b. Persistently infected individuals are known as **carriers.**

    c. Constant viral antigenic stimulation leads to high antibody titers for some antigens.

4. Latent infections occur when the infecting virus persists in the body in a noninfectious form that can periodically reactivate to an infectious virus and produce clinical disease; they are synonymous with **recurrent disease.**

    a. An antibody stimulus is produced only during the initial (**primary**) infection and during recurrent episodes.

    b. Subclinical reactivations may occur.

    c. Latent infections are difficult to detect in cells because viral antigen production is not detected and cytopathology is not observed during "silent" periods.

5. Slow infections have a **prolonged incubation** period lasting months or years.

    a. These infections do not cause clinical symptoms during incubation but can produce some infectious agents.

    b. They are most often associated with **chronic, progressive, fatal viral diseases of the central nervous system** (CNS), such as kuru and Creutzfeldt-Jakob disease.

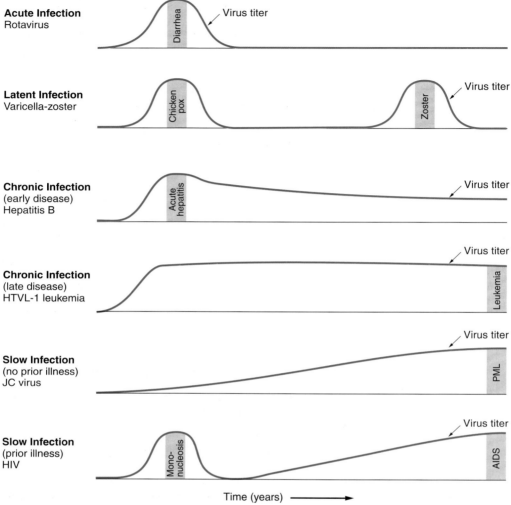

FIGURE 5.3. Patterns of viral disease. PML, progressive multifocal leukoencephalopathy.

E. Patterns of acute disease.

1. **Localized disease** occurs when viral multiplication and cell damage remain localized to the site of viral entry into the body.

   a. Localized disease has a short incubation time and may cause **systemic clinical features** (e.g., **fever**).

   b. Pronounced viremia (virions in the blood) does not usually occur.

   c. Sites include the **respiratory tract** (influenza, rhinovirus); **alimentary tract** (picornaviruses, rotaviruses); **genitourinary tract** (papillomavirus); and the **eye** (adenovirus).

   d. Disease can spread over the surface of the body to other areas where it causes another localized infection (picornavirus-induced conjunctivitis).

   e. The immune response that is induced is much weaker than the response induced by disseminated infections.

2. **Disseminated infections** involve the spread of virus from its entry site to a target organ. They involve a **primary viremia** and perhaps a **secondary viremia.**

   a. Incubation time is moderate (e.g., weeks), allowing more time for the host's immune system to eliminate the viral infection.

b. The **main clinical symptoms are associated with infection of one target organ,** although infection of other organs may be involved.

c. A substantial immune response is generated that frequently confers lifelong immunity to the host.

d. **Viral dissemination** is a major feature of disseminated infections.

    (1) Viruses may travel in other cells (red blood cells and mononuclear peripheral white blood cells), the plasma, extracellular spaces, and nerve fibers.

    (2) Viruses can be prevented from disseminating by viral-specific cytotoxic cells and neutralizing antibodies.

3. **Congenital infections** are viral infections of a fetus and are caused by maternal viremia.

a. These infections may lead to **maldeveloped organs.**

b. They are serious because of the immaturity of the fetal immune system, the placental barrier to maternal immunity, and the undifferentiated state and rapid multiplication of fetal cells.

V. HOST DEFENSES TO VIRUSES

A. **Host defense mechanisms** are responsible for the self-limiting nature of most viral infections.

1. Defense mechanisms have both immune and nonimmune aspects.

2. They operate during all stages of a viral infection and may contribute to the clinical pattern of disease (immunopathology).

B. **Nonimmune defenses.**

1. **Innate immunity** includes **anatomic barriers** (dead cells of the epidermis) and **chemical barriers** (mucous layers) that limit contact of the virus with susceptible cells. They are dependent on the complex parameters associated with the **age and physiologic status** of the host.

2. **Cellular resistance** involves **nonpermissive cells,** which lack factors (e.g., viral receptor sites) necessary for virus replication.

3. **Inflammation** limits the spread of virus from an infection site and results in unfavorable environmental conditions for viral replication (e.g., antiviral substances, low pH, elevated temperature).

4. **IFN** is a host-specific, viral-induced glycoprotein that inhibits viral replication by inducing the synthesis of several antiviral proteins including **2′,5′A synthetase** and specific protein kinases.

a. Although it is not viral specific, IFN is fairly species specific.

b. **IFN** is the **first viral-induced defense mechanism** at the primary site of infection in nonimmune individuals.

5. **Interfering RNA (RNAi).**

a. **Formation:** Double-stranded viral RNA interacts with **ribonuclease DICER** to form **short interfering** RNAs (siRNA), which interact with argonaute proteins to form **RISC (RNA-inducing silencing complexes).**

b. RISC binds to viral mRNA and inhibits viral gene expression by repressing translation or degrading the viral mRNA.

C. **Humoral immunity.** This defense mechanism involves the **production by B lymphocytes of neutralizing and nonneutralizing antibodies** against viral-specific antigens. It is the defense mechanism most important against cytolytic viral infections accompanied by viremia and viral infections of epithelial surfaces.

1. **Neutralizing antibodies** inhibit a virus's ability to replicate by inhibiting viral attachment, penetration, or uncoating, or all three processes.

a. Lesions may also be induced in the viral envelope with the aid of a complement.

b. These antibodies are most protective if they are present at the time of infection or during viremia.

2. **Nonneutralizing antibodies** enhance phagocytosis of virion degradation by acting as opsonins.

D. **Cell-mediated immunity** involves cytotoxic **T lymphocytes,** antibody-dependent cell-mediated cytotoxicity, natural killer cells, and activated macrophages.
  1. Soluble factors from T lymphocytes (**lymphokines**) and macrophages (**monokines**) regulate cellular immune responses.
  2. This form of immunity is the most important defense mechanism against noncytolytic infection in which the membrane of the virus-infected cell is antigenically altered by the virus.

E. **Viral-induced immunopathology** can result from various immunologic interactions, including immediate hypersensitivity, antibody-antigen complexes (as in hepatitis B virus [HBV]), and tissue damage due to cytotoxic cells or antibody and complement. These reactions can contribute to the disease process and are a common feature of **persistent viral infections.**

F. **Viral-induced immunosuppression** can occur during cytolytic or noncytolytic infection when infecting viruses alter the immune responsiveness or decrease the numbers of lymphocytes. It is frequently observed as a **transient consequence** of disseminated viral infections that involve lymphocyte infection by the virus.

VI. IMMUNOTHERAPY, ANTIVIRALS, AND INTERFERON

A. **Immunotherapy.**
  1. **Virus vaccines** lead to **active immunization** and are effective in preventing infections caused by viruses with few antigenic types. Vaccines may use **live virus, killed virus, virion subunits, viral polypeptides,** or **viral DNA** (Table 5.2).

table **5.2**	Viral Immunotherapy: Active Immunization (Vaccines)			
Virus	**Passive Immunization***	**Live Strain**	**Killed**	**Recombinant Viral Protein**
Adenovirus	No	Yes (previous military use; no longer available)	No	No
Hepatitis A virus	Yes	No	VAQTA or Havrix Twinrix	No
Hepatitis B virus	Yes	No	No	Engerix-B or Recombivax-HB Twinrix
Hepatitis E virus	No	No	No	Recombinant capsid protein
Human papilloma virus (types 6, 11, 16, and 18)	No	No	No	Quadrivalent Gardasil or Bivalent Cervarix (types 16 and 18)
Influenza virus	No	Yes	Yes	No
Measles virus	Yes	Enders	No	No
Mumps virus	No	Jeryl Lynn	No	No
Poliovirus	No	Sabin**	Salk	No
Rabies virus	Yes	No	Yes (human diploid cell)	No
Respiratory syncytial virus	Yes	No	No	No
Rotavirus	No	Rotarix RotaTeq	No	No
Rubella	No	Ra 27/3	No	No
Smallpox (variola) virus	No	Vaccinia	No	No
Varicella-zoster virus	Yes	Oka	No	No
Yellow fever virus	No	17D	No	No

*Commercial preparations available
**No longer recommended

    a. Live virus vaccines use **attenuated virus strains** that are relatively avirulent.
      (1) Advantages: may be administered in a single dose by the natural route of infection; induces a wide spectrum of antibodies and cytotoxic cells.
      (2) Disadvantages: limited shelf life, possible reversion to virulence, and possible production of persistent infection.
      (3) Examples include vaccines for **measles, mumps, rubella, chickenpox, rotavirus, yellow fever,** and some **adenovirus strains.**
    b. Killed virus vaccines are prepared from whole virions by **heat** or **chemical inactivation** of infectivity.
      (1) They stimulate antibodies only to surface antigens of the virus.
      (2) Advantage: easily combined into **polyvalent vaccines** (vaccines containing virions from several virus strains).
      (3) Disadvantages: lack of development of secretory immunoglobulin A (IgA), need for boosters, poor cell-mediated response, and possible hypersensitivity reactions.
      (4) Examples include vaccines for **poliovirus (Salk vaccine), rabies, influenza,** and **hepatitis A virus** (HAV).
    c. Virion subunit vaccines are purified proteins (viral receptors) obtained from virions.
      (1) Advantages and disadvantages are the same as those for killed vaccines.
      (2) Example is the **adenovirus vaccine.**
    d. Viral polypeptides are **polypeptide sequences of virion receptors** that have been synthesized or result from the purification of proteins made from cloned genes.
      (1) Advantages and disadvantages are the same as those for killed vaccines.
      (2) Examples include **HBV,** hepatitis E (**HEV**), and human papillomavirus (**HPV**) vaccines.
    e. DNA vaccines are plasmid DNA expression vectors containing **specific viral genes** (usually envelope genes).
      (1) These vaccines elicit both humoral and cell-mediated immune responses.
      (2) DNA vaccines are being evaluated for human use to protect against **human immunodeficiency virus (HIV)** and **influenza viruses.**
  2. Passive immunization is acquired by injection of pooled human plasma or gamma-globulin fractions from immune individuals into high-risk individuals.
    a. This form of immunization is valuable in the **prevention of some viral diseases but has little value after disease onset.**
    b. Passive immunity is used to prevent **rubella, measles, mumps, HAV, HBV, rabies,** and **varicella zoster virus (VZV) infections.**

B. Antiviral agents.
  1. General characteristics:
    a. Antiviral agents must selectively inhibit viral replication without affecting the viability or normal functions of the host cell (**selective toxicity**) (Fig. 5.4 and Tables 5.3, 5.4, and 5.5).
    b. They work by inhibiting the viral nucleic acid replication process, the penetration and uncoating process, or specific viral enzyme function.
    c. Only a few viral infections have antiviral agents (herpesviruses, influenza viruses, hepatitis B and C viruses, respiratory syncytial virus [RSV], and HIV).
    d. There are no broad-spectrum antivirals.
  2. Inhibitors of attachment fusion and uncoating:
    a. Raltegravir binds to CCR5 coreceptor of some HIV strains.
    b. Rimantadine and amantadine bind to the M2 protein of influenza A virus, which inhibits this ion pore in the virion envelope, thus preventing $H+$ ion influx and uncoating.
    c. Enfuvirtide inhibits HIV viral fusion protein gp41.
  3. Inhibitors of nucleic acid synthesis:
    a. Ribavirin is an **analog of the nucleoside guanosine;** its action varies for different viruses.
      (1) This drug alters cellular nucleotide pools, inhibits viral RNA synthesis, and may cause lethal RNA mutations.
      (2) It is used for severe RSV infections and in combination with IFV-α for chronic hepatitis C virus (HCV) infections.

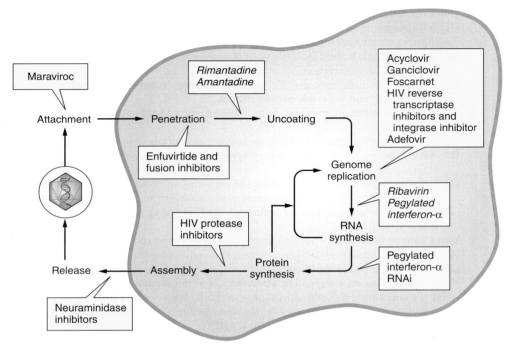

FIGURE 5.4. Sites of antiviral action.

t a b l e **5.3**	Inhibitors of Herpes Viruses		
Drug	**Administration Route**	**Mechanism of Action**	**Indications**
Acyclovir	Topical or oral	Inhibits HSV and VZV DNA synthesis	Primary genital herpes (HSV), encephalitis and keratitis Primary varicella infections Localized or ophthalmic zoster HSV and VZV in immunocompromised or transplant patients
Cidofovir	Parenteral	Inhibits CMV DNA synthesis	CMV retinitis in AIDS patients
Famciclovir	Oral	Inhibits HSV and VZV DNA synthesis	Zoster
Fomivirsen	Intravitreal	Inhibits early CMV gene transcription	CMV retinitis where other therapies failed
Foscarnet	Parenteral	Inhibits herpesvirus DNA polymerase	Acyclovir-resistant HSV and VZV infections Ganciclovir-resistant CMV retinitis
Ganciclovir	Oral and parenteral	Inhibits herpesvirus DNA synthesis	CMV retinitis Disseminated CMV infection of immunocompromised or AIDS patients Prophylaxis for disseminated CMV infections in transplant patients
Trifluridine	Topical	Inhibits herpesvirus DNA polymerase	HSV Keratoconjunctivitis
Valacyclovir	Oral	Inhibits HSV and VZV DNA synthesis	Herpes labialis, genital herpes, and zoster
Vidarabine	Topical or parenteral	Inhibits herpesvirus DNA polymerase	HSV keratitis and encephalitis (acyclovir is the drug of choice)

AIDS, acquired immunodeficiency syndrome; CMV, cytomegalovirus; HSV, herpes simplex virus; VZV, varicella-zoster virus

table 5.4 Inhibitors of Human Immunodeficiency Virus

Drug	Administration Route	Mechanism of Action	Indications
A. Nucleoside Inhibitors of Reverse Transcriptase			
Abacavir	Oral	Inhibits HIV DNA synthesis	AIDS, HIV infection
Didanosine	Oral	Inhibits HIV DNA synthesis	AIDS, HIV infection
Emtricitabine	Oral	Inhibits HIV DNA synthesis	AIDS, HIV infection
Lamivudine	Oral	Inhibits HIV DNA synthesis	AIDS, HIV infection*
Stavudine	Oral	Inhibits HIV DNA synthesis	AIDS, HIV infection
Zalcitabine	Oral	Inhibits HIV DNA synthesis	AIDS, HIV infection
Zidovudine	Oral	Inhibits HIV DNA synthesis	AIDS, HIV infection
B. Nonnucleoside Inhibitors of Reverse Transcriptase			
Delavirdine	Oral	Inhibits HIV reverse transcriptase (nonnucleoside)	AIDS, HIV infection
Efavirenz	Oral	Inhibits HIV reverse transcriptase (nonnucleoside)	AIDS, HIV infection
Etravirine	Oral	Inhibits HIV reverse transcriptase (nonnucleoside)	AIDS, HIV infection
Nevirapine	Oral	Inhibits HIV reverse transcriptase (nonnucleoside)	AIDS, HIV infection
Rilpivirine	Oral	Inhibits HIV reverse transcriptase (nonnucleoside)	AIDS, HIV infection
C. Nucleotide Inhibitor of Reverse Transcriptase			
Tenofovir	Oral	Nucleotide that inhibits HIV DNA synthesis	AIDS, HIV infection*
D. Integrase Inhibitor			
Enfuvirtide	Oral	Inhibits HIV-1 integrase	AIDS, HIV-1 infection
E. Protease Inhibitor			
Amprenavir	Oral	Inhibits HIV protease	AIDS, HIV infection
Atazanavir	Oral	Inhibits HIV protease	AIDS, HIV infection
Darunavir	Oral	Inhibits HIV protease	AIDS, HIV infection
Fosamprenavir	Oral	Inhibits HIV protease	AIDS, HIV infection
Indinavir	Oral	Inhibits HIV protease	AIDS, HIV infection
Lopinavir	Oral	Inhibits HIV protease	AIDS, HIV infection
Nelfinavir	Oral	Inhibits HIV protease	AIDS, HIV infection
Ritonavir	Oral	Inhibits HIV protease	AIDS, HIV infection
Saquinavir	Oral	Inhibits HIV protease	AIDS, HIV infection
F. Attachment Inhibitor			
Raltegravir	Oral	Binds to CCR5 coreceptor for some HIV strains	AIDS, HIV-1 infections caused by strains using CCR5 coreceptor
G. Cell Fusion Inhibitor			
Maraviroc	Parenteral	Inhibits HIV fusion protein gp41	AIDS, HIV infection

AIDS, acquired immunodeficiency syndrome; HIV, human immunodeficiency virus
*Also used for chronic HBV infections

  b. Acyclovir, valacyclovir, penciclovir, famciclovir, ganciclovir, entecavir, cidofovir, adefovir, azidothymidine (AZT), abacavir, didanosine, zalcitabine, zidovudine, tenofovir, emtricitabine, stavudine, and lamivudine are **analogues** of **nucleosides** that prevent DNA chain elongation after recognition and base pairing.
  (1) These drugs are activated by phosphorylation by cellular or viral kinases.
  (2) They are selective inhibitors because: (1) there is a higher binding affinity for viral DNA polymerase or (2) DNA synthesis is more rapid in infected cells.
  (3) Examples include many herpes simplex (HSV), VZV, cytomegalovirus (CMV), and HIV antivirals.

table 5.5	Inhibitors of Other Viruses		
Drug	**Administration Route**	**Mechanism of Action**	**Indications**
Adefovir	Oral	Inhibits HBV reverse transcriptase	Chronic hepatitis B virus infection
Amantadine	Oral	Inhibits influenza A virus penetration or uncoating	Prophylaxis for influenza A virus
Entecavir	Oral	Inhibits HBV reverse transcriptase	Chronic hepatitis B infections
Interferon-α	Parental	Induces antiviral proteins	Chronic hepatitis B and hepatitis C virus infections
Oseltamivir	Oral	Inhibits influenza A and B virus neuraminidase	Influenza A and B virus infections
Ribavirin	Oral or inhalation	Inhibits nucleic acid polymerases	Severe RSV infection Chronic HCV and IFNs Lassa fever
Rimantadine	Oral	Inhibits influenza virus penetration or uncoating	Prophylaxis for influenza A virus
Telbivudine	Oral	Inhibits HBV reverse transcriptase	Chronic hepatitis B virus infection
Zanamivir	Inhalation	Inhibits influenza A and B virus neuraminidase	Influenza A and B virus infections

HBV, hepatitis B virus; HCV, hepatitis C virus; IFNs, interferons; RSV, respiratory syncytial virus

    c. Idoxuridine, trifluorothymidine, and fluorouracil are **analogs of thymidine,** which either (1) inhibit thymidine biosynthesis or (2) replace thymidine in DNA, which leads to misreading of the DNA and mutations.

    d. Foscarnet is a nonnucleoside nucleic acid polymerase inhibitor that binds to and inhibits the DNA polymerase of all herpesviruses and the reverse transcriptase of HIV.

    e. Nevirapine, delavirdine, efavirenz, etravirine, and rilpivirine are **nonnucleoside HIV reverse transcriptase inhibitors** that are used in combination therapy with various nucleoside analog inhibitors of that enzyme.

    f. Raltegravir inhibits HIV integrase, preventing HIV provirus formation.

  4. Protease inhibitors:

    a. These drugs include **saquinavir, indinavir, ritonavir, nelfinavir, amprenavir, atazanavir, darunavir, fosamprenavir, and lopinavir.**

    b. They inhibit the action of HIV protease; used in combination with AZT and a second nucleoside analog as "cocktail" therapy for HIV.

  5. Neuraminidase inhibitors:

    a. These drugs include **oseltamivir** and **zanamivir.**

    b. They inhibit the neuraminidase of **influenza A and B** viruses; they may be used for prophylaxis as well as treatment.

  6. mRNA inhibitors:

    a. Fomivirsen is a synthetic oligonucleotide complementary to a sequence in CMV RNA (an antisense compound). It prevents transcription of early CMV genes.

    b. It is approved for intravitreal therapy of CMV retinitis after other therapies have failed.

C. Interferons.

  1. IFNs are host-coded proteins, or glycoproteins, produced in and secreted from virus-infected cells in response to virus infection, synthetic nucleotides, and foreign cells.

  2. IFNs bind to cell-surface receptors and induce antiviral proteins, including a protein kinase and 2′,5′A synthetase (which synthesizes an oligoadenylic acid), leading to the destruction of viral mRNA.

  3. They are host specific but not viral specific.

  4. Three groups or families are recognized: IFN-α, IFN-β, and IFN-γ.

  5. IFN-α (Intron-A) is licensed for treatment of chronic HBV and HCV infections and can produce adverse effects at high doses or with chronic therapy.

  6. They have toxic side effects, including bone marrow suppression.

VII. DIAGNOSTIC VIROLOGY

A. **Laboratory viral diagnosis** involves one of three basic approaches: virus isolation; direct demonstration of virus, viral nucleic acid, or antigens in clinical specimens; or serologic testing of viral-specific antibodies.

1. Because the clinical symptoms of a virus are often distinctive, lab diagnosis is frequently not necessary.

2. If done, it begins with identification of the most likely viruses based on clinical symptoms and the patient's history.

3. It is often not possible during the first few days after infection.

B. **Virus isolation.**

1. This technique identifies virus replication in susceptible cells. Tissue culture cells, embryonated eggs, or animal hosts are often used.

   a. In live infected tissue culture cells, replication may be detected by observing a characteristic **cytopathogenic effect** (CPE) such as polykaryocyte formation or hemadsorption (adhesion of red blood cells to infected cells).

   b. In fixed infected tissue culture cells, replication may be detected by observing characteristic inclusion bodies (see Table 5.1) or performing immunohistochemical staining of viral antigens.

   c. In an embryonated egg, replication is detected by pock formation; in animals, by the development of clinical symptoms.

2. Proper collection and preservation of specimens are necessary for virus isolation.

3. It is best accomplished during the onset and acute phase of disease.

C. **Direct examination of clinical specimens.**

1. **General characteristics:**

   a. Specimens may include sections of tissue biopsies, tissue imprints or smears, blood, cerebrospinal fluid, urine, throat swabs, feces, or saliva.

   b. Only those specimens likely to contain the virus (e.g., throat swabs for respiratory tract infection) should be examined.

   c. Examples include the following assays: viral-induced CPE (see 5 IV C 5), immunohistochemical staining, nucleic acid hybridization and amplification methods, and solid-phase immunoassay.

2. **Immunohistochemical staining.** This technique uses fixed or fresh specimens and chemically labeled (fluorescein) or enzymatically labeled (peroxidase) antibodies to detect viral antigens with either a direct or an indirect staining method. May use impression slides made from specific tissues.

3. **Nucleic acid hybridization and amplification** involves the detection of viral DNA or RNA sequences in nucleic acid extracted from specimens. It is highly sensitive and specific and is a popular technique for identifying adenovirus in nasopharyngeal washings, CMV in urine, and HIV in the blood of seronegative individuals.

   a. **Polymerase chain reaction** (PCR) may be used to amplify viral genes.

   b. Dot blot hybridization techniques that usually use single-stranded, complementary nucleic acid probes may be used.

4. **Solid-phase immunoassays** detect viral antigens such as rotavirus and HAV in feces. They use specific viral antibodies and radioimmunoassay (RIA) or enzyme-linked immunosorbent assay (ELISA) techniques. These assays are highly sensitive and specific.

D. **Serologic tests.**

1. **General characteristics:**

   a. Serologic tests are used to determine the **titer** of specific antiviral antibodies.

   b. Paired blood samples are taken (one sample at the onset and one sample during the recovery phase of the illness); **at least a fourfold increase in titer between the samples must be present to indicate a current infection.**

   c. The test may be diagnostic without the use of paired samples if significant levels of IgM antiviral antibodies are obtained.
   d. Techniques include virus neutralization, complement fixation, hemagglutination inhibition tests, and solid-phase immunoassays.
2. **Virus neutralization tests** are based on the principle that certain antiviral antibodies will neutralize the CPE of the virus.
   a. Constant amounts of virus are incubated with decreasing amounts of serum added to susceptible cells.
   b. These tests are expensive to perform and must be standardized for each virus.
3. **Hemagglutination inhibition tests** are based on the principle that antihemagglutinin antibodies in serum will inhibit viral agglutination of erythrocytes.
   a. These tests can be performed only on viruses with hemagglutinins on their surface (influenza, measles).
   b. They require careful standardization of erythrocytes and viral hemagglutinin preparations.
4. **Solid-phase immunoassays** are highly sensitive and specific assays used to detect specific viral antibodies.
   a. They use viral antigens in RIA and ELISA protocols.
   b. These tests are several hundred times more sensitive than other serologic tests.

VIII. DNA VIRUSES

DNA viruses that cause human disease are classified into seven families (Table 5.6). The replication of all viral DNA occurs in the nucleus except for poxviruses, which replicate entirely in the cytoplasm. Some DNA viruses can produce latent infections and all except parvoviruses can transform cells.

A. **Naked DNA viruses.**
   1. **Human adenoviruses:**
      a. Description: naked DNA viruses with an **icosahedral nucleocapsid** composed of **hexons, pentons, and fibers.**
      b. Virulence factors: toxic activity associated with pentons and hemagglutinating activity associated with pentons and fibers.
      c. Classification: are classified into nearly 50 serotypes.
      d. Genome: contains **double-stranded DNA** that replicates asymmetrically.

t a b l e **5.6**	Virion and Nucleic Acid Structure of DNA Viruses				
Virus Family	**Prominent Examples**	**Virion Structure**	**Virion Polymerase**	**Capsid Symmetry**	**DNA Structure**
Adenoviridae	Adenoviruses	Naked	No	Icosahedral	Linear, double stranded
Herpesviridae	Herpes simplex virus Varicella-zoster virus Epstein-Barr virus Cytomegalovirus	Enveloped	No	Icosahedral	Linear, double stranded
Poxviridae	Smallpox virus Vaccinia virus Molluscum contagiosum virus	Brick shaped, enveloped	Yes	Complex	Linear, double stranded
Papillomaviridae	Human papillomavirus	Naked	No	Icosahedral	Circular, double stranded
Polyomaviridae	JC virus	Naked	No	Icosahedral	Circular, double stranded
Hepadnaviridae	Hepatitis B virus	Enveloped	Yes	Icosahedral	Circular, double stranded
Parvoviridae	B19 virus	Naked	No	Icosahedral	Linear, single stranded

  e. **Replication:** replicate in the nucleus of epithelial cells.
  f. **Clinical disease:**
   (1) Cause localized infections of the eye, respiratory tract, gastrointestinal (GI) tract, and urinary bladder.
   (2) Frequently cause subclinical infections and can cause **latent infections of lymphoid tissue** (e.g., **tonsils**).
   (3) Can cause tumors in other animals because **E1A and E1B gene products bind to cellular tumor suppressor proteins p110^{Rb} and p53.**
  g. **Diagnosis:** may be diagnosed by virus isolation from the eyes, throat, or urine or ELISA procedures on fecal specimens from patients with GI infections.
2. **Papillomaviruses:**
  a. **Description: naked viruses** with an **icosahedral capsid** and **double-stranded circular DNA.**
  b. **Classification:** exist in more than 100 different subtypes.
  c. **Replication:** replicate in epithelial cells of epithelial and mucosal tissue; form **koilocytotic cells** (cytoplasmic vacuoles and enlarged nuclei) during replication.
  d. **Clinical disease:**
   (1) May cause lytic, latent, or transforming human infections depending on the host cell.
   (2) **Types 16 and 18 are associated with cervical intraepithelial neoplasia** (CIN) involving the **inactivation of tumor suppression proteins, p53 and p110^{Rb}, by early viral proteins E6 and E7,** respectively.
  e. **Prevention:**
   (1) **Gardasil,** a recombinant viral protein vaccine containing types 6, 11, 16, and 18 viruslike particles, is available for protection.
   (2) **Cervarix,** a recombinant vital protein vaccine, contains types 16 and 18 viruslike particles.
3. **Parvoviruses:**
  a. **Description: small, naked viruses** with **icosahedral capsids** containing **single-stranded DNA.**
  b. **Clinical disease:** includes one human virus (**B19**) that causes disease involving cytolytic replication in erythroid precursor cells.
4. **Polyomaviruses:**
  a. **Description: naked viruses** with an **icosahedral capsid** containing **double-stranded circular DNA.**
  b. **Clinical disease:** includes two human viruses, **BK virus** and **JC virus,** which infect the kidney where they usually do not cause disease but become **latent;** when reactivated by immunosuppression, BK causes a urinary tract infection and JC travels to and replicates in oligodendrocytes to cause a neurological disease (**progressive multifocal leukoencephalopathy**).

B. **Enveloped DNA viruses.**
1. **Hepadnaviruses** have only one representative that infects humans: **HBV.**
  a. **Description: icosahedral capsid containing a partially double-stranded DNA surrounded by an envelope; the virion of HBV is called the Dane particle.**
  b. **Replication:** have a **virion-associated multifunctional enzyme complex with reverse transcriptase, DNA polymerase, and ribonuclease activity,** which is necessary for viral DNA replication.
  c. **Clinical disease:** can cause acute and symptomatic or asymptomatic chronic liver disease and is implicated in primary hepatocellular carcinoma; induces a cell-mediated response that is responsible for symptoms and recovery from the infection.
  d. **Diagnosis:** produces unique antigens (**HBsAg, a surface antigen, and HBcAg and HBeAg core-associated antigens**) associated with infections or their antibodies that are monitored by serological tests to determine the source of HBV infections.
  e. **Treatment and prevention:**
   (1) Has been genetically manipulated to produce a **recombinant subunit vaccine (Recombivax HB and Energix-B)** or used in a combination vaccine (Twinrix) utilized for protection from HAV and HBV.
   (2) Chronic infection may be treated with INF-α or four reverse transcriptase inhibitors.

2. **Herpesviruses** are **enveloped viruses** with an **icosahedral nucleocapsid** containing **double-stranded DNA.**
   a. **Herpes simplex type 1 and 2 (HSV-1 and -2):**
      (1) **Cytopathology:** can cause cell rounding and polykaryocyte formation or inclusion bodies (**Cowdry type A inclusions**) in infected cells.
      (2) **Replication:** produce a **viral-specific thymidine kinase** necessary for DNA replication; it is the target of several antiherpes nucleoside analog drugs like acyclovir.
      (3) **Clinical disease:**
         (a) **Latently infect neurons.**
         (b) Produce both acute and latent infections whose clinical lesions occur primarily on mucosal surfaces (lip and genitals), but can cause encephalitis and eye infections as well.
      (4) **Treatment:** Infections may be treated with antivirals that affect the viral DNA polymerase (foscarnet, trifluridine, or vidarabine) or stop DNA chain elongation (acyclovir, penciclovir, famciclovir, and valacyclovir), but **none eliminate latent infections.**
   b. **Varicella-zoster virus:**
      (1) **Cytopathology:** produces similar cytopathology as HSV and also **latently infects neurons.**
      (2) **Clinical disease:** causes vesicular lesions in both acute (**chickenpox**) and recurrent (**shingles**) disease.
      (3) **Treatment and prevention:**
         (a) Infections may be treated with nucleoside analog DNA chain terminators (acyclovir, famciclovir, and valacyclovir), but latent infections are not eliminated.
         (b) An attenuated virus, the **Oka strain, is used in vaccines to prevent chickenpox and diminish shingles recurrences.**
   c. **Cytomegalovirus:**
      (1) **Cytopathology:** causes swelling of infected cells (**cytomegalic cells**) and "owl's eye" **intranuclear inclusion bodies.**
      (2) **Replication:** replicates in epithelial cells of oropharynx, but **latently infects monocytes, macrophages, and lymphocytes.**
      (3) **Clinical disease:**
         (a) May depress immune response during initial infection due to interaction of cells involved in cellular immunity.
         (b) Causes a **heterophile-negative mononucleosis** and is a potentially serious congenital infection.
         (c) Latent infections are usually reactivated to asymptomatic disease, but reactivation in immunosuppressed individuals can be serious (e.g., giant cell pneumonia in acquired immunodeficiency syndrome [AIDS] patients).
      (4) **Treatment:** does not produce its own thymidine kinase, but does produce a protein kinase that phosphorylates **ganciclovir, a nucleoside analog** that when incorporated into viral DNA inhibits replication; **cidofovir is phosphorylated by cellular kinases** and also inhibits viral DNA replication.
   d. **Epstein-Barr virus (EBV):**
      (1) **Pathobiology:** can productively infect and abortively infect human B lymphocytes; **abortive infection induces B-cell proliferation and potential transformation.**
      (2) **Virulence factors:** uses complement receptor 3 (CS-21 or CR-2) as the cellular receptor.
      (3) **Clinical disease:**
         (a) Produces several distinct antigens, including **latent membrane proteins (LMPs), nuclear antigens (EBNAs), early antigens (EAs), a membrane antigen (MA), and a viral capsid antigen (VCA).**
         (b) Usually causes clinically inapparent infections, but may cause **heterophile-positive infectious mononucleosis** and is **associated with Burkitt's lymphoma and nasopharyngeal carcinoma.**
      (4) **Diagnosis:** is associated with the production of **atypical lymphocytes (Downey cells)** and **IgM heterophile antibodies** (antibodies detected using antigens from a source different from the one used to induce them) identified by the **mononucleosis spot test.**

      e. **Human herpesviruses types 6 and 7 (HHV 6 and 7):**
         (1) **Description: T-lymphotropic viruses** associated with roseola diseases and febrile seizures in infants.
         (2) **Clinical disease:** cause latent infections of peripheral blood lymphocytes and can reactivate during immunosuppression of transplant and AIDS patients.
      f. **Human herpesvirus type 8 (Kaposi's sarcoma-associated herpesvirus; HHVS or KSHV):**
         (1) **Pathobiology:** preferentially infects B lymphocytes and appears to be sexually transmitted.
         (2) **Genome:** contains more than 10 homologues of cellular genes (e.g., cyclin D, interleukin 6, and so forth) in its genome.
         (3) **Clinical disease:**
            (a) **Associated with Kaposi's sarcoma.**
            (b) Linked to some AIDS-associated B-cell lymphomas.
            (c) Implicated in **multiple myeloma.**
  3. **Poxviruses (new family):**
    a. **General characteristics:**
      (1) **Description:**
         (a) **Complex brick-shaped virion** that consists of an **outer envelope enclosing a core containing linear, double-stranded DNA** and two lateral bodies.
         (b) Have more than 100 structural polypeptides, including many enzymes and a transcriptional system associated with the virion.
      (2) **Replication:** replicate in the cytoplasm of the cell.
      (3) **Cytopathology:** produce **eosinophilic inclusion bodies called Guarnieri bodies** and membrane hemagglutinins in infected cells.
      (4) **Classification:** include **human viruses** (vaccina, variola, and molluscum contagiosum) and **animal viruses** (cowpox virus, paravaccinia virus [in cows], and orf virus [in sheep]); the animal viruses can cause highly localized occupational infections (usually of the finger).
    b. **Variola virus** causes smallpox.
    c. **Vaccinia virus** is the variant of variola virus that generally produces only a mild disease and is used as the immunogen in smallpox vaccination. It is being studied as a **possible immunizing vector** containing foreign genes for polypeptides, which would elicit neutralizing antibodies for other viruses (e.g., HSV types 1 and 2).
    d. **Molluscum contagiosum virus** infects epithelial cells, where it causes a localized disease involving small, wartlike lesions on the face, arms, back, buttocks, and genitals that usually resolves spontaneously in several months; it also **causes a sexually transmitted disease** with papular lesions that can ulcerate and mimic genital herpes.

IX. RNA VIRUSES

Although both naked and enveloped RNA viruses exist, they are usually discussed based on the nature of their RNA genome, which may be single stranded or double stranded. Using this criterion, there are, therefore, four categories of RNA viruses: (1) **positive-sense** (virion s.s. RNA can serve as mRNA), (2) **negative-sense** (s.s. RNA complementary to the virion RNA serves as mRNA), (3) **ambisense** (virion RNA has portions of both positive-sense and negative-sense RNA), and (4) **double stranded** (virion RNA is double stranded). All of these viruses except the influenza viruses and HIV replicate entirely in the cytoplasm of the cell, and since cells lack cytoplasm RNA polymerase, they must code for and produce their own. All negative-sense RNA viruses are enveloped and an RNA polymerase acts as a transcriptase or replicase associated with the virion. Many RNA viruses have developed unique mechanisms to produce individual polypeptides from polycistronic RNA.

A. **Positive-sense viruses** (Table 5.7).
  1. **Caliciviruses:**
    a. **Description:** naked viruses with an **icosahedral nucleocapsid** that **contain positive-sense, single-stranded RNA**.

t a b l e   5.7   Virion and Nucleic Acid Structure of Positive-Sense RNA Viruses

Virus Family	Prominent Examples	Virion Structure	Virion Polymerase	Capsid Symmetry	RNA Structure
Caliciviridae	Norwalk agent	Naked	No	Icosahedral	Linear single stranded, nonsegmented
Picornaviridae	Coxsackieviruses Echoviruses Enteroviruses Hepatitis A virus Polioviruses Rhinoviruses	Naked	No	Icosahedral	Linear, single stranded, nonsegmented
Flaviviridae	Dengue virus Hepatitis C virus St. Louis encephalitis virus Yellow fever virus	Enveloped	No	Icosahedral	Linear, single stranded, nonsegmented
Togaviridae	Eastern, Western, and Venezuelan equine encephalomyelitis viruses	Enveloped	No	Icosahedral	Linear, single stranded, nonsegmented
Retroviridae	Human immunodeficiency virus Leukemia viruses Sarcoma viruses	Enveloped	No*	Helical	Linear, single stranded, nonsegmented*
Coronaviridae	Coronaviruses SARS-CoV	Enveloped	No	Helical	Linear, single stranded, nonsegmented

*Retroviruses are diploid and have reverse transcriptase

   b. Classification: have been classified in four genera, of which two infect humans to cause gastroenteritis; those belonging to the **Norovirus genus (previously called "Norwalk agents")** cause epidemics of gastroenteritis associated with contaminated food and are transmitted via the fecal-oral route.

2. Coronaviruses:
  a. Description:
    (1) Enveloped viruses with a **helical nucleocapsid that contains single-stranded RNA with positive (messenger) polarity**.
    (2) Have distinctive club-shaped surface projections that give the appearance of a solar corona to the virion.
  b. Clinical disease: most frequently associated with the common cold in adults and gastroenteritis in infants, but recently a variant strain, **SARS-CoV, emerged to cause a severe acute respiratory syndrome.**

3. Flaviviruses:
  a. General characteristics:
    (1) Description: enveloped viruses with a **single-stranded, positive-sense RNA** and **no discernible capsid structure**.
    (2) Replication: replicate in the cytoplasm of the cell, where the RNA is translated into a large polyprotein that is subsequently cleaved (by **posttranslational cleavage**) into individual proteins.
  b. Dengue virus:
    (1) Description: arbovirus transmitted from monkeys to humans by mosquitoes.
    (2) Clinical disease:
      (a) Four serotypes exist; antibodies (called **"enhancing" antibodies**) to one serotype increase efficiency of infection by another serotype, resulting in more serious disease.
      (b) Causes characteristic skin lesions as well as fever with muscle and joint pain; is sometimes called **break bone fever.**
  c. Hepatitis C virus:
    (1) Description: also known as **non-A, non-B hepatitis virus;** exist in **six genotypes** with different worldwide distribution.

    (2) Clinical disease:

        (a) Infects the body after parenteral entry and **causes 90% of blood transfusion-associated or blood product administration-associated hepatitis.**

        (b) Can cause **chronic infections** involving carrier state individuals and is **implicated in primary hepatocellular carcinoma.**

    (3) Diagnosis: diagnosed by ELISA serology and **molecular genotyping of circulating virions** to determine the patient's likelihood to respond to treatment with INF-α and ribavirin since only two genotypes respond.

  d. St. Louis encephalitis virus:

    (1) Description: an **arbovirus** with a mosquito vector that transfers the virus from wild birds to humans.

    (2) Clinical disease: usually causes inapparent infections but may produce encephalitis.

  e. Yellow fever virus:

    (1) Description: +ss RNA with envelope; arbovirus that is usually transferred from monkeys to humans by mosquitoes.

    (2) Clinical disease:

        (a) Causes a biphasic disease with clinical signs involving the vascular endothelium during initial virus replication and involving the liver during later replication.

        (b) Can cause chronic infections; therefore, individuals with the virus are in a carrier state.

    (3) Diagnosis: diagnosed by **eosinophilic hyaline masses called Councilman bodies** in the cytoplasm of infected liver cells.

    (4) Prevention: prevented by immunization with the **attenuated vaccine strain 17D.**

  f. West Nile virus:

    (1) Description: arbovirus that is transferred from a bird reservoir (especially crows and jays) to humans by a mosquito vector; **leading cause of arboviral encephalitis in the United States.**

    (2) Clinical disease: causes an encephalitis that is most serious for those older than 50 years of age.

4. Hepevirus (Hepatitis E-like viruses):

  a. Description: naked viruses with a **single-stranded, positive-sense RNA genome,** which has been divided into **four genotypes.**

  b. Clinical disease: produce a hepatitis transmitted by the fecal-oral route, but not endemic in the United States.

5. Picornaviruses:

  a. General characteristics:

    (1) Description: small, naked viruses with an **icosahedral nucleocapsid** that contains **single-stranded, positive-sense RNA covalently linked to a small protein (VPg** in poliovirus).

    (2) Replication: replicate in the cytoplasm of the cell, where RNA is translated into a large polyprotein that is subsequently cleaved (**posttranslational cleavage**).

    (3) Classification: classified into nine genera, but only five (**enteroviruses, hepatoviruses, kobuviruses, parechoviruses, and rhinoviruses) cause human disease.**

  b. Enteroviruses cause a variety of human diseases involving infections of the alimentary tract (are stable at **acidic pH 3 to 5**). They include polioviruses, coxsackie A and B viruses, and echoviruses.

    (1) Coxsackie viruses:

        (a) Classification: divided into two groups, depending on the type of paralysis they cause following inoculation into mice (**group A cause flaccid paralysis; group B cause spastic paralysis**).

        (b) Clinical disease: cause a variety of diseases involving enanthems and exanthems (rashes), the eye, and the meninges.

            1. Group B are cardiotrophic and can cause severe chest pain due to the infection of muscles between the ribs.

            2. Cause infections that tend to occur in summer and early fall.

            3. Are most often not identified during infections, but are simply classified as enteroviral disease.

- **(2) Echoviruses:**
  - **(a) Clinical disease:** cause diseases similar to coxsackie viruses except not particularly associated with heart disease or chest pain; most associated with aseptic meningitis.
  - **(b) Diagnosis:** not frequently identified during infections, but are simply classified as enteroviral infections.
- **(3) Enteroviruses** cause diseases similar to coxsackie and echoviruses, particularly CNS and eye infections.
- **(4) Polioviruses:**
  - **(a) Classification: exist in three serotypes.**
  - **(b) Pathobiology:** spreads in the body by hematogenous and neural routes.
  - **(c) Clinical disease:**
    1. Replicate in the intestine where they usually produce an asymptomatic infection, but can spread to the spinal cord and CNS via neural pathways.
    2. **Destroy anterior horn cells of the spinal cord as a result of replication there.**
    3. May cause a rare paralytic disease as a result of invasion of the CNS.
  - **(d) Prevention:** The three serotypes have been inactivated and combined in a **trivalent vaccine (Salk vaccine);** live attenuated strains were present in the Sabin vaccine, which is no longer recommended.
- **c. Hepatovirus:**
  - **(1) Description:** contains the **hepatitis A viruses** that replicate in hepatocytes where they cause a food-borne or water-borne hepatitis.
  - **(2) Treatment and prevention:** may be treated prophylactically with immune human globulin or prevented by immunization with **killed virus vaccines (Havrix or VAQTA) containing formalin-inactivated virions or a combination vaccine for HAV and HBV (Twinrix).**
- **d. Kobuviruses** are recently discovered viruses causing **gastroenteritis.**
- **e. Parechoviruses:**
  - **(1) Description:** consist of three human pathogens (HPeV-1, -2, and -3).
  - **(2) Clinical disease:** produce **gastroenteritis** and **respiratory disease;** may occasionally cause aseptic meningitis and encephalitis.
- **f. Rhinoviruses:**
  - **(1) Description:** exist in more than 100 serotypes; are **acid labile.**
  - **(2) Replication:** bind to ICAM-1 and replicate best at 33°C/91°F; replication may be inhibited by **pleconaril,** an experimental compound that binds to the capsid and prevents viral attachment to cells.
  - **(3) Clinical disease:** are the leading cause of the **common cold.**
- **6. Retroviruses (new family):**
  - **a. General characteristics:**
    - **(1) Description: enveloped viruses with an icosahedral capsid.**
    - **(2) Genome:**
      - **(a)** Contain **two identical copies of single-stranded positive-sense RNA (diploid genome)** with a host tRNA bound to the 5' end and a viral specified **reverse transcriptase enzyme complex** (RNA-dependent DNA polymerase and RNase activity), integrase enzyme, and protease enzyme.
      - **(b)** Have three notable gene regions: *gag* **(structural proteins),** *pol* **(reverse transcriptase),** and *env* **(envelope glycoproteins),** which are flanked by **long terminal repeat sequences** with regulatory functions.
      - **(c)** Use posttranslational cleavage processes during the synthesis of *gag* and *env* gene products.
      - **(d)** Need the host-cell transfer RNA to interact with reverse transcriptase before the reverse transcriptase complex can bind to RNA and initiate DNA synthesis.
    - **(3) Classification:**
      - **(a)** Divided morphologically into four types (A, B, C, and D).
      - **(b)** Classified into three groups: **lentiviruses (visna and maedi viruses** of sheep, HIV); **spumaviruses;** and **oncoviruses** (types B, C, and D RNA tumor viruses).

(4) Clinical disease: cause mostly "slow" diseases of animals and various cancers, except for HIV, which causes MDS.
b. **Human immunodeficiency virus type 1 and 2 (HIV-1 and -2):**
   (1) Description: members of the lentivirus subfamily and exist as **lymphotropic and macrophage trophic strains.**
   (2) Pathobiology:
   (a) Initiate infection by interaction of an envelope glycoprotein (gp120) with the cellular T4 (CD4) lymphocyte surface receptor.
   (b) Synthesize core **proteins (p18, p24, and RT) and transregulatory proteins (*tat rev,* and *nef*).**
   (c) Have **regulatory genes (TRE and *rre*).**
   (d) Infect and kill T-helper cells, resulting in depression of both humoral and cell-mediated immunity.
   (3) Clinical disease: causes immunosuppression, leading to opportunistic infections, cancers, and neurologic disorders.
   (4) Treatment: replication may be inhibited by **six classes of antivirals: nucleoside analogs and nonnucleoside inhibitors of reverse transcriptase; integrase inhibitor; protease inhibitors; attachment inhibitor; and fusion inhibitor.**
c. **Human T-cell lymphotropic viruses (HTLV-1 and -2)** belong to the oncovirus subfamily and are associated with human cancers (**adult T-cell leukemia** [HTLV-1], **hairy cell leukemia** [HTLV-2]), and a neurologic myelopathy (**tropical spastic paraparesis** [HTLV-1]).
7. **Togavirus:**
   a. **General characteristics:**
      (1) Description: enveloped viruses with an **icosahedral nucleocapsid** containing **single-stranded, positive-sense RNA;** have **hemagglutinins** associated with their envelope.
      (2) Classification: divided into four groups of which two (alphaviruses and rubiviruses) are human pathogens.
   b. **Alphaviruses:**
      (1) Description: arboviruses with mosquito vectors and animal reservoirs.
      (2) Clinical disease:
      (a) Cause encephalitis or moderate systemic disease following the bite of a mosquito that has fed on an animal viral reservoir.
      (b) Lead to more serious encephalitis than do flaviviruses.
      (c) Include **Eastern equine encephalomyelitis virus, Western equine encephalomyelitis virus, and Venezuelan equine encephalomyelitis virus.**
      (3) Diagnosis: diagnosed by serologic tests, usually ELISA for IgM, because virus isolation is difficult.
   c. **Rubivirus—(Rubella virus):**
      (1) Clinical disease: causes **German measles** in children and **congenital infections with serious consequences** to fetuses infected during the first 10 weeks of pregnancy.
      (2) Diagnosis: done by ELISA tests for IgM and immunity determined by ELISA to IgG.
      (3) Prevention: strain RA 27/3 has been attenuated for use in a live vaccine.

B. **Negative-sense viruses (Table 5.8).**
   1. **Bunyaviruses:**
      a. **Description:**
         (1) Enveloped arboviruses with **three circular helical nucleocapsids,** each containing a unique piece of **single-stranded, negative-polarity RNA** (L, M, and S segments), viral nucleoprotein, and transcriptase enzyme.
         (2) Can interact with viruses that are closely related serologically to produce recombinant viruses by genetic reassortment.
      b. **Replication:** replicate within the cytoplasm and bud from the membranes of the Golgi apparatus.
      c. **Clinical disease:**
         (1) Have rodent hosts and infect humans during an arthropod bite.

table 5.8	Virion and Nucleic Acid Structure of Negative-Sense RNA Viruses				
Virus Family	**Prominent Example**	**Virion Structure**	**Virion Polymerase**	**Capsid Symmetry**	**RNA Structure**
Paramyxoviridae	Mumps virus Measles virus Parainfluenza virus Respiratory syncytial virus	Enveloped	Yes	Helical	Linear, single stranded, nonsegmented
Rhabdoviridae	Rabies virus Vesicular stomatitis virus	Enveloped	Yes	Helical	Linear, single stranded, nonsegmented
Filoviridae	Ebola virus Marburg virus	Enveloped	Yes	Helical	Linear, single stranded, nonsegmented
Orthomyxoviridae	Influenza viruses	Enveloped	Yes	Helical	Linear, single stranded, eight segments
Bunyaviridae	California encephalitis virus Hantavirus	Enveloped	Yes	Helical	Circular, single stranded, three segments
Unclassified (genus: delta virus)	Hepatitis D virus	Naked	No	Helical	Circular, single stranded

    (2) Cause **mosquito-borne encephalitis (California and LaCrosse encephalitis viruses); sand-fly and mosquito-borne fever (sandfly fever virus and Rift Valley fever virus); rodent-borne hemorrhagic fever (Hantaan virus); and respiratory distress syndrome (Hantavirus).**

    (3) **Hantavirus (Sin Nombre virus) causes an acute, potentially fatal, pulmonary syndrome** initiated by inhaling the virus contained in dried deer mouse saliva, urine, or feces.

2. Orthomyxoviruses (influenza):

  a. General characteristics:

    (1) **Description: enveloped,** spherical or filamentous viruses with **eight helical nucleocapsids** containing a unique single-stranded, **negative-sense RNA.**

    (2) **Components:** have a **hemagglutinin (H),** a **neuraminidase (N),** a **matrix protein (M)** associated with the envelope, a **transcriptase (P)** that is associated with the nucleocapsid, and a **nucleoprotein (NP)** associated with the RNA.

      (a) **Influenza virus hemagglutinin:**

        1. This **envelope glycoprotein contains a virus receptor that binds to the cellular receptor site.** Agglutinates many species of red blood cells.

        2. It induces neutralizing antibodies and has fusion activity that allows the virion envelope to fuse with the host-cell plasma membranes.

        3. Antigenic changes are **responsible for influenza epidemics.** Frequent minor mutations result in antigenic changes, leading to **antigenic drift**; major antigenic changes resulting from reassortment between the hemagglutinin-coding RNA segments of animal or human viruses (see Fig. 5.2) cause **antigenic shift.**

      (b) **Influenza virus neuraminidase:**

        1. This envelope glycoprotein removes terminal sialic acid residues from oligosaccharide chains, resulting in less viscous mucous secretions, thereby facilitating virus spread.

        2. It is involved in the release of virions from infected cells.

        3. It can undergo antigenic shift and drift mutations; however, epidemics do not result from these changes.

        4. Its activity is **inhibited by the antivirals oseltamivir and zanamivir.**

  b. Influenza virus M2 protein:

    (1) This protein forms a proton channel during replication that **facilitates uncoating** and is rendered nonfunctional in influenza A virus infections by the antivirals amantadine and rimantadine.

(2) They are assembled in the cytoplasm but **have a nuclear phase since they depend on host nuclear functions,** including RNA polymerase II, for transcription.

(3) Classification:

  (a) Are classified as type A, B, or C, depending on a nucleocapsid antigen; A is the only one infecting both animals and humans.

  (b) Are designated by the nomenclature, which indicates virus type, species isolated from (unless human), site of isolation, strain number, year of isolation, and hemagglutinin and neuraminidase subtype; for example, A/swine/NewJersey/8/76 (H1N1) and A/Phillippines/2/82 (H3N2).

c. Influenza is a localized infection of the respiratory tract that may result in **pandemics** due to reassortment of the hemagglutinin.

d. Avian flu is a contagious disease of animals caused by influenza A viruses that normally infect birds and occasionally pigs, but have rarely crossed species lines to infect humans.

  (1) It is caused by influenza A viruses with H_5 or H_7 hemagglutinins.

  (2) Prevention: may be prevented with a vaccine containing an inactivated reassortment strain of an H5N1 avian virus.

3. Paramyxoviruses:

a. General characteristics:

  (1) Description: spherical, enveloped viruses with a **single helical nucleocapsid** containing **single-stranded, negative-sense RNA;** exist in few antigenic types.

  (2) Components: have a **hemagglutinin-neuraminidase (HN), a fusion protein (F), a matrix protein (M) associated with the envelope, and a nucleocapsid-associated transcriptase (P).**

    (a) Paramyxovirus HN:

      1. This large surface glycoprotein has both hemagglutinating and neuraminidase activity, except in measles virus, which lacks neuraminidase activity, and in RSV, in which both activities have been lost.

      2. HN **is responsible for virus adsorption.**

      3. It stimulates the production of neutralizing antibodies.

    (b) Paramyxovirus fusion protein:

      1. This surface glycoprotein has fusion and hemolysin activities, except in RSV, in which hemolysis activity is lost.

      2. It is **responsible for virus penetration into the cell.**

  (3) Replication: replicate in the cytoplasm of the cell.

  (4) Clinical disease: cause acute and persistent infections.

  (5) Classification: divided into three genera on the basis of chemical and biologic properties: **paramyxoviruses (parainfluenza and mumps viruses), morbilliviruses (measles virus), and pneumoviruses (RSV and metapneumovirus).**

b. Parainfluenza viruses:

  (1) Classification: exist in four serotypes.

  (2) Clinical disease: cause a **variety of fall and winter upper and lower respiratory tract illnesses; croup** (type 2 virus) is a well-known infant disease.

  (3) Diagnosis: may be diagnosed using fluorescent antibody (FA) techniques on nasopharyngeal washes or swab to detect viral antigens.

c. Mumps virus:

  (1) Classification: exists in **one serotype.**

  (2) Clinical disease: often causes asymptomatic infections, but can cause a generalized disease involving enlargement of the parotid glands.

  (3) Diagnosis: usually diagnosed clinically.

  (4) Prevention: Infections are inhibited by a **live attenuated vaccine containing the Jeryl Lynn strain of virus** (usually included with live attenuated measles and rubella virus strains).

d. Measles virus:

  (1) Description: exists in **one serotype.**

  (2) Components: has hemagglutinin, but no neuraminidase activity (H protein rather than HN protein).

  (3) Pathobiology: uses the CD46 molecules as its cellular receptor.

(4) Replication: frequently **forms giant multinucleated cells (syncytia)** as part of its replication process (called **Warthin-Finkeldey cells in nasal secretions**).

(5) Clinical disease: causes an acute generalized disease characterized by a maculopapular rash, fever, respiratory distress, and Koplik's spots on the buccal mucosa.

(6) Prevention: infections can be prevented by a **live attenuated measles vaccine (Moraten strain)** that is part of the trivalent (measles, mumps, and rubella) vaccine given to children.

   e. Respiratory syncytial virus:

   (1) Description: exists in **one serotype.**

   (2) Components: has only hemagglutinin activity (H protein), no neuraminidase activity.

   (3) Replication: induces syncytia formation during replication.

   (4) Clinical disease: causes a **potentially serious respiratory tract pathogen of infants.**

   (5) Diagnosis: diagnosed by enzyme immunoassay (EIA) for viral antigens in nasopharyngeal washes.

   f. Human metapneumovirus (hMNV) is a newly discovered virus that causes bronchiolitis and pneumonia in infants and lower respiratory tract infection in the elderly.

   g. Newcastle disease virus:

   (1) Description: natural respiratory tract pathogen of birds, particularly chickens.

   (2) Clinical disease: causes an **occupational disease of poultry workers** presenting as a mild conjunctivitis without corneal involvement.

4. Rhabdoviruses:

   a. General characteristics:

   (1) Description: enveloped, bullet-shaped viruses with a **helical nucleocapsid** containing **single-stranded, negative-sense RNA.**

   (2) Replication: have a **virion-associated transcriptase** and replicate in the cytoplasm.

   (3) Classification: includes the human pathogen rabies virus and the bovine pathogen vesicular stomatitis virus.

   b. Rabies virus:

   (1) Replication: has a virion-associated transcriptase or replicase.

   (2) Cytopathology: produces specific **cytoplasmic inclusion bodies, called Negri bodies,** in infected cells.

   (3) Pathobiology:

   (a) Uses acetylcholine receptors on muscle cells to initiate infection.

   (b) Has a **predilection for the hippocampus (Ammon's horn cells).**

   (c) Can travel throughout the nervous system in nerve fibers.

   (4) Clinical disease:

   (a) Produces disease after inoculation by an animal bite (**zoonotic disease**) or, occasionally, inhalation.

   (b) Causes fatal disease unless the infected person previously received immunization or receives postexposure prophylaxis consisting of passive immunization with human rabies immune globulin and immunization with a vaccine.

   (5) Diagnosis: identified in suspected tissues by a direct immunofluorescent test for viral antigens.

   (6) Treatment and prevention:

   (a) Grown in human MRC-5 diploid cell cultures (Pitman-Moore strain of virus) before inactivation and used in active immunization.

   (b) Has been grown (Flury LEP strain) in primary chicken fibroblasts before inactivation and inclusion in a PCEC (purified chick embryo cell culture) vaccine used for postexposure vaccination.

   (c) Has been attenuated by growth in a chick embryo for use as an animal, not human, vaccine (Flury vaccine).

5. Filoviruses:

   a. Classification: include Marburg and Ebola viruses.

   b. Description: enveloped viruses with a **helical nucleocapsid** containing **single-stranded, negative-sense RNA.**

   c. Clinical disease: cause African hemorrhagic fevers, which then lead to death.

table 5.9   Virion and Nucleic Acid Structure of Other RNA Viruses

Virus Family	Prominent Example	Virion Structure	Virion Polymerase	Capsid Symmetry	RNA Structure
Arenaviridae	Lassa fever virus Lymphocytic choriomeningitis virus	Enveloped	Yes	Helical	Circular, single stranded, two ambisense segments
Reoviridae	Colorado tick fever virus: Reoviruses Rotaviruses	Naked	Yes	Icosahedral	Linear, double stranded, 10 to 12 segments

C. Ambisense viruses: arenaviruses (Table 5.9).

 1. **Description: enveloped viruses** with **two string-of-beads nucleocapsids, each containing a unique single-stranded, circular RNA.**
 2. **Genome:** have two molecules (L, or large, and S, or small) of single-stranded, ambisense RNA.
 3. **Replication:** replicate in the cytoplasm and **have host-cell ribosomes in their virion.**
 4. **Clinical disease:**
    a. Infect mice, rats, or both as their natural hosts; are initially passed from rodents to humans but can be transferred by direct human contact.
    b. Cause highly contagious hemorrhagic fevers (Junin, Machupo, and Lassa viruses) that are not endemic to the United States and a meningitis or finlike illness (**lymphocytic choriomeningitis virus**) that is endemic.

D. Double-stranded RNA viruses.

 1. **Reoviruses (see Table 5.9):**
    a. **General characteristics:**
       (1) **Description: naked** viruses with a **double-shelled (outer shell and core) icosahedral capsid containing 10, 11, or 12 segments of double-stranded RNA.**
       (2) **Replication:** replicate in the cytoplasm; have a **core-associated transcriptase or replicase.**
       (3) **Classification:** classified into five groups; reoviruses, orthoreoviruses, rotaviruses, orbiviruses, and coltiviruses have strains that infect humans.
    b. **Coltiviruses:**
       (1) **Genome:** have **12 segments of double-stranded RNA.**
       (2) **Clinical disease:**
          (a) Infect insects, which transfer the virus to humans.
          (b) Cause mild fevers in humans.
          (c) Represented by **Colorado tick fever virus,** which is carried by the wood tick *Dermacentor andersoni.*
    c. **Orthoreoviruses:**
       (1) **Genome:** have **10 segments of double-stranded RNA.**
       (2) **Components:** have an outer shell-associated hemagglutinin (d 1) that agglutinates human or bovine erythrocytes; is the viral receptor, therefore determining tissue tropism and is the determinant for the three serotypes of reoviruses.
       (3) **Clinical disease:** produce minor upper respiratory tract infections and gastrointestinal disease, but also are frequently recovered from healthy people.
       (4) **Diagnosis:** may be diagnosed by ELISA for viral antigens in clinical specimens.
    d. **Rotaviruses:**
       (1) **Genome:** have **11 segments of double-stranded RNA;** virion has wheel-and-spoke morphology.
       (2) **Classification:** exist in at least **seven serotypes, with type A being involved in most human infections.**
       (3) **Clinical disease:** cause infantile diarrhea and are the most common cause of gastroenteritis in children; are frequent causes of **nosocomial infections.**

   (4) Diagnosis: diagnosed by demonstrating virus in the stool or by serologic tests, particularly ELISA.

   (5) Prevention: have been modified and genetically manipulated for preparation of live attenuated vaccines **(RotaTeq and Rotarix)**.

   e. Orbiviruses:

   (1) Description: arboviruses, transmitted by biting flies, mosquitoes, or ticks.

   (2) Genome: contain **10 segments of double-stranded RNA.**

   (3) Classification: classified into 14 serotypes, four cause human disease.

   (4) Clinical disease: basically a domestic animal disease, but may cause a febrile illness and occasionally encephalitis in humans in Africa, Central America, Russia, and Eastern Europe.

E. Viroid-like agents: hepatitis D virus (delta-associated virus).

   1. Description: virus with **circular, single-stranded RNA molecules (viroid-like) and an internal core δ antigen surrounded by an HBV envelope.**

   2. Replication: is **defective** and can replicate only in the presence of HBV.

   3. Clinical disease: is associated with both acute and chronic hepatitis and always with HBV; causes more severe hepatitis than does HBV alone.

   4. Diagnosis: may be diagnosed serologically with an ELISA test.

X. SLOW VIRUSES AND PRIONS

A. Subacute sclerosing panencephalitis virus.

   1. Description: variant or close **relative of measles virus**.

   2. Clinical disease: causes **subacute sclerosing panencephalitis,** a rare, fatal, slowly progressive demyelinating CNS disease of teenagers and young adults; may result from improper synthesis or processing of the matrix (M) viral protein.

B. JC virus.

   1. Description: a **papovavirus** that frequently infects humans but rarely produces disease unless the host is immunosuppressed.

   2. Clinical disease:

   a. Has been isolated from patients with **progressive multifocal leukoencephalopathy,** a rare CNS disease.

   b. Causes demyelination by infecting and killing oligodendrocytes.

C. Animal lentiviruses.

   1. Description: retroviruses that cause slow, generalized infections of sheep (**visna** and **progressive pneumonia virus**) and goats (**caprine arthritis virus**); undergo considerable **antigenic variation** in their host due to mutations in envelope glycoproteins.

   2. Replication: produce minimal amounts of infective viruses in their hosts.

D. Prions.

   1. Description:

   a. Not viruses but are **proteinaceous material lacking nucleic acid** that may be acquired or inherited and **is identical or closely related to a 30 to 35 kDa host membrane glycoprotein (PrPᶜ).**

   b. PrPᶜ can undergo a change in its tertiary structure (e.g., the PrP of scrapie [PrPˢᶜ] that causes an aggregation of itself and PrPᶜ on neuronal cell surfaces); the aggregates (amyloid) are released and cause slow diseases called spongiform encephalopathies.

   2. Clinical disease: associated with several degenerative CNS diseases (subacute spongiform virus encephalopathies): kuru and Creutzfeldt-Jakob disease of humans, scrapie of sheep, bovine spongiform encephalopathy (or mad cow disease), and transmissible encephalopathy of mink.

XI. ONCOGENIC VIRUSES

A. **General characteristics:**
  1. Oncogenic viruses **cause cancers** when they infect appropriate animals. They are classified as DNA or RNA tumor viruses.
  2. **Pathobiology:**
     a. Oncogenic viruses **transform infected cells** by altering cell growth, cell-surface antigens, and biochemical processes.
     b. When they enter cells, these viruses introduce "transforming'" genes or induce expression of quiescent cellular genes, which results in the **synthesis of one or more transforming proteins.**
     c. The RNA viral genome is converted to DNA by reverse transcriptase and integrated into the host-cell chromosome, forming a **provirus.**

B. **DNA tumor viruses.**
  1. **General characteristics:**
     a. Cause **transformation** in **nonpermissive cells** (infected cells that do not support total virus replication).
     b. **Classification:**
        (1) Human viruses include human papillomaviruses: adenoviruses, HBV, EBV, molluscum contagiosum virus, JC and BK viruses, and possibly HSV-2.
        (2) Animal viruses include chicken **Marek's disease virus** (a herpesvirus), mouse **polyomavirus** (a papovavirus), and monkey SV40 virus (a papovavirus).
     c. Protein products of some DNA tumor viruses (e.g., adenovirus, papillomavirus, and polyomavirus) interact with cellular **tumor suppressor gene products** that suppress oncogene expression.
  2. **SV40 virus:**
     a. **Replication:** undergoes productive replication in monkey cells but transforms nonpermissive hamster and mouse cells.
     b. **Pathobiology:**
        (1) Synthesizes an early protein called **large tumor (T) antigen,** which associates with two antioncogene proteins, p53 and $p110^{Rb}$, and the retinoblastoma gene product; establishes and maintains **SV40-induced transformation.**
        (2) Synthesizes two other tumor antigens: middle T and small T antigen.
  3. **Polyomavirus** grows permissively in mouse cells but transforms nonpermissive hamster and rat cells. It synthesizes a **transforming large T antigen.**
  4. **Human adenovirus** may be highly oncogenic (types 12, 18, and 31) or weakly oncogenic (types 3, 7, 14, 16, and 21) when injected into hamsters. It synthesizes an **E1B** protein that binds to cellular p53 and **E1A** protein that binds to cellular $p110^{Rb}$ if highly oncogenic.
  5. **Human papillomavirus** may have a strong association (types 16 and 18) or a moderate association (types 31, 33, 35, 45, 51, 52, and 56) with cervical carcinoma. HPV synthesizes an **E6 protein** that binds to cellular **p53** and **E7 protein** that binds to cellular $p110^{Rb}$.
  6. **EBV** is a cofactor in the etiology of **Burkitt's lymphoma** and **nasopharyngeal carcinoma.** It can immortalize and transform B lymphocytes due to specific EBNA and LMP proteins.
  7. **HBV** is associated with primary hepatocellular carcinoma. It synthesizes an X protein, which binds to cellular p53.

C. **RNA tumor viruses.**
  1. **General characteristics:**
     a. **Description:** retroviruses (oncovirus group); are also called **oncornaviruses.**
     b. **Pathobiology:** infect permissive cells, but transform rather than kill.
     c. **Clinical disease:** cause tumors of the reticuloendothelial and hematopoietic systems (leukemias), connective tissues (sarcomas), or mammary gland.
  2. **Type B tumor viruses** have an eccentric electron-dense core structure in their virion. They are best exemplified by **mouse mammary tumor virus,** also called **Bittner virus.**

3. Type C tumor viruses have electron-dense cores in the center of the virion. They include most RNA tumor viruses.

   a. Genome: may contain a cellular-derived **oncogene** (which codes for a cancer-inducing product) as well as **virogenes** (*gag,* pol, and *env*); however, a few nondefective murine leukosis viruses (AKR and Moloney viruses) and HTLV-1 and -2 lack oncogenes.

     (1) Oncogenes are genes that cause cancer.

       (a) Copies are found in viruses (**v-onc**) and cells (**c-onc** or **proto-oncogene**).

       (b) In normal cells, oncogenes are "switched off" or down-regulated by antioncogene proteins (e.g., p53 and $p110^{Rb}$).

       (c) Their products are essential to normal cell function or development and include:

         1. Tyrosine protein kinases (*src* gene-Rous sarcoma virus, abl gene-Abelson leukemia virus).

         2. Guanine-nucleotide-binding proteins (Ha-*ras*-Harvey sarcoma virus).

         3. Chromatin-binding proteins (*myc*-MC29 myclocytomatosis virus and *fos*-FBJ osteosarcoma virus).

         4. Cellular surface receptors such as epidermal growth factor receptor (*erb*-B product of avian erythroblastosis virus).

         5. Cellular growth factors such as platelet-derived growth factor (SIS gene product of simian sarcoma virus).

   b. Classification: are classified as nondefective or defective based on replicative ability.

     (1) Nondefective viruses:

       (a) Have all their virogenes and can therefore replicate themselves.

       (b) Have high oncogenic potential if they also contain an oncogene (e.g., **Rous chicken sarcoma virus**).

       (c) Have low oncogenic potential if they do not have an oncogene (e.g., **AKR** and **Moloney murine leukemia viruses** and **human T-cell leukemia viruses [HTLV]-1 and -2**).

     (2) Defective viruses:

       (a) Have a virogene or part of a virogene replaced by an oncogene.

       (b) Need **helper viruses** to provide missing virogene products for replication.

       (c) Have high oncogenic potential, for example, murine sarcoma viruses (**Kirsten** and **Harvey viruses**) and murine leukemia viruses (**Friend** and **Abelson viruses**).

4. HTLV-1 and -2:

   a. Are nondefective human retroviruses with no identifiable oncogene that transform T4 antigen-positive cells.

   b. Are associated with **human adult acute T-cell lymphocytic leukemia** and tropical spastic paraparesis (HTLV-1) and some forms of **hairy cell leukemia** (HTLV-2).

Review Test

1. Clinical viral disease

(A) Is most frequently due to toxin production
(B) Usually follows virus infection
(C) Can result without infection of host cells
(D) Is associated with target organs in most disseminated viral infections

2. The eclipse period of a one-step viral multiplication curve is defined as the period of time between the

(A) Uncoating and assembly of the virus
(B) Start of the infection and the first appearance of extracellular virus
(C) Start of the infection and the first appearance of intracellular virus
(D) Start of the infection and uncoating of the virus

3. HTLVs

(A) Are associated with leukemias
(B) Are defective RNA tumor viruses
(C) Carry tyrosine protein kinase oncogenes
(D) Synthesize early proteins that interact with p53 Rb

4. Amantadine inhibits

(A) Influenza A and B virus hemagglutinin binding activity
(B) Influenza A virus M2 protein activity
(C) Influenza A and B virus neuraminidase activity
(D) Influenza B virus RNA-dependent RNA polymerase activity

5. Passive immunization is available for protection from

(A) Influenza A virus
(B) Hepatitis A virus
(C) Parainfluenza type 2 virus
(D) Rubella virus

6. Linear, single-stranded DNA is the genetic material of

(A) Caliciviruses
(B) Flaviviruses
(C) Papillomaviruses
(D) Parvoviruses

7. Host-cell tRNAs are involved in the genome replication of

(A) Influenza A virus
(B) Retroviruses
(C) Respiratory syncytial virus
(D) Rhinovirus

8. An RNA virus that has a nuclear phase to its replication process is

(A) Coronavirus
(B) Rhabdovirus
(C) Retrovirus
(D) Togavirus

9. Negri bodies are associated with

(A) Cytomegalovirus infections
(B) Herpes simplex virus infections
(C) Rabies virus infections
(D) Rubella virus infections

10. Persistent virus infections

(A) Are usually confined to the initial site of infection
(B) Are preceded by acute clinical disease
(C) Elicit a poor antibody response
(D) May involve infected carrier individuals

11. A killed virus vaccine is

(A) Jeryl Lynn mumps vaccine
(B) Enders measles vaccine
(C) Salk poliovirus vaccine
(D) Oka varicella-zoster vaccine

12. The first viral-induced defense mechanism in a nonimmune individual is the

(A) Generation of cytotoxic T lymphocytes
(B) Production of interferon
(C) Synthesis of lymphokines
(D) Synthesis of neutralizing antibodies

13. Localized viral disease

(A) Is a major feature of congenital viral infections
(B) Is associated with a pronounced viremia
(C) Can be associated with carrier individuals
(D) May have systemic clinical features such as fever

14. Lymphotropic and macrophage trophic designation is important in the pathogenesis of

(A) Cytomegalovirus
(B) Herpes simplex virus
(C) Human immunodeficiency virus
(D) JC virus

15. Viral oncogenes are present in

(A) JC virus
(B) Human T-cell lymphotropic virus type 1
(C) Rous sarcoma virus
(D) Simian virus 40

16. Dane particles are associated with

(A) Hepatitis A virus
(B) Hepatitis B virus
(C) Hepatitis C virus
(D) Hepatitis E virus

17. The exchange of homologous segments of RNA between two different influenza type A viruses is called

(A) Complementation
(B) Genetic reassortment
(C) Phenotypic masking
(D) Phenotypic mixing

18. The Monospot test is based on

(A) Destruction of Downey cells
(B) Heterophile antibodies
(C) Syncytia inhibition
(D) Viral capsid antigen antibodies

19. Disinfection of day care center play tables with 70% ethanol is least likely to affect the viability of

(A) Cytomegalovirus
(B) Parainfluenza virus
(C) Respiratory syncytial virus
(D) Rotavirus

20. The nanogram level of antigen in serum is detected by

(A) Dot blot tests
(B) Enzyme-linked immunosorbent assay
(C) Fluorescent antibody staining
(D) Protein-protein hybridization tests

21. A virus that infects and lyses progenitor erythroid cells causing aplastic crises in patients with hemolytic anemia is

(A) California encephalitis virus
(B) Epstein-Barr virus
(C) Parvovirus B19
(D) Yellow fever virus

22. A viral protein that is thought to induce tumors by binding to a cellular tumor suppressor protein is

(A) Adenovirus E1A
(B) Epstein-Barr nuclear antigen proteins
(C) Hepatitis B virus e protein
(D) Human immunodeficiency virus *gag* protein

23. Viruses whose genomes have a messenger (positive-sense) polarity are

(A) Adenoviruses
(B) Papovaviruses
(C) Paramyxoviruses
(D) Polioviruses

24. Antiviral nucleoside analogs

(A) Are effective only against replicating viruses
(B) Include foscarnet
(C) Inhibit replicases
(D) May block viral penetration

25. A commercial vaccine consisting of virion subunits prepared by recombinant technology exists for

(A) Hepatitis B virus
(B) Rabies virus
(C) Rotavirus
(D) Varicella-zoster virus

Answers and Explanations

1. **The answer is D.** Many viral infections are asymptomatic or subclinical. Clinical disease, however, is often associated with viral replication in target organs during disseminated viral infections.

2. **The answer is C.** The period of time between the adsorption and penetration of the virus until the first appearance of intracellular virus is the eclipse phase.

3. **The answer is A.** Human T-lymphotropic virus type 1 (HTLV-1) is associated with adult T-cell leukemia; HTLV-2 is implicated in human hairy cell leukemia.

4. **The answer is B.** Amantadine binds to the M2 protein of influenza A virus, which inhibits this ion pore and prevents uncoating of the virus.

5. **The answer is B.** A commercially available human immune globulin preparation is available for pre-exposure and postexposure prophylaxis for hepatitis A virus.

6. **The answer is D.** Parvoviruses have linear, single-stranded DNA, while papovaviruses have circular, double-stranded DNA. Caliciviruses and flaviviruses are RNA viruses.

7. **The answer is B.** Host-cell tRNAs act as primers for the synthesis of retrovirus DNA by reverse transcriptase.

8. **The answer is C.** The reverse transcriptase of retroviruses makes a DNA copy of the genomic RNA. This DNA must be integrated into the host-cell DNA in the nucleus for the remaining steps in the replication process to occur.

9. **The answer is C.** Negri bodies are intracytoplasmic inclusion bodies found in rabies virus-infected neurons and are important in the diagnosis of infected animals.

10. **The answer is D.** Some persistent virus infections, such as serum hepatitis caused by hepatitis B virus, involve carrier individuals who may or may not have clinical signs of the disease.

11. **The answer is C.** Although many of the childhood vaccines like measles, mumps, and chickenpox contain live, attenuated virus, the Salk poliovirus vaccine contains killed virus.

12. **The answer is B.** The production of interferons that induce the synthesis of antiviral replication proteins in neighboring cells occurs before the appearance of any other viral-induced immune defense mechanisms.

13. **The answer is D.** Although localized infections are not associated with pronounced viremia, they can have clinical features similar to viremic systemic infections.

14. **The answer is C.** Strains of human immunodeficiency virus are classified as lymphotropic or macrophage trophic depending on their preferred site of latency.

15. **The answer is C.** Viral oncogenes are found in many RNA tumor viruses. Both Rous sarcoma virus and human T-cell lymphotropic virus type 1 are RNA tumor viruses, but only Rous sarcoma virus carries an oncogene (*v-src*).

16. **The answer is B.** The spherical virion of hepatitis B virus is called the Dane particle.

17. **The answer is B.** Genetic reassortment is the name given to the process whereby homologous pieces of RNA are exchanged between two different strains of influenza viruses replicating in the cell.

18. **The answer is B.** IgM antibody produced in response to most Epstein-Barr virus infections agglutinates sheep and beef erythrocytes and forms the basis for the Monospot test used in diagnosing infectious mononucleosis caused by EBV.

19. The answer is D. Since rotavirus is a naked virus, it is least susceptible to inactivation by 70% alcohol, a lipid solvent disrupting the envelope of the three enveloped viruses.

20. The answer is B. Enzyme-linked immunosorbent assay (ELISA) is the most sensitive method of detecting antigens in the serum.

21. The answer is C. The target cells of human parvovirus B19 are progenitor erythroid cells; infections in patients with hemolytic anemia can be serious.

22. The answer is A. In permissive cells, adenovirus E1A protein is involved in the replication process, but in nonpermissive cells it can bind to cellular tumor suppressor protein p110Rb and inactivate its normal cellular function, which results in cellular transformation.

23. The answer is D. The genetic material of poliovirus is single-stranded RNA, which can be translated into a large polyprotein that is subsequently cleaved into the individual viral proteins.

24. The answer is A. Nucleoside analogs inhibit viral replication by inhibiting viral DNA synthesis or function; they do not affect RNA replicases or block penetration.

25. The answer is A. Both the Recombivax-HB and Engerix-B vaccines for protection from hepatitis B virus contain the virus surface antigen prepared from yeast using recombinant DNA technology.

chapter 6

System-Based and Situational Viral Infections

In this chapter, the diseases associated with viral infections are divided into three categories: system based, location based, or situation based. The majority of the information for a specific virus is found under the system- or situation-based disease section with which it is most closely associated. Viruses causing clinical signs and symptoms within more than one system or situation are noted in all sections, but only important aspects of virus interactions relevant to that occasion are noted. Treatment for viral infections is supportive unless noted. The viruses listed under each heading are the most prominent ones; comprehensive lists are found in virology infectious disease textbooks.

SYSTEM-BASED DISEASE

I. EYE INFECTIONS

Viruses are the most common cause of conjunctivitis. Adenovirus and enterovirus are the most common and are highly contagious. These infections are usually self-limiting and resolve in 1 to 3 weeks. Herpes simplex viruses (HSV) and varicella zoster virus (VZV) infections are rare but more serious.

A. **Adenoviruses.**
1. Adenoviruses are involved in respiratory tract infections but can cause a conjunctivitis known as **pinkeye,** which resolves spontaneously in a few days.
2. They can cause a serious **epidemic keratoconjunctivitis,** which may be transmitted by contaminated ophthalmologic instruments.

B. **Enterovirus type 70** is associated with a hemorrhagic conjunctivitis.

C. **Herpes simplex virus.**
1. **HSV** can produce a **conjunctivitis** that may progress to a **keratitis** involving the formation of a **dendritic ulcer,** which, if untreated, can lead to visual impairment; it may cause a neonatal conjunctivitis originating from an infected birth canal.
2. **Treatment:** treated with topical acyclovir.

D. **VZV** is estimated to cause **conjunctivitis** in 4% of chickenpox cases; it may reactivate in the ophthalmic branch of the trigeminal nerve to cause **herpes zoster ophthalmicus.**

II. EAR INFECTIONS

Viral upper respiratory tract infections that cause colds and pharyngitis often lead to otitis media and sinusitis. Common respiratory viruses like **rhinovirus, respiratory syncytial virus (RSV),** and **adenoviruses** may cause 50% of these infections.

III. UPPER RESPIRATORY TRACT (MOUTH AND THROAT) INFECTIONS

Viral diseases included here range from infections largely confined to the mouth (herpangina) and nose and throat (colds) to systemic infections with pharyngitis as a major symptom (infectious mononucleosis). Many viruses whose prominent clinical symptoms originate farther down the respiratory tract (RSV and influenza viruses) begin their infectious process in the mouth and throat.

A. **Coxsackie A viruses** are members of the enterovirus genera of the Picornavirus family. These viruses cause:
   1. **Herpangina,** a disease characterized by sudden fever, sore throat, vomiting, and discrete vesiculopapular lesions on the tongue, tonsils, and the roof of the mouth.
   2. **Hand, foot, and mouth disease,** a febrile illness producing vesicular lesions or blisters on the palate, hands, and feet. Coxsackie A 16 is the usual cause.

B. **Herpes simplex viruses (HSV-1 and -2).**
   1. These viruses may cause a clinically apparent primary infection (e.g., **gingivostomatitis** by HSV-1 in children and HSV-2 in young adults) or recurrent infection (e.g., **cold sores**).
   2. Progression to a severe, fatal encephalitis (HSV-1) or meningitis (HSV-2) can occur.
   3. Virus latently infects neurons and may be reactivated to travel to peripheral tissue by physical or emotional stress, or immune suppression.
   4. **Diagnosis:** cause vesicular lesions with an erythematous base that contain cytopathology visualized by a **Tzanck smear** for rapid identification of the virus.
   5. **Treatment:** can be treated by acyclovir, penciclovir, famciclovir, or valacyclovir, but drug-resistant strains can arise; the virus is **not eliminated by treatment once latency has been established.**

C. **Epstein-Barr virus (EBV)** usually causes a clinically inapparent systemic infection but may cause infectious mononucleosis and is associated with Burkitt's lymphoma and nasopharyngeal carcinoma.
   1. **Infectious mononucleosis:**
      a. This **systemic disease** of children and young adults (sometimes called the kissing disease) is characterized by sore throat, fever, enlarged lymph nodes and spleen, and sometimes hepatitis.
      b. **Diagnosis:**
         (1) Associated with the production of atypical reactive T lymphocytes (**Downey cells**) and **IgM heterophile antibodies** (IgM interacts with Paul-Bunnell antigen on sheep, horse, or bovine erythrocytes, causing agglutination) and may be identified by the **Monospot test.**
         (2) Can also be diagnosed by serologic tests involving immunofluorescence procedures on fixed EBV-producing cells or enzyme-linked immunosorbent assay (ELISA) tests.
   2. Burkitt's lymphoma and nasopharyngeal carcinoma is characterized by cells that express EBV nuclear antigen (EBNAs) and latent membrane protein (LMPs) and carry multiple copies of viral DNA.

D. **Cytomegalovirus (CMV)** usually causes an asymptomatic infection in children and adults. It causes approximately 10% of mononucleosis cases that are clinically similar to those caused by EBV except that no heterophile antibodies are produced.

E. **Rhinoviruses.**
   1. These viruses are the most frequent cause of the **common cold.**
   2. **Treatment and prevention:**
      a. Because there are more than 100 serotypes, a vaccine is improbable.
      b. Rhinoviruses can be inhibited with **pleconaril** (not FDA approved), which binds to capsid and prevents uncoating.

F. **Coronaviruses** cause 5% to 10% of colds (second to rhinoviruses); a recently identified strain (SARS-CoV) causes a serious lower respiratory tract disease.

G. **Adenoviruses.**
   1. Respiratory diseases caused by adenoviruses range from acute febrile pharyngitis to **pharyngoconjunctival fever** and occasionally acute pneumonia (types 4 and 7).
   2. Adenoviruses may contaminate swimming pools and lead to pharyngoconjunctival fever.
   3. They may cause latent infections of human tonsils.

H. **Enteroviruses.**
   1. Several groups including Coxsackie viruses and echoviruses can cause **summer and autumn epidemics of pharyngitis.**
   2. Enteroviruses that are also involved in pharyngitis are not identified, although rapid diagnosis by reverse transcription-polymerase chain reaction (RT-PCR) is available.

I. **Parainfluenza and respiratory syncytial viruses** can cause mild upper respiratory tract infections similar to colds, but are more noted for diseases farther down the respiratory tract.

J. **Human papillomaviruses (HPV)** can cause **laryngeal papillomas** or warts.

IV. LOWER RESPIRATORY TRACT INFECTIONS

Many of these diseases are manifestations of upper respiratory viruses' progression down the respiratory tract. They include some notable childhood infections like croup and some serious interstitial viral pneumonias that set up in the lungs for secondary bacterial infection. Viral pneumonias are classified as atypical pneumonias. Coxsackie B virus causing pleurodynia is also included here.

A. **Parainfluenza viruses.**
   1. These viruses cause the following diseases:
      a. **Laryngotracheobronchitis,** called **croup,** that usually occurs in the fall in 2- to 5-year-old children and is characterized by a **distinctive "barking" cough.**
      b. **Pneumonia in infants and elderly and nosocomial disease** in facilities dedicated to these groups.
   2. **Diagnosis:** rapidly diagnosed by detection of viral antigens in nasopharyngeal washings or swabs by immunofluorescent techniques.

B. **Respiratory syncytial virus.**
   1. RSV is the **most important infant respiratory virus.**
   2. It causes **75% to 80% of bronchiolitis cases, 70% of which** progress to pneumonia.
   3. Serious disease occurs in premature infants, elderly, and immunosuppressed people.
   4. It is a frequent cause of **nosocomial infections.**

5. **Diagnosis:** may be diagnosed by several laboratory techniques including immunofluorescent and enzyme immunoassays for viral antigens in nasopharyngeal washings or swabs.

6. **Treatment:** may be treated with **ribavirin** aerosols in severe cases; high-risk children and infants treated prophylactically with **RSV-IGIV (RespiGam) or palivizumab (Synagis).**

C. **Influenza.**
   1. Influenza is a localized infection of the respiratory tract with symptoms ranging from a mild rhinotracheitis to a fatal pneumonia.
      a. In healthy individuals, influenza is usually not serious; in the elderly or in patients with a secondary bacterial pneumonia, it may cause serious complications.
      b. It may rarely progress to encephalitis a few weeks postinfection.
      c. It is associated with Guillain-Barré syndrome (influenza virus types A and B) and Reye's syndrome (influenza virus type B).
   2. **Pandemics may result due to reassortment of the hemagglutinin.**
   3. **Diagnosis:** can be diagnosed by enzyme immunoassay (EIA), direct immunofluorescence, or RT-PCR of respiratory secretions or serologically.
   4. **Prevention:** may be prevented by either an **inactivated trivalent vaccine** (whole, split, and subunit vaccines exist) or a **live attenuated trivalent vaccine** containing recent A/H_1N_1 A/H_3N_2, and B strains.
   5. **Treatment:** may be prevented chemoprophylactically and treated (both A and B strains) by administration of **zanamivir** or **oseltamivir** (viral neuraminidase inhibitors); amantadine and rimantadine (M2 ion channel inhibitors) are no longer recommended for treatment of influenza A and are ineffective against influenza B.

D. **Adenoviruses.**
   1. These viruses are associated with acute respiratory disease (**ARD**), a term referring to certain clinical signs, symptoms, and pathology in military recruits.
   2. Adenovirus types 4 and 7 are used in an oral bivalent vaccine that is administered to prevent ARD in the military.

E. **Hantavirus (Sin Nombre virus).**
   1. Hantavirus causes a pulmonary disease that starts with flulike symptoms and leads to interstitial pulmonary edema and respiratory failure (**hantavirus pulmonary syndrome**).
   2. It is transmitted by infected rodent urine and feces to humans.

F. **SARS coronavirus (SARS-CoV)** causes a severe acute respiratory syndrome (**SARS**) last reported in Asia in April 2004.

G. **Human metapneumovirus (hMPV)** is a recently discovered virus causing bronchiolitis and pneumonia in infants and lower respiratory tract disease in the elderly. It may also cause winter epidemics and is a possible nosocomial disease.

H. **Coxsackie B virus** causes **epidemic pleurodynia (Bornholm disease)** characterized by sudden onset of severe paroxysmal chest pain, fever, headache, and fatigue. It is more likely to occur in teenagers and young adults.

V. GASTROINTESTINAL INFECTIONS

Viruses have been estimated to cause **two-thirds of all infective diarrheas.** Viral gastroenteritis is the second most common viral illness after upper respiratory infections. They are clinically similar (vomiting, fever, abdominal pain, and watery diarrhea) to some bacterial gastroenteritis, but no blood or pus appears in the stool.

A. **Rotaviruses** account for 50% to 80% of all cases of **viral gastroenteritis,** with more severe symptoms in **neonates and infants** and asymptomatic infections in older children and adults.
  1. It also causes **possible nosocomial disease** and outbreaks in day care centers.
  2. When infection occurs in malnourished children, the mortality rate is 30%.
  3. **Diagnosis:** usually diagnosed by EIA for rotavirus antigens in the feces.
  4. **Prevention:** have been genetically manipulated and attenuated to prepare two live, oral vaccines.
     a. **Rotarix vaccine** contains attenuated subtypes G1, 3, 4, and 9 human viruses.
     b. **RotaTeq vaccine** contains five reassortment viruses with WC3 bovine parent and G1, G2, G3, G4, and PL human VP7 outer protein subtypes.

B. **Adenoviruses** are the second most common cause of gastroenteritis in neonates and young children. They may be associated with small outbreaks.

C. **Astroviruses** produce a disease similar to rotaviruses, as well as adenoviruses in neonates and young children.

D. **Noroviruses (Norwalk and similar viruses)** cause **gastroenteritis associated with contaminated water or shellfish and other food in adults and school-age children.**
  1. Infections occur most frequently in contained settings like schools, cruise ships, camps, hospitals, and so forth.
  2. Noroviruses are the cause of **winter vomiting disease,** a disease involving school and family outbreaks.

VI. LIVER INFECTION

Viruses are the major cause of infectious liver disease. The virus may be transmitted enterically, parenterally, or in one case by a mosquito bite. Clinically, the diseases range from asymptomatic or mild to severe acute disease to chronic disease (types B, C, and D). B and C viruses are associated with primary hepatocellular carcinoma. **Acute infections by these viruses cannot be distinguished from each other clinically,** but serum enzyme increases in aspartate aminotransferase (AST) and alanine aminotransferase (ALT) allow differentiation from other liver disease. Vaccines, antivirals, and human gamma globulin preparation are available for protection or treatment of some viruses. Other viruses like **HSV, CMV, EBV, and rubella can cause acute hepatitis as part of their systemic disease.**

A. **Enterically transmitted viruses.**
  1. **Hepatitis A virus (HAV):**
     a. HAV causes **"infectious hepatitis,"** an acute disease that is clinically milder or asymptomatic in young children.
     b. It is transmitted by close personal contact between individuals in places like homes and child day care centers and shed in the feces for 2 weeks before symptoms are apparent.
     c. **Diagnosis:** usually identified by EIA for HAV immunoglobulin M (IgM) or ELISA for HAV antigen in feces.
     d. **Prevention:** inactivated by formalin for inclusion in **Havrix and VAQTA vaccines** that can be used to protect children 12 months or older. Havrix is combined with Energix-B to form **Twinrix** for use in individuals 18 years or older, which protects against HAV and hepatitis B virus (HBV).
  2. **Hepatitis E virus (HEV):**
     a. HEV causes disease in endemic areas (not in the United States) and is transmitted by drinking fecally contaminated drinking water.

   b. It causes a clinical disease similar to HAV but is more severe in pregnant women (15% to 25% mortality rate when a woman is infected during the third trimester).
   c. **Prevention: Genotype 1 recombinant protein vaccine** has been effective in preventing clinical disease.

B. Parenterally transmitted viruses.
   1. Hepatitis B virus:
   a. HBV causes acute clinical disease previously called **serum hepatitis** in approximately 25% of infected individuals. Between 5% to 10% of HBV infections lead to chronic disease; 10% of these individuals develop cirrhosis and permanent liver damage.
   b. **Progression to chronic disease is inversely related to the age of infection** (approximately 90% in infected neonates).
   c. It is transmitted by body fluids (blood, saliva, semen, vaginal secretions, and breast milk) and can be considered a sexually transmitted disease (**STD**); it can be transmitted by asymptomatic **chronic carriers.**
   d. It is associated with the development of **primary hepatocellular carcinoma (PHC).**
   e. Serological markers indicate the course of infection:
      (1) HBeAg—infectious virus and transmissibility
      (2) IgM HBc—recent infection
      (3) IgG HBc—recovery and lifelong immunity
      (4) HBeAg and HBsAg—chronic infection if no antibodies to them are present
   f. **Treatment and prevention:**
      (1) Disease can be prevented by immunization with two recombinant subunit **vaccines (Recombivax HB and Energix-B)** containing HBsAg: one **HAV/HBV combination vaccine (Twinrix** for those 18 years of age or older), and two **pediatric vaccines (Comvax and Pediarix).**
      (2) Chronic infections can be treated with six drugs: standard and pegylated interferon-α and four reverse transcriptase inhibitors (lamivudine, cidofovir, dipivoxil, and entecavir) to improve survival and reduce progression to PHC.
   2. Hepatitis D virus (HDV):
   a. HDV is a **defective virus** that contains the **delta antigen** and requires HBV for replication.
   b. It can cause a **coinfection** (infection by both HBV and HDV in a naive individual) or a **super-infection** (HDV infection of a person chronically infected with HBV).
   c. Coinfection may cause a more severe acute disease than HBV alone but carries a lower risk of chronic infection.
   d. **Superinfection may develop into a chronic infection with a high risk of severe chronic liver disease.**
   e. **Treatment and prevention:** may be treated and prevented using the antivirals and vaccines directed against HBV.
   3. Hepatitis C virus (HCV):
   a. HCV is a common cause of **transfusion and liver transplant-associated hepatitis** if the patient's blood and liver are not prescreened. It can also be considered an **STD** and can be transmitted at birth from a HCV-infected mother.
   b. Acute disease is usually mild or asymptomatic disease, but up to **70% of those infected develop chronic disease.** A high percentage of these individuals have asymptomatic disease that leads to cirrhosis and liver failure or PHC.
   c. RNA levels in the blood are monitored by PCR techniques to diagnose chronic HCV infections and monitor response to antiviral therapy.
   d. **Treatment:** Infections are treated with a combination of subcutaneous pegylated interferons and oral ribavirin, but **only genotypes 2 and 3 of the six genotypes are likely to respond.**

C. Mosquito-transmitted virus: Yellow fever virus.
   1. Yellow fever virus is acquired through the bite of a mosquito; therefore, it is an **arboviral disease.**
   2. It causes an acute disease in Africa and Central and South America.
   3. **Prevention:** may be prevented from causing disease by vaccination with the **live, attenuated vaccine strain 17D** of the virus.

VII. URINARY TRACT INFECTIONS (UTIs)

Viral UTIs are rare, but acute and latent infections occur. Some viral systemic diseases shed virus in the urine during symptoms; for example, CMV in congenitally infected children.

A. **Adenoviruses** cause a **hemorrhagic cystitis** with dysuria and hematuria, predominantly in young boys.

B. **BK virus** causes an asymptomatic infection early in childhood, but establishes a **latent infection** in the kidney and ureter epithelium, which can reactivate during immunosuppression.

VIII. CARDIOVASCULAR INFECTIONS

Viruses are the most common infectious cause of myocarditis and pericarditis. Sore throats, fever, and malaise frequently precede cardiac signs and symptoms. In addition to the following viruses, several viruses causing multisystem infections such as influenza, EBV, mumps, and adenovirus can cause myocarditis as part of other infectious processes. Some arboviruses cause hemorrhagic fevers in endemic areas.

A. **Coxsackie B virus** is the main viral cause of acute infection **myocarditis and pericarditis.**

B. **Other enteroviruses (Coxsackie A and echoviruses)** are less common causes of pericarditis and myocarditis.

C. **Dengue virus and several other arboviruses** can cause **hemorrhagic fever,** occasionally leading to **shock syndrome.**

IX. NERVOUS SYSTEM INFECTIONS

Viruses cause acute, latent, and slow infections of the nervous system. Some acute infections lead to acute postinfection syndromes. Acute disease varies from mild meningitis to fatal encephalitis. Blood-borne invasion is most common, although entrance to the central nervous system (CNS) via the cerebrospinal fluid (CSF) or retrograde axoplasmic flow from peripheral nerves also occurs. Viral penetration of the blood-brain barrier results in **perivascular cuffing involving sensitized T cells, B cells, and macrophages.** Meningitis and encephalitis should first be considered viral rather than bacterial disease. Arboviruses can be involved in acute disease and unconventional agents called prions in slow infections.

A. **Aseptic meningitis.** Viral (aseptic) meningitis is milder and more common than bacterial meningitis except in children younger than 10 years of age, where bacterial meningitis is more common.
   1. **Enteroviruses (Coxsackie and echoviruses):**
      a. These viruses **cause 90% of aseptic meningitis.**
      b. Infection occurs primarily in late summer and early fall.
      c. **Diagnosis:** may be rapidly diagnosed by PCR tests for viral RNA in the CSF.
   2. **Mumps virus** causes a spring infection in unvaccinated individuals.
   3. **Lymphocytic choriomeningitis (LCM) virus** is transferred to humans through contact with urine of infected mice, guinea pigs, or hamsters (**zoonotic infection**).

4. **HSV type 2** almost always causes meningitis during a primary genital infection.
5. **Human immunodeficiency viruses (HIVs)** cause meningitis in 5% to 10% of cases during initial infection.

B. **Meningoencephalitis/encephalitis.** These diseases, if of an infectious origin, are primarily viral diseases with HSV-1, arboviruses, and rabies causing life-threatening disease. **Cerebral dysfunction occurs.** Several childhood illnesses like measles, mumps, and chickenpox may have a meningoencephalitis component. Prognosis usually depends on the agent, but antiviral therapy is available for HSV infections and immune globulins for rabies.
1. **Herpes simplex viruses:**
   a. HSVs are the most common cause of severe sporadic meningoencephalitis.
   b. They cause disease following primary infection of infants (usually HSV-2) or due to reactivation of HSV-1 following some type of immunosuppression in adults.
   c. The infection is **localized to the temporal lobes** so computed tomography (CT) scans and electroencephalograms (EEGs) are diagnostic aids.
   d. **Treatment:** may be treated with high-dose, intravenous acyclovir, or with ganciclovir or foscarnet in acyclovir-intolerant patients. The mortality rate is 70% in untreated patients.
2. **Rabies virus:**
   a. Rabies virus is usually acquired through the bite of an infected animal (**zoonotic infection**) and is always fatal if the patient is untreated or unimmunized.
   b. It may be acquired from aerosols containing the virus.
   c. The virus travels by retrograde axoplasmic flow in peripheral nerves to the brain.
   d. The incubation time may last several months depending on the initial site of infection.
   e. **Diagnosis:** diagnosed by epidemiology and clinical findings including fever, headache, muscle spasms, and convulsions.
   f. **Prevention:** prevented by vaccination with a **killed vaccine** (**HDCV,** commercially called **Imovax-Rabies**) or treated with rabies **immunoglobulin** (**RIG,** commercially called **Imogam-Rabies**).
3. **Arboviruses:**
   a. **West Nile virus:**
      (1) West Nile virus is the **leading cause of arboviral encephalitis in the United States.**
      (2) Birds, particularly **crows and jays, are natural hosts.**
      (3) The virus is normally transmitted by mosquito bite, but can be transferred by blood transfusions, breastfeeding, and through the placenta.
      (4) It causes asymptomatic disease in 80% of those infected, but 20% develop **West Nile fever,** and less than 1% develop **West Nile neurologic disease (WNND),** which is more likely to occur in individuals older than 60 years of age.
   b. **Other arboviruses (St. Louis, LaCrosse, California, Eastern equine [EEE], and Western equine encephalitis [WEE] viruses):**
      (1) These viruses cause **mosquito-borne infections with bird or mammal reservoirs.**
      (2) Diseases vary in severity depending on the virus (California virus infection rarely results in fatalities, while the EEE virus is estimated to have a 50% mortality rate).

C. **Poliomyelitis/poliovirus.**
1. Poliovirus usually causes an asymptomatic (95%) or minor upper respiratory tract (4%) infection. In rare cases, it can cause an aseptic meningitis that can progress to a paralytic disease by destroying the lower motor neurons of the spinal cord and brainstem, resulting in paralysis of the lower limbs and occasionally respiratory paralysis.
2. **Prevention:** may be prevented by a **trivalent inactivated vaccine (Salk vaccine);** an effective World Health Organization (WHO) vaccine program has eliminated this disease from most parts of the world.

D. **Transverse myelitis/human T-lymphotropic virus type 1 (HTLV-1).**
1. HTLV-1 causes a disease known as **tropical spastic paraparesis** (TSP), which is a slowly progressive disease in which 30% of those infected are bedridden and 45% are unable to walk after 10 years.
2. TSP is endemic in the Caribbean.

E. **Acute postinfectious encephalomyelitis.** In this rare disease, the neurological signs and symptoms develop late during the clinical infection or weeks after recovery. The symptoms include personality and behavior changes, which may proceed to convulsions and coma. **Immunopathological mechanisms** perhaps involving autoimmune reactions to CNS antigens are thought to be responsible.

1. **HIV, CMV, and EBV** are frequently associated with **Guillain-Barré syndrome.**
2. **Influenza B, VZV, and adenovirus** have been implicated in conjunction with salicylates in **Reye's syndrome.**
3. **Various childhood viruses** like measles, mumps, rubella, and VZV have been implicated.
4. **Rabies virus** vaccine has been observed to cause this disease.

F. **Latent or recurrent infections.** After primary systemic infection with some viruses, the virus becomes latent in neurons and reactivates to cause disease under conditions of immunosuppression induced by drug treatment, advancing age, and so forth.

1. **Herpes simplex viruses:**
   a. **HSVs** can **latently infect neurons** in the trigeminal ganglia and reactivate to cause **fever blisters or cold sores.**
   b. **Treatment:** may be treated with topical or oral acyclovir, but the **virus** is **not eliminated.**
2. **Varicella zoster virus:**
   a. VZV **reactivates from the neurons** of sensory ganglia (usually in areas supplied by the trigeminal nerve and thoracic ganglion) to cause **herpes zoster or shingles.**
   b. **Postherpetic neuralgia (PHN)** may occur after skin lesions of shingles have crusted.
   c. **Treatment and prevention:**
      (1) Shingles may be treated with oral acyclovir and famciclovir; PHN may be treated with famciclovir.
      (2) The incidence of both diseases is decreased by immunization of the elderly (age 60 or older) with **Zostavax vaccine** (contains a higher dose of live attenuated virus than childhood VZV vaccines).
      (3) Shingles may also be treated or infection prevented by **varicella zoster immune globulin (VZIG)** preparations.

G. **Slow CNS infections.** Two of these infections involve rare complications of common viruses, while the spongiform encephalitis involves "unconventional" infectious agents called prions.

1. **Measles virus** can cause a rare **subacute sclerosing panencephalitis (SSPE)** that develops 1 to 10 years after apparent recovery from acute measles.
2. **JC virus:**
   a. JC virus can reactivate to cause a rare syndrome known as **progressive multifocal leukoencephalopathy (PML).**
   b. **Diagnosis:** may be diagnosed by PCR techniques for viral DNA in the CSF.
3. **Kuru and variant Creutzfeldt-Jakob disease (vCJD) prions:**
   a. These prions cause progressive brain disorders involving typical spongiform histological changes in affected areas of the brain.
   b. They are transmitted by cannibalism practices (kuru) or consumption of beef containing the prion associated with bovine spongiform encephalopathy (**vCJD**).

X. SKIN, MUCOSAL, AND SOFT TISSUE INFECTIONS

Some viruses cause acute localized infections (e.g., HPV [warts]), while others produce exanthems and enanthems as part of their systemic disease process (e.g., VZV [chickenpox]). The exanthems are manifested as a vesicular or maculopapular rash, which may act as diagnostic aids. Those viruses that cause lesions in the mouth and throat were previously covered and those that produce lesions in the genitalia will be discussed under STD. Those viruses that mainly affect children are included in the childhood infections section.

A. Human papillomaviruses.
   1. HPV causes **cutaneous warts** (common, plantar, and flat), which can be curetted or ablated by freezing with liquid nitrogen.
   2. The warts or papilloma lesions contain **koilocytotic cells.**

B. Molluscum contagiosum virus causes wartlike lesions that typically occur in groups on the arms and face.

C. Orf virus.
   1. This virus causes a sheep or goat disease that can be transferred to humans (**zoonotic infection**).
   2. It causes papulovesicular lesions that usually begin on the finger, but can also occur on the face.

D. HSV, VZV, human herpes viruses 6 and **7, human parvoviruses, measles virus, rubella virus, Coxsackie** and **echoviruses,** and other rash-producing viruses are covered in other sections.

SITUATION-BASED DISEASES

XI. CHILDHOOD INFECTIONS

This section describes the viruses associated with the common childhood diseases that occur in unvaccinated children. Important congenital and neonatal infections are covered later.

A. Measles virus.
   1. Measles virus causes an infection producing a **maculopapular rash** (first seen below the hairline and behind the ears) and produces a high fever, cough, coryza, conjunctivitis, and **Koplik spots** on buccal mucosa (12 to 24 hours before the rash).
   2. Measles may cause complications including a postinfectious encephalitis, giant cell pneumonia, atypical measles (disease in those previously vaccinated), and, after many years, SSPE.
   3. **Temporary immunosuppression** occurs due to lymphocyte infection.
   4. **Diagnosis:** has a clinical diagnosis.
   5. **Prevention:** may be prevented by **vaccination with the live attenuated Enders-Edmonston strain** by itself or in combination with attenuated strains of mumps and rubella viruses (MMR vaccine).

B. Mumps virus.
   1. Mumps virus is often associated with asymptomatic disease but can cause a late winter or early spring disease characterized by sudden onset, fever, and parotitis; it is sometimes accompanied by orchitis, pancreatitis, and meningoencephalitis (50% have involvement, but only 10% have symptoms).
   2. **Diagnosis:** has a clinical diagnosis or ELISA for IgM.
   3. **Prevention:** Disease is prevented by vaccination with the **live attenuated Jeryl Lynn strain** or in combination with attenuated strains of measles and rubella viruses (MMR vaccine).

C. Rubella virus.
   1. Rubella virus causes a benign disease in children, which may be subclinical or symptomatic. Symptoms include a 3- to 5-day rash consisting of macules that coalesce to a "blush," fever, malaise, and swollen neck and suboccipital lymph nodes. It causes a more severe disease in adults that may be complicated by arthralgia, arthritis, and a postinfectious encephalitis (1 in 5,000 cases).
   2. It can produce a **severe congenital infection,** leading to severe teratogenic effects in fetuses of nonimmune mothers.

3. **Diagnosis:** Infections are diagnosed by ELISA for IgM and immune status of individuals by ELISA for IgG.
4. **Prevention:** Disease is prevented by vaccination with the **live, attenuated RA 27/3 strain** of the virus or in combination with attenuated strains of measles and mumps viruses (MMR vaccine).

D. **Varicella zoster virus.**
1. VZV causes a disease (**chickenpox**) characterized by fever and vesicular rash on the trunk, face, and scalp, which is usually benign and self-limiting in healthy children but more severe in adults (potential for pneumonia).
2. VZV latently infects neurons; the virus can reactivate to cause herpes zoster or shingles later in life.
3. **Diagnosis:** diagnosed clinically.
4. **Prevention:** may be prevented by **vaccination with the live, attenuated Oka strain** or treatment of high-risk or immunosuppressed individuals with **VZIG.**

E. **Human parvovirus B-19.**
1. Although these infections are usually asymptomatic, this virus can cause **erythema infectiosum (fifth disease),** a biphasic illness first presenting as flulike, but progressing in several weeks to arthralgia accompanied by a **"slapped cheek" rash,** which first appears on the face and then spreads to the arms and legs.
2. It may cause **aplastic crises** in individuals suffering from chronic hemolytic anemia.
3. **Diagnosis:** may be diagnosed by ELISA for IgM.

F. **Human herpes viruses 6 and 7** cause a benign disease of young children called **exanthem subitum (roseola),** which is characterized by a rapid onset fever and an immune-mediated generalized rash.

XII. CONGENITAL AND NEONATAL INFECTIONS

Several viruses can infect the fetus with results that vary from inconsequential effects to death. **Disease is frequently dependent on the time of fetal infection.** Infection during the first 5 months of pregnancy may have serious consequences. Other viruses like HSV can infect infants during travel through an infected birth canal or shortly after birth (HBV). All of the following viruses except HBV can cross the placenta. Primary disease in children and adults has been discussed previously.

A. **Rubella virus.**
1. Rubella virus causes a 90% chance of multiple **defects in fetuses** infected during the first 10 weeks of pregnancy.
2. It causes some reversible effects like hepatitis and meningoencephalitis in the neonate, but permanent auditory and other CNS-related problems are common.
3. There is no treatment and a baby infected during the first 3 months is likely to be severely affected.

B. **Cytomegalovirus.**
1. CMV causes the **most common congenital infection** that almost always accompanies a primary infection in a pregnant woman.
2. Infections are usually asymptomatic at birth, but approximately 25% will develop deafness and neurological problems.
3. CMV can infect neonates during delivery through an infected birth canal or via breastfeeding, but infants usually remain healthy.

C. **Parvovirus B-19** can infect both mother and fetus during epidemics, but the outcome is good for both, unless the infection of the fetus occurs during the first 20 weeks of pregnancy, when a severe anemia resulting in death can occur.

D. **Varicella zoster virus.**
  1. VZV can cause deformities in fetuses exposed during weeks 13 to 20 of pregnancy, but administration of VZIG to the mother offers protection.
  2. VZV may have a 40% mortality rate in neonates born to mothers with an active chickenpox infection at the time of birth; VZIG given to the newborn can help minimize the effect of VZV infection.

E. **Herpes simplex virus.**
  1. HSV can be transferred to the fetus transplacentally from the mother. It results in a severe disease with high mortality; treatment with acyclovir is helpful.
  2. Transmission at the time of delivery can cause a serious disseminated disease, and intravenous acyclovir should be administered.

F. **Human immunodeficiency virus (HIV).**
  1. HIV may be transmitted transplacentally, during vaginal birth, or after birth through breast milk of an HIV-infected mother. Maternal treatment during pregnancy reduces transmission during birth and transplacentally by almost 99%. Women with HIV are advised not to breastfeed.
  2. It can be diagnosed in newborns by detecting HIV RNA in the blood.

G. **HBV** can be transmitted by fluids including breast milk to infants born to chronically infected mothers (HBeAg$^-$ in 10% to 25% and HBeAg$^+$ in 90%). It usually causes an asymptomatic disease with a high probability of becoming a chronic infection.

XIII. SEXUALLY TRANSMITTED DISEASES

HIV, HSV-1, HSV-2, and HPV are the main viruses emphasized in this section. Although not known for their genital signs and symptoms, HIV and HBV are well known as STDs. Both HSV and HPV are associated with distinctive genital lesions. HBV and CMV may be acquired through sexual contact but have no genital signs or symptoms. The diseases associated with these viruses are described elsewhere in this chapter.

A. **Human immunodeficiency virus.**
  1. HIV causes an **asymptomatic or infectious mononucleosis-like primary infection** that is followed by a variable, but frequently long (years) **latent period** before progressing to acquired immunodeficiency syndrome **(AIDS)-related complex (ARC) disease and then finally AIDS.**
  2. It may be transmitted intrauterinely, perinatally, or through breast milk.
  3. It can be inhibited by several classes of antivirals:
     a. Inhibitors of reverse transcriptase (both nucleoside analogs and nonnucleosides).
     b. Viral protease inhibitors.
     c. Fusion inhibitors.
  4. **Treatment:** treated with **highly active antiretroviral therapy** (HAART), a combination of two nucleoside analogs and a protease inhibitor.

B. **Herpes simplex viruses.**
  1. HSV causes the most common infections that lead to genital ulcers.
  2. A mild meningitis may be associated with the genital disease and frequently leads to **latent infections with recurrent disease.**
  3. **Treatment:** can be treated with oral acyclovir, valacyclovir, or famciclovir to shorten disease associated with primary infection and recurrences, but **antiviral resistant strains** can emerge during prolonged therapy and the virus is never eliminated from the infected ganglion by antiviral treatment.

C. **Human papillomavirus.**
  1. Several strains of HPV cause **venereal warts, the most common STD.**
  2. Some types (most commonly 16 and 18) are *also* associated with cervical dysplasia and **cervical intraepithelial neoplasia** (CIN).

3. **Treatment and prevention:**
   a. Genital warts may be treated with podophyllin or cryotherapy.
   b. A **recombinant quadrivalent vaccine (Gardasil)** containing virus-like particles of types 6, 11, 16, and 18, the causes of 90% of genital warts and 70% of CIN, and **Cervarix**, a bivalent vaccine containing L1 proteins from type 16 and 18 viruses, is available.

D. **HBV.** Although it does not produce genital signs or symptoms, HBV is considered an STD (see VI B 1 for clinical diseases).

XIV. POSTINFECTIOUS DISEASE

A number of viruses are associated with postinfectious disorders. Most have been mentioned in the nervous system section. They include VZV, measles, influenza, and mumps viruses (meningoencephalitis), CMV (Guillain-Barré syndrome), influenza B, and VZV (Reye's syndrome). Possible mechanisms include persistent low-grade infection, autoantibodies, and immune complexes.

A. **EBV** sometimes causes **erythema multiforme** following virus infection of toddlers.

B. **HSV** can cause **erythema multiforme** during recurrences of cold sores.

XV. ORGAN TRANSPLANT-ASSOCIATED DISEASES

Two mechanisms are involved in initiating these infections: the virus in the transplanted organ and reactivation of the virus during immunosuppressive therapy of the patient.

A. **HBV** can cause chronic asymptomatic infections involving the pancreas and the liver, and a donor should be serologically monitored for this virus before being deemed acceptable.

B. **CMV** can be reactive in AIDS and other immune-suppressed patients to cause a life-threatening pneumonitis.

XVI. ARBOVIRAL AND ZOONOTIC DISEASES

A. The majority of important arboviral diseases have been discussed: West Nile virus and encephalitis viruses in the nervous system and yellow fever virus in the gastrointestinal system.

B. The **four important zoonotic infections—hantavirus, rabies virus, LCM virus, and orf virus**—have been discussed in the respiratory, nervous, and skin sections, respectively.

C. **Dengue virus** is transmitted by a mosquito bite in the Caribbean or Southeast Asia.
   1. It causes **"breakbone fever"** consisting of high fever, headache, rash, and back and bone pain.
   2. It is particularly dangerous in children where reinfection by a different serotype can result in a severe hemorrhagic fever and can lead to a **fatal dengue shock syndrome.**

Review Test

Directions: Each of the numbered items or incomplete statements in this section is followed by answers or completions of the statement. Select the ONE lettered answer that is BEST in each case.

1. An 8-year-old boy is brought to your office by his mother. He has had a slight fever and a sore throat for the past 2 days. He has eight ulcerative lesions in his mouth, three vesicular lesions on his left hand, and five similar lesions on his right foot. The most probable cause of his disease is

(A) Coxsackie A virus
(B) Human herpes virus 6
(C) HSV
(D) HPV

2. A 16-year-old boy presents at your office with a sore throat, fever, and enlarged lymph nodes. His tonsils are enlarged, the pharynx is inflamed, and splenomegaly is observed. He complains of severe fatigue. Confirmation of the causative agent is best done by observing

(A) A positive Tzanck smear
(B) IgM heterophile antibodies
(C) Koilocytotic cells
(D) RT-PCR for enterovirus

3. The most common cause of congenital infections is

(A) CMV
(B) HSV
(C) Parvovirus
(D) Rubella virus

4. A 23-year-old medical student on the Caribbean island of Dominica presents at the Student Health Clinic complaining of an increasingly severe headache and back and bone pain. Yesterday she was nauseated and vomited several times during the night. She has a 39.5°C/103°F fever, which appeared suddenly, and a generalized rash that blanches under pressure. She had been hiking in the rainforest 1 week earlier and was particularly bothered by mosquitoes at that time. The most likely infectious agent causing her symptoms is

(A) Dengue virus
(B) LCM virus

(C) West Nile virus
(D) Yellow fever virus

5. A 4-year-old girl is brought to your rural clinic office by her mother who states the child has a runny nose, barking cough, and a sore throat. Your examination indicates respiration is labored. None of her three siblings is sick. The most probable viral cause of her symptoms is

(A) Adenovirus
(B) Influenza virus
(C) Parainfluenza virus
(D) RSV

6. The individual most likely to develop chronic liver disease is a

(A) 1-month-old infant infected with HBV
(B) 22-year-old coinfected with HBV and HDV
(C) 26-year-old alcoholic intravenous drug abuser infected with HBV
(D) 30-year-old infected with yellow fever virus

7. A 64-year-old man living on a farm in southern Minnesota is brought on July 15 to the emergency room by his brother. The brother said the man had a 2-day history of fever, headache, and some vomiting, but today he appeared confused. He is confused by some of the simple questions you ask him. His spinal tap is clear with 75% PMNs and a head CT is normal. The most likely cause of his symptoms is

(A) California encephalitis virus
(B) Enterovirus
(C) HSV
(D) West Nile virus

8. A mother brings her 18-month-old son to your office. She was called by her day care center who reported he had vomited twice during the morning and had diarrhea as well.

She noted he had a slight fever the past 2 days and had not been very hungry. The most likely cause of his illness is

(A) Adenovirus
(B) Astrovirus
(C) Norovirus
(D) Rotavirus

9. A vaccine is available for protection against the disease observed in review question 8. The immunizing agent(s) for this vaccine is a(n)

(A) Attenuated virus
(B) Formalin-inactivated virus
(C) Preparation of reassortment viruses
(D) Viral attachment protein preparation

10. Donors for liver transplants must be monitored and determined to be serologically negative for previous

(A) CMV infections
(B) EBV infections
(C) HBV infections
(D) HEV infections

11. On September 17, a 22-year-old male college student appears at the Student Health Clinic complaining of moderate headache, nausea, and vomiting. His temperature is 38.5°C/101°F and his physical examination shows stiffness in the neck. What is the most likely viral cause of the symptoms?

(A) CMV
(B) Enterovirus
(C) EBV
(D) HSV type 1

12. Knowing the genotype of the causative virus is important for determining the treatment of chronic

(A) CMV infections
(B) HCV infections
(C) IC virus infections
(D) VZV infections

Answers and Explanations

1. **The answer is A.** Coxsackie A virus causes hand, foot, and mouth disease, which is characterized by vesicular lesions in the mouth and extremities.

2. **The answer is B.** This boy's symptoms are consistent with infectious mononucleosis caused by EBV. During its pathogenesis, this virus produces an IgM heterophile antibody that is the basis for the Monospot test.

3. **The answer is A.** CMV is the most common cause of congenital infections that can lead to various symptoms in the newborn.

4. **The answer is A.** Dengue virus, which is transmitted by mosquito bites, is present in the Caribbean and causes "breakbone fever," which is consistent with these symptoms.

5. **The answer is C.** The child's symptoms are those found with croup caused by parainfluenza virus.

6. **The answer is A.** The potential for chronic liver disease following HBV infection is inversely proportional with the age of infection. The probability is over 90% with neonates.

7. **The answer is D.** The symptoms are most consistent with West Nile neurologic disease, a rare complication of West Nile virus infections.

8. **The answer is D.** Rotaviruses are the most likely cause of infant gastroenteritis.

9. **The answer is C.** The segmented double-strand RNA genome of rotaviruses formed the basis for the preparation of a pentavalent rotavirus vaccine (RotaTeq) consisting of reassortment viruses.

10. **The answer is C.** Donors for liver transplants are serologically monitored for evidence of previous HBV and HCV infections since they can be asymptomatic yet transfer the virus to the liver recipients.

11. **The answer is B.** Enteroviral meningitis, for which there is only supportive treatment, is frequently seen in late summer or early fall.

12. **The answer is B.** Only genotypes 2 and 3 of HCV are likely to respond to the currently recommended combination treatment with pegylated interferon-α and ribavirin for chronic HIV infections.

I. OVERVIEW OF FUNGI

A. **Fungi are eukaryotic organisms** so they have many similarities to our cells. **Differences targeted by antifungals include:**

1. Fungal cells have **cell walls** (CWs).

   a. Fungal CWs **protect cells from osmotic shock, determine cell shapes,** and have components that **are antigenic.**

   b. Fungal CWs are composed primarily of **complex carbohydrates** such as **chitin with glucans and mannose-proteins.** The **CW glucan** (not found in humans) is the **antifungal target of the echinocandins like caspofungin.**

2. **Ergosterol** is the dominant **fungal membrane sterol** rather than cholesterol, which is **an important difference targeted by imidazoles, triazoles, and polyenes antifungals.**

B. **Types.** Fungi **include** organisms called **molds, mushrooms,** and **yeasts.**

1. **Hyphae** are **filamentous (tubelike) cells of molds (also known as the filamentous fungi)** and **mushrooms.** Hyphae grow at the tips (apical growth).

   a. **Septae or septations are cross walls of hyphae** and occur in the hyphae of the great majority of the disease-causing fungi. They are referred to as septate (Fig. 7.1).

   b. **Nonseptate or aseptate hyphae lack regularly occurring cross walls.** These cells are multinucleate and are also called **coenocytic.** They often are **quite variable in width** with **broad branching angles** (Fig. 7.2).

   c. Hyphae may be **dematiaceous (dark colored)** or **hyaline (colorless).**

   d. Fluffy surface masses of hyphae and their "hidden" growth into tissue or lab medium are called **mycelia.**

2. **Yeasts** are **single-celled fungi,** generally round to oval shaped (Fig. 7.3). They **reproduce by budding** (blastoconidia).

3. **Pseudohyphae** (hyphae with sausagelike constrictions at septations) are formed by some yeasts when they elongate but remain attached to each other. *Candida albicans* **is notable for** developing into **pseudohyphae and true hyphae** when it invades tissues (Fig. 7.4).

4. **Thermally dimorphic fungi** are fungi capable of converting from a **yeast or yeastlike form to a filamentous form** and vice versa.

   a. Environmental conditions such as temperature and nutrient availability trigger changes.

   b. They exist in the **yeast or a yeastlike form in a human** and as the **filamentous form in the environment.** "Yeastie beasties in body heat; bold mold in the cold."

   c. They include the major pathogens: ***Blastomyces, Histoplasma, Coccidioides,*** and ***Sporothrix*** in the United States and *Paracoccidioides* in South and Central America. Compare *Blastomyces'* two forms (Fig. 7.5).

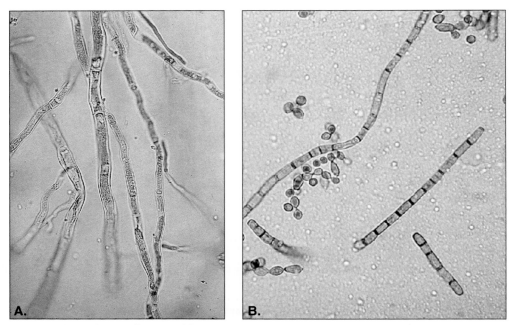

FIGURE 7.1. **Septate hyphae.** (Courtesy of Glenn D. Roberts, PhD, Mayo Clinic, Rochester, MN.)

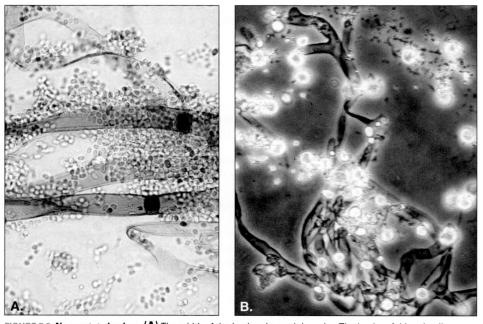

FIGURE 7.2. **Nonseptate hyphae. (A)** The width of the hyphae is much broader. The hyphae fold and collapse on themselves. **(B)** The other material in the field (creating the bright dots of light) are debris from human cells that have been lysed by mounting the necrotic tissue in KOH (potassium hydroxide). (Courtesy of Glenn D. Roberts, PhD, Mayo Clinic, Rochester, MN.)

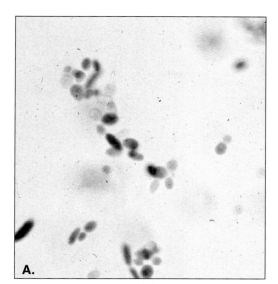
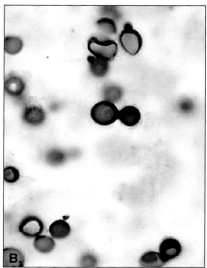

FIGURE 7.3. **Budding yeasts. (A)** Lactophenol blue stained budding yeasts. **(B)** Budding yeasts stained with silver stain. This fungus is *Cryptococcus neoformans* but the capsule cannot be seen well with the silver stain. (Courtesy of Glenn D. Roberts, PhD, Mayo Clinic, Rochester, MN.)

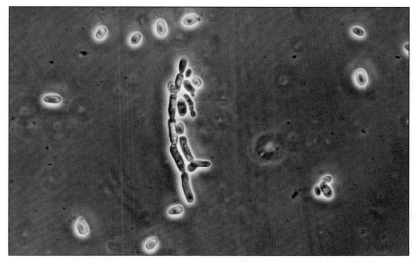

FIGURE 7.4. **Pseudohyphae.** When yeasts like *Candida albicans* bud but do not separate and continue to elongate, the result is pseudohyphae. Note the sausagelike constrictions between the cells. (Courtesy of Glenn D. Roberts, PhD, Mayo Clinic, Rochester, MN.)

5. **Fungal spores** are formed either asexually or by a sexual process involving nuclear fusion and then meiosis. Fungal morphology including spores may be used in identification.
   a. **Conidia are asexual spores** of filamentous fungi (molds) or mushrooms (Fig. 7.6A).
   b. **Blastoconidia** are the new yeast **"buds"** (Fig. 7.6B).
   c. **Arthroconidia are conidia formed by laying down joints** in hyphae followed by fragmentation of the hyphal strand (Fig. 7.6C).

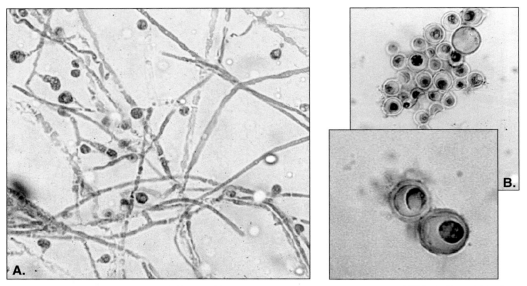

FIGURE 7.5. *Blastomyces* **is a dimorphic fungus.** Shown here are the hyphal and tissue forms. **(A)** Hyphal form. This photo shows the environmental hyphae and conidia of *Blastomyces dermatitidis*. **(B)** Tissue form of the budding yeast. Note *Blastomyces*' big yeasts with the thick cell wall and the broad base between the mother cell and the bud (seen in the inset). (Courtesy of Glenn D. Roberts, PhD, Mayo Clinic, Rochester, MN.)

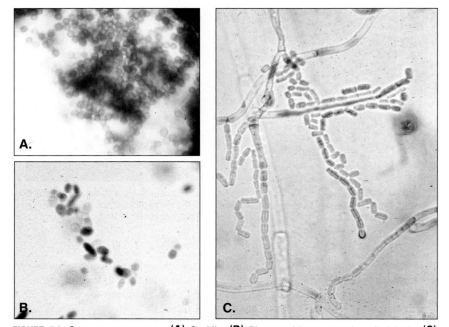

FIGURE 7.6. **Common spore types. (A)** Conidia. **(B)** Blastoconidia, commonly called buds. **(C)** Strands of hyphae breaking up into arthroconidia. Arthroconidia may be seen when dermatophytes grow in skin, where they often reproduce without a lot of branching and produce arthroconidia. Distinctive barrel-shaped conidia may also be produced by *Coccidioides immitis* (see Fig. 7.3A). (Courtesy of Glenn D. Roberts, PhD, Mayo Clinic, Rochester, MN.)

C. **Fungal nutrition. Fungi require preformed organic compounds** derived from their environment.

1. **Saprobes** live on **dead organic material.** Some are opportunistic, causing disease if traumatically implanted into tissue.

2. **Commensal colonizers** generally **live in harmony on humans,** deriving their nutrition from compounds on body surfaces. Some are **opportunists** because under certain conditions (e.g., reduced immune responsiveness) they may invade tissue or vasculature and cause disease.

3. **Pathogens** infect the healthy but cause more severe disease in the compromised hosts. The damage to living cells provides nutrition. Most of these are also environmental saprobes.

II. FUNGAL GROUPS

A few general **group names** are important.

A. **Zygomycetes (phycomycetes)** are the **nonseptate fungi.** Common genera are *Mucor* and *Rhizopus.* (Most fungi have cross walls.)

B. **Dermatophytes** are **three genera of filamentous fungi causing cutaneous infections:** *Trichophyton, Epidermophyton,* and *Microsporum.*

C. **Thermally dimorphic fungi** in the United States are *Histoplasma, Blastomyces, Coccidioides,* and *Sporothrix.*

D. **Dematiaceous fungi** are **darkly pigmented fungi.**

III. OVERVIEW OF FUNGAL DISEASES

Individual infections are covered in Chapter 8.

A. **Fungal allergies** are common. Molds grow on *any* damp organic surface, and spores are constantly in the air. Spores (and, in some cases, volatile fungal metabolites) play a role in sick building syndrome, allergies, farmer's lung, silo worker's disease, and allergic bronchopulmonary aspergillosis and can become a major problem following flooding.

B. **Mycotoxicoses** may result from ingestion of fungal-contaminated foods (e.g., St. Anthony's fire from ergot-contaminated rye bread or aflatoxin [a carcinogen]-contaminated peanuts) or the ingestion of psychotropic (*Psilocybe*) or toxic (*Amanita*) mushrooms.

C. **Fungal infections (mycoses).**

1. Mycoses range from superficial to overwhelming systemic infections that are rapidly fatal in the compromised host.

2. Mycoses are increasing in prevalence as a result of increased use of antibiotics, corticosteroids, and cytotoxic drugs.

3. Mycoses are commonly classified as superficial, cutaneous, mucocutaneous, subcutaneous, and systemic infections. The systemic infections are subdivided into those caused by pathogenic or opportunistic fungi.

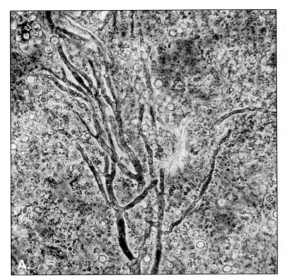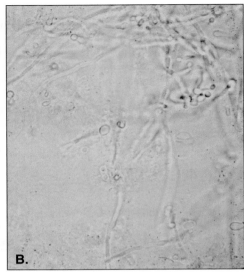

FIGURE 7.7. Wet mounts. **(A)** Dichotomously branching hyphae released by tissue by KOH (potassium hydroxide) digestion. (Courtesy of Glenn D. Roberts, PhD, Mayo Clinic, Rochester, MN.) **(B)** Wet mount of mucosal scrapings for vaginitis
showing pseudohyphae and some yeasts.

IV. DIAGNOSIS OF FUNGAL INFECTIONS

A. Clinical manifestations suggestive of fungal infection trigger special orders to the mycology unit.

B. Microscopic examination: rapid methods.
   1. Potassium hydroxide in a wet mount (**KOH mount**) of skin scrapings breaks down the human
      cells, enhancing the visibility of the unaffected fungus (Fig. 7.7).
   2. A nigrosin or **India ink** wet mount of cerebrospinal fluid (**CSF**) highlights the **capsule of Cryp-
      tococcus neoformans** but is very **insensitive** (misses 50% of cases).
   3. A **Giemsa** or Wright's stain of **thick blood or bone marrow smear** may detect the **intracellular
      Histoplasma capsulatum.**
   4. **Calcofluor white stain** "lights up" fungal elements in exudates, small skin scales, or frozen sec-
      tions under a fluorescent microscope, giving the fungus a fluorescent blue-white appearance
      on a black background.

C. Histologic staining: special fungal stains for fixed tissues are necessary because fungi are not
   distinguished by color with hematoxylin and eosin (H & E) stain.
   1. **Gomori methenamine-silver stain: Fungi are dark gray to black.**
   2. Periodic acid-Schiff (**PAS**) reaction: **Fungi are hot pink to red.**
   3. **Gridley** fungus stain: **Fungi are purplish rose** with a yellow background.
   4. **Calcofluor white** stain: as above.
   5. **Immunofluorescent** stains are available for some fungal pathogens.

D. DNA probes and nucleic acid amplification (NAATs) are now available for some systemic
   pathogens.

E. Cultures for fungi must be specially ordered. They use special media (e.g., **Sabouraud's** dextrose
   medium), enriched media (e.g., blood agar) with antibiotics to inhibit bacterial growth, and enriched media with both antibiotics and cycloheximide (which inhibits many saprobic fungi).

1. **Identification (ID) of *yeast* cultures:**
   a. Identification traditionally has been based on morphologic characteristics (presence of capsule, formation of germ tubes in serum, and morphology on cornmeal agar) and biochemical tests (urease, nitrate reduction, and carbohydrate assimilations and fermentations).
   b. Some yeast cultures may be identified with DNA probes.
   c. Speciation should be done for serious yeast infections as certain species carry drug resistance.
2. **Identification of *filamentous fungal* cultures:**
   a. Identification is based on morphologic criteria or uses an immunologic method called exoantigen testing, in which antigens extracted from the culture to be identified are immunodiffused against known antisera.
   b. DNA probes/nucleic acid amplification kits are available for some systemic pathogens.

F. **Fungal antigen detection** uses known antibodies to identify circulating fungal antigens in a patient's serum, CSF, or urine. Antibodies are available for *Histoplasma* and *Cryptococcus*. These tests are important when patients are compromised and antibodies may not be reliably detected.

G. **Serologic testing** done to identify patient antibodies specific to a fungus generally requires acute and convalescent sera and is complicated by some cross-reactivity among pathogenic fungi and some patients' inability to produce antibody.

V. ANTIFUNGAL DRUGS

Fungi have ergosterol as their dominant membrane sterol; humans have cholesterol. In ergosterol synthesis, squalene is converted to lanosterol, which is converted to ergosterol. Human cells have no CWs and do not synthesize glucans. Because fungi are eukaryotic and their ribosomes and many pathways resemble those of humans, drugs that inhibit ribosomal function or inhibit common pathways cannot be used. Instead, the unique fungal pathways have to be targeted.

A. **Polyene antifungals.**
   1. **General characteristics:**
      a. Polyenes **bind to ergosterol** in fungal membranes, creating ion channels, **leading to leakage** and cell death. Additionally, polyene membrane damage through an oxidative process may be responsible for the rapid killing.
      b. Because polyenes also bind to cholesterol (but less avidly than ergosterol), they are quite toxic. The toxicity is reduced by the use of liposomal formulations.
      c. They have poor gastrointestinal absorption.
   2. **Amphotericin B (AMB):**
      a. AMB is administered intravenously (IV) for serious fungal infections and has been the drug of choice for most life-threatening fungal infections. Lipid formulations have reduced toxicity.
      b. Resistance is infrequent, but there is some reduced AMB sensitivity among some *Candida* species. Resistance is associated with lower membrane levels of ergosterol.
      c. AMB is used in combinations with 5-fluorocytosine or fluconazole but only with very specific fungi in specific body locales.
   3. **Nystatin** is not absorbed from the gastrointestinal tract, so it is used topically, intravaginally, or orally to treat *Candida* overgrowth or infections of cutaneous or mucosal surfaces.

B. **5-Fluorocytosine (5-FC, flucytosine).**
   1. 5-FC is an **antimetabolite** converted in fungal cells to 5-fluorouradylic acid, which competes with uracil to **cause miscoding and disruption of RNA, protein, and DNA synthesis.**
   2. Because **resistance develops quickly** if used alone, 5-FC is used **in combination with amphotericin B or fluconazole** for cryptococcal meningitis.

C. **Imidazole drugs** are azole drugs with two nitrogens in the azole ring. They inhibit the lanosterol 14-α-demethylase interfering with ergosterol synthesis.
   1. **Ketoconazole** may be orally administered but is used only in non-life-threatening fungal infections.
   2. **Miconazole** is used topically against dermatophytes and *Candida* spp.

D. **Triazoles** are azole drugs with three nitrogens in the azole ring. They have better systemic activity than the imidazoles.
   1. **Fluconazole:**
      a. Fluconazole has excellent oral bioavailability.
      b. It is used for systemic infections, most commonly with *Candida* and *Coccidioides,* including coccidioidal meningitis in acquired immunodeficiency syndrome (AIDS), and as maintenance therapy after cryptococcal meningitis.
      c. It is used in combination with other drugs in specific situations for specific fungi.
   2. **Itraconazole:**
      a. This lipophilic imidazole drug is administered orally.
      b. It is used for treatment of mucocutaneous *Candida* infections, non-life-threatening *Aspergillus* infections, moderate or severe histoplasmosis or blastomycosis, and sporotrichosis.
   3. **Voriconazole:**
      a. This drug has a **broad spectrum of activity** with the exception of the nonseptate fungi (Zygomycetes) but may be effective against other fungi that have developed AMB resistance.
      b. It is now a **primary drug for the treatment of invasive aspergillosis** as an alternative to AMB.
   4. **Posaconazole** is a newer azole licensed for treatment of Zygomycetes (nonseptate fungi) infections.

E. **Echinocandins** inhibit fungal glucan synthesis, thus leading to a weakened cell wall and cell lysis.
   1. Echinocandins include caspofungin, micafungin, and anidulafungin.
   2. They are effective against *Aspergillus* spp., *Candida* spp., *Pneumocystis jiroveci,* and a variety of other fungi.

F. **Topical antifungals** (including imidazoles, allylamines: terbinafine and naftifine, tolnaftate, and many others) may be used for dermatophytes and mucosal yeast infections.

Review Test

Please note that all fungal questions follow Chapter 8.

Table 8.1 is a summary of the common or serious major fungal diseases seen in the United States.

I. SUPERFICIAL SKIN INFECTIONS

A. **Pityriasis (tinea) versicolor.**
   1. This disease is a fungal overgrowth in the stratum corneum epidermidis, which disrupts melanin synthesis and manifests as **hypopigmented or hyperpigmented skin patches,** usually on the trunk of the body. There is usually little tissue response.
   2. **Epidemiology:** caused by overgrowth of the lipophilic fungus, ***Malassezia furfur,*** part of the normal flora. *M. furfur* also causes **fungemia in premature infants on intravenous (IV) lipid supplements.**
   3. **Diagnosis:** diagnosed by potassium hydroxide **(KOH) mount** of skin scales showing short, curved, septate hyphae and yeastlike cells (spaghetti and meatballs appearance).

t a b l e **8.1**	Important Fungal Infections (Common or Serious)	
Type	**Disease**	**Causative Organism**
Superficial mycoses	Tinea nigra	Dematiaceous fungi
	Pityriasis versicolor	*Malassezia furfur*
Cutaneous mycoses	Dermatophytic infections (a.k.a., dermatophytoses)	Dermatophytes: *Trichophyton, Epidermophyton, Microsporum*
Mucocutaneous mycoses	Candidiasis	*Candida albicans, Candida* spp.
Subcutaneous mycoses	Sporotrichosis	*Sporothrix schenckii*
Systemic mycoses: Pathogens	Coccidioidomycosis	*Coccidioides immitis*
	Histoplasmosis	*Histoplasma capsulatum*
	Blastomycosis	*Blastomyces dermatitidis*
Systemic mycoses: Opportunists	Cryptococcal meningitis	*Cryptococcus neoformans*
	Malassezia fungemia	*Malassezia furfur*
	Aspergillosis	*Aspergillus fumigatus, Aspergillus* sp.
	Zygomycosis (phycomycosis)	*Mucor, Absidia, Rhizopus, Rhizomucor*
	Candidiasis, systemic and local	*Candida albicans* and *Candida* spp., which have greater drug resistance, especially to fluconazole
	Pneumocystis pneumonitis/pneumonia	*Pneumocystis jiroveci* (a.k.a., *P. carinii*)

B. Tinea nigra.

1. Tinea nigra is a superficial infection of the stratum corneum epidermidis on the palmar or plantar surfaces causing benign, **flat, dark, melanoma-like lesions.**
2. It is caused by a **dematiaceous** (darkly pigmented) **fungus** that produces melanin, which colors the skin.

II. CUTANEOUS MYCOSES

A. General aspects of cutaneous mycoses.

1. **Cutaneous mycoses may be caused by any of the dermatophytes or *Candida* spp. The dermatophytes are** a homogeneous group of **filamentous fungi** with **three genera, *Epidermophyton*, *Microsporum*, and *Trichophyton*.** Most cutaneous infections are dermatophytic. ***Candida* infections are more frequently mucocutaneous or in skin folds and sometimes disseminate. Dermatophytes do not disseminate.**
2. Skin, hair, or nails may be affected; infections are classified by the area of the body involved.
3. **Epidemiology:**
   a. Diseases acquired from animals (**zoophilic**) cause lesions that are **significantly inflammatory.** Two common zoophilic species are *Microsporum canis* and *Trichophyton rubrum*.
   b. Diseases acquired from humans (**anthropophilic**) cause lesions that are **less inflammatory.** Two common anthropophilic species are *Epidermophyton floccosum* and *Microsporum audouinii*.
4. **Diagnosis:** often treated empirically or diagnosed by microscopic examination of skin, hair, or nail material mounted in 10% KOH. **Dermatophytes will show up as relatively unbranched hyphae sometimes with arthroconidia (Fig. 7.6C).** Selection of areas to sample in *Microsporum* infections may be aided by the use of a Wood's (ultraviolet [UV]) lamp.
5. **Treatment:**
   a. Lesions may become superinfected with bacteria that also must be treated. Pus, when present, is a solid indication of superinfection with bacteria.
   b. These diseases require treatment with oral drugs if hair (and hair follicles) are involved.
   c. **ID reaction:** New **sterile lesions** may arise during treatment. This **hypersensitive state** is known as the **dermatophytid (or "id") reaction, a reaction to circulating fungal antigens** that indicates treatment response.

Because dermatophytic infections are not life-threatening even in compromised hosts, you do not need to memorize the specific specie for each dermatophytic infection with the exception of favus caused by ***Trichophyton schoenleinii.*** Just learn the tissues infected by each genus of dermatophytes (see Table 8.2).

B. Tinea capitis (ringworm of the scalp, skin, and hair).

1. **Anthropophilic tinea capitis (gray patch):**
   a. Occurs in **prepubescent children** and is epidemic, spread by head gear, combs, and so forth.
   b. It is caused by *Microsporum audouinii*.
   c. It is usually noninflammatory and produces **gray** patches of hair.

| table 8.2 | Tissues Commonly Infected by Dermatophytes and *Candida* |

		Tissue Infected			
Group	*Genus*	*Hair*	*Skin*	*Nails*	*Fluoresces*
Dermatophytes	*Trichophyton*	Yes	Yes	Yes	—
	Epidermophyton	—	Yes	Yes	—
	Microsporum	Yes	Yes	—	Yes
Yeasts	*Candida*	—	Yes	Yes	—

2. **Zoophilic tinea capitis** (nonepidemic):
   a. Is transmitted by **pets or farm animals.**
   b. It is most commonly caused by *Microsporum canis* or by *Trichophyton mentagrophytes.*
   c. It is **inflammatory,** often with boggy tender areas called **kerion.**
   d. **Temporary alopecia, kerion, keloid, and inflammation** may result.
3. **Black-dot tinea capitis:**
   a. This chronic infection occurs in **adults** and is characterized by **hair breakage, followed by filling of follicles with dark conidia.**
   b. It is caused by *Trichophyton tonsurans.*

C. Tinea barbae.
   1. This infection is an **acute or chronic folliculitis of the beard, neck, or face** most commonly caused by *Trichophyton verrucosum.*
   2. It may produce pustular or dry, scaly lesions.

D. Tinea corporis.
   1. This **dermatophytic infection affects glabrous skin** and is commonly caused by *T. rubrum, T. mentagrophytes,* or *M. canis.*
   2. It is characterized by **annular lesions** with an active border that may be pustular or vesicular.

E. Tinea cruris.
   1. This **acute or chronic fungal infection of the groin** is commonly called jock itch.
   2. It is often accompanied by athlete's foot or nail infections, which also must be treated.
   3. It is caused by *E. floccosum, T. rubrum, T. mentagrophytes,* or yeasts like *Candida.*

F. Tinea pedis.
   1. This acute to chronic **fungal infection of the feet** is commonly called athlete's foot.
   2. It is most commonly caused by *T. rubrum, T. mentagrophytes,* or *E. floccosum.*
   3. There are three common clinical presentations:
      a. Chronic intertriginous tinea pedis (usually white macerated tissue between the toes)
      b. Chronic dry, scaly tinea pedis (hyperkeratotic scales on the heels, soles, or sides of the feet)
      c. Vesicular tinea pedis (vesicles and vesiculopustules)

G. Favus (tinea favosa).
   1. It is a **highly contagious** and severe form of **tinea capitis with scutula** (crust) **formation** and **permanent hair loss caused by scarring. Prophylaxis of all close contacts** is needed.
   2. It is caused by ***Trichophyton schoenleinii.*** (Know this species! Permanent hair loss!)
   3. Favus occurs in both children and adults.

III. MUCOCUTANEOUS CANDIDIASIS/*C. ALBICANS* (AND, INCREASINGLY, OTHER SPECIES OF *CANDIDA*)

A. General aspects of mucocutaneous candidiasis.
   1. *Candida* **spp.** are part of the **normal flora** of the skin, mucous membranes, and gastrointestinal tract. (The spp. means species; sp. is an unknown specie. You will see the latter on lab reports.)
   2. *Candida* **spp.** are **seen as yeasts on body surfaces.** Normal colonization must be distinguished from infection when *Candida* overgrows or invades the tissues.
   3. *Candida albicans* is seen in infected tissues as **pseudohyphae, true hyphae, blastoconidia, and yeast** cells but is still referred to as a yeast.

B. Oral thrush is a yeast infection of the oral mucocutaneous membranes.
   1. It manifests as white curdlike patches in the oral cavity.
   2. It occurs in premature infants, babies on antibiotics, asthmatics not using spacers with inhalers, immunosuppressed patients on long-term antibiotics, and acquired immunodeficiency syndrome (AIDS) patients. In the last two, it may extend through the gastrointestinal (GI) tract, causing a painful gastritis.

C. **Vulvovaginitis or vaginal thrush.**
1. **Vulvovaginitis** is a yeast (*Candida* spp.) infection of the vagina that tends to recur.
2. It manifests with a thick yellow-white discharge, a burning sensation, curdlike patches on the vaginal mucosa, and inflammation of the peritoneum.
3. It is predisposed by diabetes, antibiotic therapy, oral contraceptive use, and pregnancy.
4. Diagnosis: KOH mount of "curd" (see Fig. 7.7).

D. **Cutaneous candidiasis** involves the nails (increases with prolonged use of false nails), skin folds of babies, obese individuals (visible as creamy growth), or groin (but generally also the penis).
1. Lesions may be eczematoid or vesicular and pustular.
2. It is predisposed by moist conditions.

IV. SUBCUTANEOUS MYCOSES

These mycoses begin with traumatic implantation fungus but **remain localized in the cutaneous/ subcutaneous tissues** and are **uncommon in the United States except for sporotrichosis in gardeners, florists, and agriculture workers.**

A. **Sporotrichosis** ("rose gardener's disease") is caused by the **dimorphic fungus *Sporothrix schenckii.***
1. **At 37°C *S. schenckii*** grows as **cigar-shaped to oval, budding yeasts;** at 25°C *S. schenckii* grows as sporulating hyphae.
2. *S. schenckii* is found in or on **plant materials** such as roses, plum trees, or sphagnum moss and is **traumatically introduced** by florist's wires, splinters, or rose or plum tree thorns into subcutaneous tissues.
3. This **subcutaneous, nodular, fungal disease** is generally not painful. **When it spreads via the lymphatics** (lymphocutaneous sporotrichosis), it produces a chain of lesions on the extremities, with the older (lower) lesions ulcerating and the newer (upper) ones starting nodular.
4. **Diagnosis:** Clinical diagnosis is confirmed by culture; histology is generally negative.
5. **Treatment:** treated with itraconazole.

B. **Eumycotic mycetoma.**
1. **Eumycotic mycetoma** is a subcutaneous fungal disease characterized by (1) swelling (**tumefaction**), (2) **sinus tracts** erupting through the skin (if not treated), and (3) presence of "sulfur" **granules** (microcolonies) in the exudate.
2. It is caused by *Pseudallescheria boydii* and *Madurella* species, which are filamentous true fungi found in soil or on vegetation; entry is by traumatic implantation.
3. It usually occurs in **rural, third-world agricultural workers** in the tropics.

C. **Chromoblastomycosis.**
1. **Chromoblastomycosis is one of a group of infections caused by dematiaceous (dark) fungi** and seen in tissues as pigmented, yeastlike bodies.
2. It has **colored lesions** that start out scaly and become raised, cauliflower-like lesions. (Blastomycoses may have similarly raised lesions.)

V. PNEUMONIAS/SYSTEMIC MYCOSES (CAUSED BY FUNGAL PATHOGENS)

A. **General aspects of pneumonias/systemic mycoses.** In the United States, the three dimorphic fungal pathogens *are **Histoplasma, Coccidioides,** and **Blastomyces.***
1. During the saprobic phase, these fungi are filamentous, grow in **specific environments,** and produce **airborne spores** that are inhaled into alveoli to start infection.

2. **These pathogens are also** acquired in **specific geographic regions,** but **reactivated clinical disease can occur long after someone has left the area.** Also, dust with spores can travel on cars or archaeological artifacts and infect the immunologically naive outside the endemic zone.
3. These fungi have true **virulence factors** and can cause disease in healthy individuals.
4. They cause a spectrum of disease in three basic forms:
   a. **Acute self-limited pneumonia, asymptomatic to severe, but generally self-resolving** occurs in healthy people. However, some organisms may survive in granulomas (as also happens in tuberculosis) and can reactivate when the immune system becomes compromised later in life.
   b. Chronic (generally pulmonary) disease generally occurs in debilitated people.
   c. Disseminated infection occurs commonly in immunocompromised people or where a large spore dose overwhelms the immune system.

B. Histoplasmosis/*Histoplasma capsulatum* (see Fig. 8.1A, B).
   1. *Histoplasma* **is a thermally dimorphic, facultative intracellular, fungal pathogen** (with NO capsule).
   2. **Epidemiology:**
      a. The organism is endemic in the **great river plains of the Ohio, Missouri, and Mississippi Rivers** and the St. Lawrence Seaway plus Latin America.
      b. It is found in **soil enriched with bat or bird guano** as **hyphae** with **distinctive tuberculate macroconidia** and nondescript **microconidia.** The microconidia are of small enough size to enter the alveoli to start infection. Bat caves, old chicken coups, starling roosts, and so on, have high levels of spores.
   3. **Pathogenesis:**
      a. Inhaled conidia convert to small yeast cells that are phagocytosed but are able to survive and replicate in these phagocytic cells, including circulating monocytes.

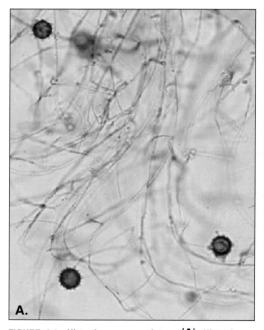
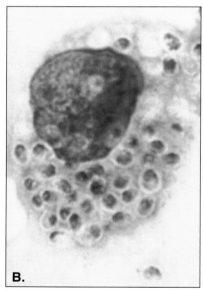

FIGURE 8.1. *Histoplasma capsulatum.* **(A)** *Histoplasma capsulatum* showing hyphae and tuberculate macroconidia characteristically found in bird-feces or bat-feces-enriched soils of the Ohio, Missouri, and Mississippi River plains. (Courtesy of Glenn D. Roberts PhD, Mayo Clinic.) **(B)** *Histoplasma capsulatum* in a single histiocyte (greatly enlarged). Each phagocytic cell can have hundreds of the tiny intracellular yeasts. Note the prominent presence of the histiocyte nucleus that distinguishes it from a spherule. (Spherules also have a cell wall.) (CDC Public Health Image Library/Dr. T. McClenan.)

    b. The yeast form appears to modulate the pH of the phagolysosome and trap calcium; both mechanisms interfere with phagocytic killing. Additionally, glucan in the cell wall appears to play a role in the fungus killing the phagocytic cells, aiding in its spread.

    c. *Histoplasma capsulatum* **has no capsule** so it is misnamed. In stained smears, the yeasts' cytoplasm shrinks away from the cell wall leaving a clear space resembling a capsule.

4. Histoplasmosis clinical symptoms:

    a. Acute histoplasmosis ranges from subclinical to severe pneumonia but self-resolves with bed rest and good nutrition. Because *Histoplasma*'s yeast cells are phagocytosed by alveolar macrophages and polymorphonuclear neutrophils (PMNs), the infected PMNs circulate in the blood so **thick blood smears and blood cultures are extremely useful for diagnosis,** even in an infection limited to lungs. Likewise, hilar lymphadenopathy and splenomegaly are often prominent. A Th1 response and granuloma formation are critical to resolution, but as in TB, some viable organisms may remain in granulomas.

    b. Disseminated histoplasmosis occurs in people with heavy spore exposure, underlying immune cell defects (e.g., patients with AIDS, T-cell deficits, or lymphoma), and children younger than 1 year of age who appear to have a defect in dendritic cell function. Symptoms include **mucocutaneous lesions** and Addison's disease (in approximately 50% of fulminant cases).

C. Blastomycosis/*Blastomyces dermatitidis* (North America) (Fig. 8.2).

  1. Description of agent and epidemiology:

    a. *Blastomyces* **is a thermally dimorphic fungus** found as a **filamentous fungus with small conidia in rotting organic material including wood.**

    b. *Blastomyces* is found in the *Histoplasma* endemic areas *plus* the southeastern U.S. sea-coast (excluding Florida) and north through Minnesota into Canada.

    c. Conidia are inhaled into alveoli where they transform into *Blastomyces*'s **big, budding yeasts with thick walls and broad bases on buds.**

  2. Pathogenesis: found in the **tissues as a large yeast with a double refractile wall and broad-based buds.** Strains shedding high levels of cell wall glycoprotein WI-1 are not

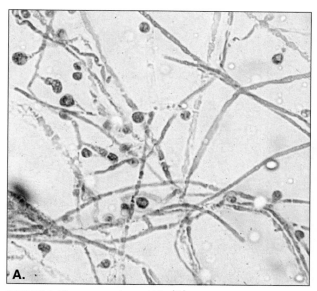
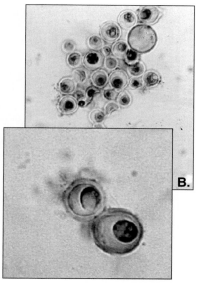

FIGURE 8.2. *Blastomyces dermatitidis.* **(A)** Nondescript *Blastomyces dermatitidis* hyphae and conidia characteristically found in highly organic soil (often with rotting wood) in the endemic area. (Courtesy of Glenn D. Roberts, PhD, Mayo Clinic.) **(B)** The more distinctive *Blastomyces dermatitidis* budding yeast. Note the thick cell wall and the broad base between the mother cell and the blastoconidium (bud). One budding pair has been enlarged in the inset for detail. (Courtesy of Glenn D. Roberts, PhD, Mayo Clinic.)

recognized by the macrophages; these strains continue to replicate, probably triggering a Th2 response.

3. Blastomycosis clinical symptoms: Outcome depends on the patient's underlying state of health, inhaled dose, and strain of *Blastomyces*.

  a. Acute pulmonary blastomycosis may not self-resolve, so even acute infections are treated with itraconazole.

  b. Chronic pulmonary blastomycosis (coin lesions) may be misdiagnosed as carcinoma.

  c. Disseminated blastomycosis may have bone and skin lesions, the latter useful for rapid diagnosis by the demonstration of **broad-based, budding yeasts in KOH** mounts of scrapings of active edges of a **skin lesion.**

D. Coccidioidomycosis (nicknamed valley fever)/*Coccidioides immitis* (Fig. 8.3).

  1. Description of agent and epidemiology:

   a. *Coccidioides immitis* is a thermally dimorphic pathogen that is endemic in California's **San Joaquin Valley** and the **Lower Sonoran Desert of the southwestern United States and Mexico.**

   b. Arthroconidia are found in alkaline desert sand. When inhaled, they resist phagocytosis due to their extremely hydrophobic nature.

   c. In the lungs, inhaled arthroconidia develop into larger spherical, walled structures called **spherules** with internal **endospores.**

  2. Coccidioidomycosis clinical symptoms:

   a. Acute, self-limiting coccidioidomycosis is similar to acute histoplasmosis except that erythema nodosum or multiforme are more likely. Persons with AIDS, pregnant women in the third trimester, Filipinos, African and Native Americans, and certain other ethnic groups have an increased risk of dissemination. Itraconazole or fluconazole is used to treat individuals at high risk of dissemination.

   b. Chronic coccidioidomycosis does not self-resolve.

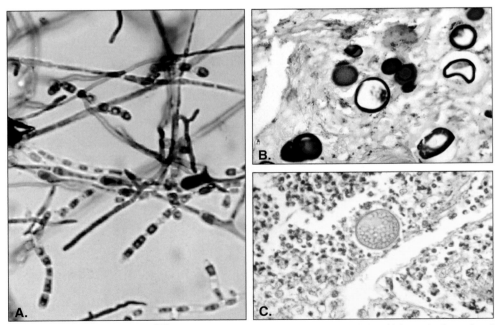

FIGURE 8.3. *Coccidioides immitis.* **(A)** *Coccidioides immitis* hyphae and arthroconidia, which are the forms found in the southwestern United States. (Courtesy of Glenn D. Roberts, PhD, Mayo Clinic.) **(B)** *Coccidioides immitis* spherules (some of them empty) from lung stained with silver stain. (Courtesy of Glenn D. Roberts, PhD, Mayo Clinic.) **(C)** *Coccidioides immitis* single spherule in tissue showing endospores inside the spherule. (CDC Public Health Image Library/Dr. Lucille K. Georg.)

    c. Disseminated coccidioidomycosis occurs under conditions of reduced cell-mediated immunity and high complement fixing antibody (a Th2 response). The clinical presentation is similar to disseminated histoplasmosis, with dissemination frequently to the meninges and mucous membranes.

VI. OPPORTUNISTIC MYCOSES

A. General aspects of opportunistic mycoses.

    1. These infections range from annoying or painful mucous membrane or cutaneous infections in mildly compromised patients to serious disseminated infections in severely immunocompromised patients.

    2. They are caused by endogenous or ubiquitous organisms of low inherent virulence that cause infection in debilitated, compromised patients.

    3. They are caused most commonly by **Candida, Cryptococcus, Aspergillus, Pneumocystis, Rhizopus, Mucor,** and **Pneumocystis,** but any fungus may cause an opportunistic infection if a patient is immunocompromised.

    4. Incidence is increasing as the number of compromised patients increases.

    5. Although these infections may be life-threatening in compromised patients, they are rarely serious in well-nourished, drug-free, healthy persons.

B. Candidiases are the most common opportunists.

    1. *Candida* spp. may cause mucocutaneous infections (see 8 III B) or more serious infections involving the bronchi or lungs, alimentary tract, bloodstream, urinary tract, and, less commonly, the heart or meninges.

    2. The most common cause is **C. albicans,** but incidence of infections due to other species of *Candida* is increasing.

    3. Predisposed individuals include very young or very old, those with wasting or nutritional diseases, those who are pregnant or immunosuppressed, and those who have diabetes, a history of long-term antibiotic and steroid use, indwelling catheters, or AIDS. Areas with excessive moisture like skin folds are also susceptible.

    4. Systemic candidiases are generally treated with fluconazole, lipid-based amphotericin B, or capsofungin.

    5. Candidiasis clinical signs and symptoms.

        a. Alimentary (see 8 III B).

        b. Candidemias or blood-borne infections occur most commonly in patients with indwelling catheters or GI tract overgrowth and minor bowel defects; these infections are manifested by fever, macronodular skin lesions, and endophthalmitis, leading to **endocarditis** or **cerebromeningitis.**

        c. Bronchopulmonary infection occurs in patients with chronic lung disease; it is usually manifested by persistent cough.

C. *Malassezia furfur* **septicemia** occurs primarily in premature neonates on intravenous lipid emulsions; it usually resolves if lipid supplements are stopped.

D. Cryptococcal meningitis or meningoencephalitis/*Cryptococcus neoformans.*

    1. Description of agent and epidemiology:

        a. C. neoformans is a **yeast** that possesses an **antigenic polysaccharide capsule.**

        b. It is found in weathered pigeon droppings.

        c. Central nervous system (CNS) disease occurs most commonly in patients with Hodgkin's lymphoma, diabetes, AIDS (where it is the dominant meningitis), leukemias, or leukocyte enzyme deficiency disease.

    2. Cryptococcal meningitis or meningoencephalitis clinical symptoms: Initial symptoms include headache of increasing severity, usually with fever, followed by typical signs of meningitis and sometimes personality changes.

   3. **Diagnosis:** diagnosed by cerebrospinal fluid (CSF) latex particle agglutination test for *Cryptococcus,* India ink wet mount, and culture following lysis of white blood cells in CSF.
   4. **Treatment:** treated with amphotericin B plus 5-fluorocytosine or fluconazole.

E. **Aspergilloses** are a variety of infections and allergic diseases that are caused *by Aspergillus fumigatus* and other species of *Aspergillus.*
   1. **Description and epidemiology:**
      a. ***A. fumigatus* is a ubiquitous, filamentous fungus** (one of our major recyclers) whose airborne spores (conidia) are constantly in the air.
      b. **Aspergilli** have characteristic **septate hyphae branching dichotomously at acute angles** (so it is **monomorphic**).
   2. **Forms of aspergillosis:**
      a. **Allergic bronchopulmonary aspergillosis** is an allergic disease in which the organism colonizes the mucous plugs formed in the lungs but does not invade lung tissues. It is diagnosed by the finding of high titers of immunoglobulin E (IgE) to *Aspergillus.*
      b. **Aspergilloma (fungus ball)** is a roughly spherical growth of *Aspergillus* in a preexisting lung cavity; growth does not invade the lung tissues. It presents clinically as recurrent hemoptysis and is diagnosed by radiologic methods; an "air sign" shift will be seen with a change in the position of the patient.
      c. **Invasive aspergillosis** is most common in patients with severe neutropenia starting in the lungs or spreading from sinus colonization. It requires aggressive treatment with voriconazole or lipid formulation of amphotericin B.

F. **Rhinocerebral zygomycoses** (also called **phycomycoses** or **mucormycoses**) are infections caused by **nonseptate fungi** (phylum Zygomycota, genera *Rhizopus, Absidia, Mucor,* and *Rhizomucor*).
   1. It occurs in patients with **acidotic diabetes or leukemia;** in these patients, it is **very invasive,** having a predilection for **invading blood vessels and the brain** and causing rapid decline to death.
   2. **Clinical symptoms:** presents with **facial swelling** and blood-tinged exudate in the turbinates and eyes, **mental lethargy,** blindness, and fixated pupils.
   3. **Diagnosis:** must be diagnosed rapidly, usually by a KOH mount of necrotic tissue or exudates from the eye, ear, or nose.
   4. **Treatment:** must be rapid! Management consists of (1) control of diabetes, (2) surgical debridement, and (3) aggressive treatment with amphotericin B or posaconazole.

G. *Pneumocystis* **pneumonitis/pneumonia** are infections caused by ***Pneumocystis jiroveci*** (formerly *Pneumocystis carinii*).
   1. ***Pneumocystis jiroveci*** has been reclassified as a fungus based on molecular biologic techniques such as ribotyping and DNA homology. It is an **obligate fungal organism** of humans (cannot be grown in vitro) but is extracellular, growing on the surfactant layer over the alveolar epithelium. **Trophozoites** and the larger **cysts** are seen in alveoli by **methenamine-silver** or calcofluor white stain of tissue.
   2. **Interstitial plasma cell pneumonitis** occurs in malnourished infants, transplant patients, patients on antineoplastic chemotherapy, and patients on corticosteroid therapy. Radiographs show a patchy, diffuse appearance, sometimes referred to as a ground-glass appearance.
   3. ***Pneumocystis jiroveci* pneumonia (PCP):**
      a. This pneumonia is responsible for approximately one-third of deaths in AIDS patients.
      b. PCP causes morbidity and mortality when $CD4^+$ counts decrease to less than $200/mm^3$ unless prevented with prophylaxis.
      c. Unlike the pneumonitis, PCP lacks plasma cells in the alveolar spaces.
      d. The organism causes a partial pressure of oxygen (PO_2) decline that is out of proportion to radiologic appearance.
      e. Radiographs show a characteristic ground-glass appearance.

4. **Diagnosis:** diagnosed by microscopy of biopsy specimen or alveolar fluids (Giemsa, specific fluorescent antibody, toluidine blue, methenamine-silver, or calcofluor stains). Presence of serum antibodies is not a useful indicator of infection because almost all healthy and immunocompromised individuals have antibodies to *Pneumocystis,* suggesting exposure is common.

5. **Treatment:** treated prophylactically with trimethoprim-sulfamethoxazole or trimethoprim and dapsone.

VII. TABLES FOR SELF-TESTING

The following tables present fungal infections in a format useful for solving case-history questions on the USMLE. For optimal use, cover the last column, which has the answers, and use these to test yourself *the first time* you use them. In the first two the patients are immunocompetent (Tables 8.3 and 8.4). In Table 8.5, the patients are compromised.

A. Table 8.3 summarizes superficial, cutaneous, mucocutaneous, subcutaneous, and allergic fungal diseases in the basically healthy individual.

B. Table 8.4 summarizes systemic infections in immunocompetent patients.

C. Table 8.5 summarizes opportunistic infections in compromised patients.

table 8.3 Symptoms and Clues to Diagnosis of Fungal Diseases in Generally Healthy Patients with Superficial, Cutaneous, Mucocutaneous, Subcutaneous, or Allergic Fungal Diseases*

Presenting Symptoms	Clues	Fungal Agent/Disease
Scattered small hypo- or hyperpigmented areas of skin, generally on the trunk of the body	KOH: yeastlike cells and short, curved, septate hyphae	*Malassezia furfur*/pityriasis versicolor
Cutaneous lesions with various degrees of inflammation; lesions spread from the periphery and may be spread by scratching	KOH: hyphae and arthroconidia KOH: pseudohyphae and yeasts	Dermatophytes: *Epidermophyton, Trichophyton, Microsporum*/tineas *Candida albicans* and *Candida* spp./candidiasis
Mucocutaneous lesion (vaginitis or diaper rash)	KOH: pseudohyphae and yeast	*Candida albicans* and *Candida* spp./candidiasis
Subcutaneous lesions following lymph nodes or solitary nodule	KOH: sparse cigar-shaped yeast in tissue Hyphae and conidia at 25°C	*Sporothrix schenckii* (*most* likely in the United States)/sporotrichosis
Colorful subcutaneous lesions, often pedunculated	KOH: dark, yeastlike cells with planar septations (sclerotic bodies) in giant cells	*Fonsecaea pedrosoi* and related forms/chromoblastomycosis
Subcutaneous swelling with sinus tracts and granules in exudate	Granules that are microcolonies of fungus	*Pseudallescheria boydii*/eumycotic mycetoma
Chronic cough; reduced lung capacity; mucous plugs in bronchus	High IgE levels against *Aspergillus*	*Aspergillus* sp./allergic bronchopulmonary aspergillosis

*Examination of skin scrapings or other tissue mounted in and cleared with potassium hydroxide (KOH) and examined microscopically

| t a b l e **8.4** | Symptoms and Clues to Diagnosis of Fungal Diseases in Generally Healthy Patients with Systemic Symptoms |

Presenting Symptoms	Clues	Fungal Agent/Disease
Acute pulmonary disease (cough, fever, night sweats) not responsive to antibacterials	Tissue: small, intracellular yeast Environmental form or 25°C culture: hyphae with micro-conidia and large tuberculate macroconidia Exposure to dusty environments such as bat-infested attics or caves, old chicken coops, construction in the Great Plains around the Ohio, Mississippi, and Missouri riverbeds	*Histoplasma capsulatum/* histoplasmosis
	Environmental form or 25°C culture: hyphae with microconidia Tissue: large, budding yeast with double retractile wall Exposure to dust/soil containing rotting organic material/ wood in the Great Plains around the Ohio, Mississippi, and Missouri riverbeds plus southeastern seaboard of the United States and up through Minnesota to Canada	*Blastomyces dermatitidis/* blastomycosis
	Environmental form: hyphae with arthroconidia Tissue form: spherules with endospores Exposure to blowing sand with arthroconidia in the southwestern United States (sand storms, dirt biking, rodeos)	*Coccidioides immitis/* coccidioidomycosis
Chronic pulmonary disease (cough, fever, night sweats, weight loss, protracted)	Same as for all three acute pulmonary diseases but with long-term symptoms and elevated sedimentation rate	Same as above
Disseminated disease (extrapulmonary sites such as skin, mucous membrane lesions, brain)	Same as for acute pulmonary disease but with poor immune response as demonstrated	Same as above

| t a b l e **8.5** | Symptoms and Conditions Associated with Opportunistic Mycoses |

Symptoms	Common Underlying Condition	Fungal Disease
Vaginitis (erythema and pain)	Antibiotic use; pregnancy, diabetes, AIDS	*Candida* vaginitis
Facial swelling; lethargy; red exudate from eyes and nares; necrotic tissue	Ketoacidotic diabetes, leukemia	Rhinocerebral mucormycosis
Fever without pulmonary symptoms	Neonates with IV lipid supplements Indwelling IV catheters	Fungemia: *Malassezia* Fungemia: *Candida*
Fever; pain on urination	Urinary catheter	Urinary candidiasis
Difficulty in swallowing	AIDS	Esophageal candidiasis
Meningeal symptoms	AIDS Severe neutropenia Hodgkin's lymphoma; diabetes	Cryptococcal meningitis, *Histoplasma* or coccidioidal meningitis, *Candida* cerebritis *Aspergillus* central nervous system infection Cryptococcal meningitis (chronic)
Pulmonary symptoms	Immunocompromised patient, particularly if neutropenic AIDS Urban homeless alcoholics	Invasive *Aspergillosis* *Pneumocystis* pneumonia Histoplasmosis, coccidioidomycosis Sporotrichosis (pulmonary)
Cough without upper respiratory symptoms, hemoptysis	Previous lung damage, especially cavities	Aspergilloma (fungus balls)
Endocarditis	Intravenous drug abuse	*Candida* or *Aspergillus* endocarditis
Enteritis (often with anal pruritus)	Antibiotic use	*Candida* enteritis
Whitish covering in mouth	Premature infants, children on antibiotics	*Candida* thrush
Corners of mouth sore	Elderly suffering from malnourishment	Perlèche
Sore gums	Dentures	Denture stomatitis
Skin lesions; endophthalmitis	Indwelling catheter	Candidemia

Review Test

Directions: Each of the numbered items or incomplete statements in this section is followed by answers or completions of the statement. Select the ONE lettered answer that is BEST in each case.

1. A florist presents with a subcutaneous lesion on the hand, which she thinks resulted from a jab wound she received while she was making a sphagnum moss-wire frame for a floral wreath. The nodule has ulcerated and not healed despite use of antibacterial cream, and a new nodule is forming above the original lesion. What is most likely to be an appropriate treatment for this infection?

(A) Oral itraconazole or potassium iodide
(B) Miconazole cream
(C) Cortisone cream
(D) Oral griseofulvin
(E) Penicillin

2. Although hard to find in the above mentioned nodule, what form would be present in the tissue?

(A) Lots of hyphae
(B) Long, branching hyphae with acute angles
(C) Yeasts with broad-based buds
(D) Cigar-shaped to oval yeasts
(E) Yeast with multiple buds (mariner's wheel)

3. A patient presents with paranasal swelling and bloody exudate from both his eyes and nares, and he is nearly comatose. Necrotic tissue in the nasal turbinates show nonseptate hyphae consistent with *Rhizopus, Mucor,* or *Absidia* (phylum Zygomycota, class Phycomycetes). What is the most likely compromising condition underlying this infection?

(A) AIDS
(B) Ketoacidotic diabetes
(C) Neutropenia
(D) B-cell defects
(E) Chronic sinusitis

4. A patient presents with a circular, itchy, inflamed skin lesion that is slightly raised; it is on his left side where his dog sleeps next to him. His dog has had some localized areas of hair loss. The patient has no systemic symptoms. What would you expect to find in a KOH of skin scrapings?

(A) Clusters of yeastlike cells and short curved septate hyphae
(B) Hyphae with little branching but possibly with some hyphae breaking up into arthroconidia
(C) Filariform larvae
(D) Budding yeasts with some pseudohyphae and true hyphae
(E) Large budding yeast cells with broad bases on the buds and thick cell walls

5. A severely neutropenic patient presents with pneumonia. Bronchial alveolar fluid shows dichotomously branching (generally with acute angles), septate hyphae. What is the most likely causative agent?

(A) *Aspergillus*
(B) *Cryptococcus*
(C) *Candida*
(D) *Malassezia*
(E) *Rhizopus*

6. What is a mass of fungal filaments called?

(A) Pseudohyphae
(B) Hyphae
(C) Mycelium
(D) Septum
(E) Yeast

7. A premature infant on intravenous nutrients and high-lipid fluids has developed septicemia that cultures out on blood agar only when overlaid with sterile olive oil. What is the most likely causative agent?

(A) *Aspergillus*
(B) *Candida*
(C) *Cryptococcus*
(D) *Malassezia*
(E) *Sporothrix*

8. A filamentous fungus subunit is a

(A) Coenocyte
(B) Hypha

(C) Mycelium
(D) Septum
(E) Yeast

9. To treat a patient with a life-threatening fungal infection, you choose an antifungal drug that causes pore formation in the fungal membrane and actually kills the cells. Which drug would this be?

(A) Amphotericin B
(B) Griseofulvin
(C) Ketoconazole
(D) Miconazole
(E) Nystatin

10. A 15-year-old dirt-bike rider visiting southern California the first time has developed pneumonia. The causative organism has environmental form that consists of hyphae that break up into arthroconidia, which become airborne. What is the agent?

(A) *Aspergillus fumigatus*
(B) *Blastomyces dermatitidis*
(C) *Coccidioides immitis*
(D) *Histoplasma capsulatum*
(E) *Sporothrix schenckii*

11. Which of the following drugs inhibits ergosterol synthesis, is important in treating *Candida* fungemias, and is used orally to suppress relapses of cryptococcal meningitis in AIDS patients?

(A) Amphotericin B
(B) Fluconazole
(C) Griseofulvin
(D) Echinocandins
(E) Nystatin

12. A patient has splotchy hypopigmentation on the chest and back with only slight itchiness. What is most likely to be seen on a KOH mount of the skin scraping?

(A) Yeasts, pseudohyphae, and true hyphae
(B) Filaments with lots of arthroconidia
(C) Clusters of round fungal cells with short, curved, septate hyphae
(D) Darkly pigmented, round cells with sharp interior septations
(E) Cigar-shaped yeasts

13. A patient has a dry, scaly, erythematous penis. Skin scales stained with calcofluor white show fluorescent blue-white yeasts and a few pseudohyphae. What is the causative agent of this dermatophytic look-alike?

(A) *Candida*
(B) *Trichosporon*
(C) *Trichophyton*
(D) *Malassezia*
(E) *Microsporum*

14. A recent immigrant from rural Brazil presents with a swollen face and extremely poor dental hygiene, including loss of an adult tooth, which appears to be the focus of the current infection. There are two open ulcers on the outside of the swollen cheek. Small yellow "grains" are seen in one of the ulcers. Gram stain shows purple-staining fine filaments. What is the most likely disease?

(A) Actinomycotic mycetoma
(B) Chromomycosis
(C) Eumycotic mycetoma
(D) Sporotrichosis
(E) Paracoccidioidomycosis

15. A patient who is a recent immigrant from a tropical, remote, rural area with no medical care is now working with a group of migrant crop harvesters. He has a large, raised, colored, cauliflower-like ankle lesion. Darkly pigmented, yeastlike sclerotic bodies are seen in the tissue biopsy. Which of the following is the most likely diagnosis?

(A) Actinomycotic mycetoma
(B) Chromoblastomycosis
(C) Eumycotic mycetoma
(D) Sporotrichosis
(E) Tinea nigra

16. A premature baby, now 4 days old, has developed a white coating on her buccal mucosa extending onto her lips. It appears to be painful. What is the most likely causative agent?

(A) *Actinomyces*
(B) *Aspergillus*
(C) *Candida*
(D) *Fusobacterium*
(E) *Microsporum*

17. Which of the following stains allows differentiation of fungus from human tissue by staining the fungus a pink-red color?

(A) Calcofluor white stain
(B) Gomori methenamine-silver stain
(C) Periodic acid-Schiff stain
(D) Hematoxylin and eosin stain

18. A normally healthy 8-year-old boy from Florida is visiting friends on a farm in Iowa during the month of July. He presents on July 28 with a fever, cough, and lower respiratory symptoms (no upper respiratory tract symptoms). He has been ill for 4 days. His chest sounds are consistent with pneumonia, so a chest radiograph is obtained. The radiograph shows small, patchy infiltrates with hilar adenopathy. His blood smear shows small, nondescript yeast forms inside monocytic cells. What is the most likely causative agent?

(A) *Aspergillus fumigatus*
(B) *Blastomyces dermatitidis*
(C) *Coccidioides immitis*
(D) *Histoplasma capsulatum*
(E) *Pneumocystis jiroveci*

19. Which of the following is a polyene antifungal agent used for many life-threatening fungal infections?

(A) Amphotericin B
(B) Griseofulvin
(C) Itraconazole
(D) Miconazole
(E) Nystatin

20. A logger undergoing chemotherapy for cancer has developed pneumonia and skin lesions. Biopsy of the skin lesions demonstrates the presence of large yeasts with thick cell walls and broad-based buds. What is the most likely causative agent?

(A) *Aspergillus fumigatus*
(B) *Blastomyces dermatitidis*
(C) *Coccidioides immitis*
(D) *Histoplasma capsulatum*
(E) *Sporothrix schenckii*

21. What is the scientific name for a fungal cross wall?

(A) Coenocyte
(B) Hypha
(C) Mycelium
(D) Septum
(E) Yeast

22. A noncompliant, human immunodeficiency virus (HIV)-positive patient has been complaining of a stiff neck and a severe headache. The headache was initially lessened by analgesics, but the analgesics are no longer effective. His current $CD4^+$ count is $180/mm^3$. He is not on any prophylactic drugs. What is the most likely causative agent?

(A) *Aspergillus*
(B) *Cryptococcus*
(C) *Candida*
(D) *Malassezia*
(E) *Sporothrix*

23. Which of the following features differentiates fungal cells from human cells?

(A) 80S ribosomes
(B) Presence of an endoplasmic reticulum
(C) Ergosterol as the major membrane sterol
(D) Enzymes that allow them to use carbon dioxide as their sole carbon source
(E) Presence of chloroplasts

Answers and Explanations

1. **The answer is A.** This is a classic case of lymphocutaneous sporotrichosis in which a gardener or florist is infected via a puncture wound. The drug of choice is either itraconazole or potassium iodide (administered orally in milk). Topical antifungals are not effective, and the cortisone cream would probably enhance the spread of the disease. Griseofulvin localizes in the keratinized tissues and would not halt the subcutaneous spread of this infection. Penicillin would have no effect because *Sporothrix* is not a bacterium.

2. **The answer is D.** This is a classic case of lymphocutaneous sporotrichosis. *Sporothrix schenckii* is dimorphic; the tissue form is cigar-shaped yeasts, but they are hard to find by histology.

3. **The answer is B.** Zygomycota are aseptate fungi that cause serious infections, primarily in ketoacidotic diabetic patients and cancer patients. Fungal infections common in AIDS patients include *Candida* infections (ranging from oral thrush early to fungemias later), cryptococcal meningitis, and disseminated histoplasmosis and coccidioidomycosis. Severely neutropenic patients are most likely to have invasive *Aspergillus* infections.

4. **The answer is B.** The case is ringworm acquired from a dog. In tissue, any of the dermatophytes would show hyphae and arthroconidia. Pityriasis versicolor would have the clusters of yeasts with short, septate, curved hyphae (spaghetti and meatballs appearance). A filariform larvae would only be characteristic of dog hookworm, which is usually acquired from walking barefoot where there are dog feces. It would not be acquired from sleeping with the dog, and would not cause hair loss in the dog. Choice D describes *Candida,* which does not fit the case. Choice E would describe *Blastomycosis,* which is highly unlikely.

5. **The answer is A.** *Aspergillus* spores are commonly airborne. Invasive infections with *Aspergillus* are controlled by phagocytic cells. In severe neutropenia, risk of infection is high.

6. **The answer is C.** A mycelium is a mass of hyphae (fungal filaments).

7. **The answer is D.** *Malassezia furfur* is a lipophilic fungus that is found on skin. It causes fungemia, primarily in premature infants on high-lipid intravenous supplements.

8. **The answer is B.** The fungal subunit, called a hypha, is a filamentous structure with or without cross walls (septae).

9. **The answer is A.** Although both amphotericin B and nystatin are polyenes, only amphotericin B is used systemically. The imidazoles inhibit ergosterol synthesis, and griseofulvin, which localizes in the keratinized tissues, inhibits the growth of dermatophytes by inhibiting microtubule assembly.

10. **The answer is C.** *Coccidioides immitis* is found in desert sand, primarily as arthroconidia and hyphae.

11. **The answer is B.** Fluconazole is an imidazole; all imidazoles inhibit ergosterol synthesis. Fluconazole has become the mainstay in the treatment of serious *Candida* infections, and it is used to prevent relapse of fungal CNS infections in compromised patients. Amphotericin B and nystatin both bind to ergosterol and create membrane pores, causing cell leakage and death. Echinocandins inhibit the fungal cell wall synthesis. Griseofulvin is not used against *Candida* as it may make the infection worse.

12. **The answer is C.** *Malassezia furfur* is seen in tissues as clusters of round fungal cells with short, curved septate hyphae (spaghetti and meatballs appearance) and is the causative agent of pityriasis or tinea versicolor; *M. furfur* overgrowth causes pigmentation disturbances.

13. **The answer is A.** *Candida* may cause skin infections that resemble some dermatophytic infections. The patient described in the question has *Candida* balanitis. In tinea cruris, the penis is not usually involved.

14. **The answer is A.** The disease syndrome is lumpy jaw, which is a form of mycetoma. The location of the lesions and presenting signs seen in this patient suggest actinomycotic mycetoma, a bacterial infection caused by the *Actinomyces* part of the gingival crevices flora. (Students: You needed a nonfungal question!) Yeasts will also stain Gram-positive. Remember that *Actinomyces* is a Gram-positive anaerobic bacterium that is not acid-fast.

15. **The answer is B.** The finding of dematiaceous (dark), yeastlike sclerotic bodies that have sharp planar division lines and the clinical presentation are both characteristic of chromoblastomycosis. Tinea nigra would show dematiaceous hyphae in flat palmar or plantar lesions.

16. **The answer is C.** The disease described is thrush, and it is caused by *Candida*.

17. **The answer is C.** Calcofluor white stain, Gomori methenamine-silver stain, and periodic acid-Schiff stain are all differential stains, but only the periodic acid-Schiff stain turns fungi a pink-red color. The hematoxylin and eosin stain turns fungi a pink-red color also but does not differentiate between the fungi and human tissue, so it is not a correct answer.

18. **The answer is D.** *Histoplasma* and *Blastomyces* are both endemic in Iowa (central United States bordering the Mississippi River), but only *Histoplasma* fits the description of a facultative intracellular parasite circulating in the reticuloendothelial system.

19. **The answer is A.** Amphotericin B, a polyene, is the most effective treatment for many life-threatening fungal infections. Nystatin, also a polyene, is used topically or orally, but is not absorbed.

20. **The answer is B.** *Blastomyces* has a double refractile wall and buds with a broad base of attachment to the mother cell. The environmental association appears to be rotting wood.

21. **The answer is B.** The cross wall of a hypha is called a septum or septation.

22. **The answer is B.** *Cryptococcus,* an encapsulated yeast, is the major causative agent of meningitis in patients with AIDS.

23. **The answer is C.** Ergosterol is the major fungus membrane sterol, and its presence is important in chemotherapy of fungal infections. For example, amphotericin B binds to ergosterol, producing pores that leak out cellular contents, killing the fungus. Imidazole drugs inhibit the synthesis of ergosterol. Both fungi and humans have 80S ribosomes and endoplasmic reticulum. Fungi are heterotrophic rather than autotrophic and thus cannot use carbon dioxide as their carbon source; instead, fungi break down organic carbon compounds. Fungi are also not photosynthetic.

I. CHARACTERISTICS OF PARASITES AND THEIR HOSTS

A. Parasites
1. **Ectoparasites** live on the skin or hair (e.g., lice); **endoparasites** live in the host. The rest of the chapter covers human endoparasites.
2. They may be **obligate parasites (entirely dependent on the host)** or **facultative parasites** (free living or associated with the host).
3. They rival malnutrition as the major cause of morbidity and mortality worldwide.
4. Parasites may be present in a host as a commensal organism. Factors such as a low protein diet may favor virulence and growth of organisms such as *Entamoeba histolytica*. Parasite numbers also influence the severity and progression of disease. Any decrease in immune functioning (particularly cell-mediated) is likely to cause both increased susceptibility to infection and more severe infections.

B. Hosts may be one of three types:
1. A host in which either eggs (usually ingested) or very early larval forms develop into larval or intermediate parasite stages is by convention called an **intermediate host.**
2. A host in which the larval stages infect and mature into the sexually mature adult parasites is called a **definitive host.**
3. A **reservoir host is any host** essential to parasite survival and a focus for spread to other hosts (e.g., pigs (swine) for the pig roundworm *Trichinella spiralis*).

C. Vectors are living transmitters of disease and are classified as one of the following:
1. **Mechanical vectors** are nonessential to the life cycle of the pathogen (e.g., flies who track *Chlamydia trachomatis* from one child's eye to another).
2. **Biological vectors,** by contrast, serve as the site of some developmental events in the life cycle of the parasite, such as mosquitoes in malaria.

II. PROTOZOAN PARASITES

A. General characteristics. Protozoan parasites are single-celled animals and therefore have no multicellular stages such as larvae. There are often two distinctive forms:
1. **Trophozoites** are the actively motile forms, which are delicate and do not survive long outside the body; if ingested, they rarely withstand normal stomach acid, so they are generally considered noninfectious.

2. **Cysts** are sturdy resting stages and the most common infective form in fecal-oral spread as they survive at least a while in the environment and passage through normal stomach acid.

B. Amebas move by **pseudopods created by streaming protoplasm** and include *Entamoeba, Acanthamoeba,* and *Naegleria.*

C. Flagellates move by the action of **flagella** and include *Giardia, Trichomonas, Trypanosoma,* and *Leishmania.*
   1. *Giardia* and *Trichomonas* have simple trophozoites and cysts.
   2. *Trypanosoma* and *Leishmania* species are **hemoflagellates** that infect blood and tissues. They have life cycles involving several forms:
      a. **Trypomastigotes** are free living, elongated, flagellated forms with an undulating membrane. They are seen extracellularly in blood in *Trypanosoma* infections.
      b. **Amastigotes** are "oval" cells that do not have a flagellum or an undulating membrane. They are seen in infected tissue (e.g., heart tissue infected with *Trypanosoma cruzi*) or macrophages (*Leishmania*).

D. *Ciliates* move by the action of **cilia. *Balantidium coli,*** a rare cause of dysentery, is the only human ciliate of note.

E. Apicomplexa (also called sporozoa or coccidia) are intracellular protozoans with complex life cycles involving more than one host, a gliding ("tractor") motility, and an apical complex that allows them to be taken up by host cells. They include *Plasmodium, Toxoplasma, Pneumocystis, Cryptosporidium, Cyclospora, Isopora,* and *Babesia.*

III. WORMS

A. Trematodes are the **flatworms (Platyhelminthes),** informally called **flukes.** Depending on the fluke, **human acquisition requires either being in water or ingestion of the parasites found in or on aquatic plants, fish, or crabs.**
   1. **Flukes** have complex life cycles involving two or three sequential hosts (depending on the fluke) but always **involving water and mollusks.**
   2. **Adult flukes** develop in **vertebrate hosts, including humans.** Adult flukes:
      a. Are **flat** and **fleshy.**
      b. Are **hermaphroditic except for the genus *Schistosoma,*** which has separate males and females; thus, there is the schistosome and non-schistosomal fluke division.
      c. **Lay eggs** in the vertebrate host; the eggs pass outside.
   3. **If fluke eggs land in water,** they develop a motile **early larval form,** which when released enters the **first intermediate host (aquatic snails or clams) by ingestion or invasion.** They increase in number and are released from the first host as **cercaria,** the second motile-stage larvae form.
   4. The **cercaria of the schistosomes invade the skin of people in water.** For the other trematodes (depending on which one), the late larval **cercaria either encyst on aquatic plants or infect crabs or fish.** Humans are accidently infected by non-schistosomal flukes through the **ingestion of the plants, crabs, or fish.**

B. Cestodes are **flatworms (Platyhelminthes)** informally called **tapeworms.**
   1. **Adult tapeworms** develop in their definitive host.
      a. The **adult tapeworm** has the following **parts:**
         (1) **Scolex (head),** a knobby structure with suckers or a sucking groove **used to adhere to the vertebrate host's small intestinal mucosa.**
         (2) **Neck, which produces the segments, or proglottids, producing the worm.**

      (3) Proglottids, which mature as they move away from the scolex. **Each proglottid is hermaphroditic,** with both male and female reproductive organs developing in each section (proglottid) and **mature eggs produced in the most distal proglottids.**

  b. Adult cestodes (tapeworms) inhabit the small intestines of humans or their other **vertebrate definitive host.** Lacking a gastrointestinal tract, they absorb nutrients from the host's gastro-intestinal tract.

2. Eggs from proglottids are released in the feces from the vertebrate definitive host and may contaminate soil or food. **Ingested eggs** develop into invasive larval forms that migrate through tissues and **may cause serious** disease such as **neurocysticercosis. Hosts ingest-ing the larvae,** generally in undercooked fish or meat, **develop intestinal tapeworms, which generally cause mild disease.**

3. Cestode infections:

  a. When humans are the definitive host, the presence of the adult tapeworm in the small in-testine does not cause major symptoms, but it may affect nutrition. Human adult tapeworms include *Taenia saginata* (beef), *Taenia solium* (pork flatworm), *Diphyllobothrium latum* (broad fish tapeworm found in fish in some lakes in cold regions, such as, Canada, Alaska), *Hymenolepis nana* (humans and rodents), and *Dipylidium caninum* (dogs and cats).

  b. When humans serve as the intermediate host, more serious disease results. Symptoms de-pend on the **migration of the larval forms.** Diseases include cysticercosis (*Taenia solium*), sparganosis (*Diphyllobothrium latum*), unilocular hydatid cyst disease (*Echinococcus granulosus*), and alveolar hydatid cyst disease (*Echinococcus multilocularis*).

  c. Infection can be diagnosed by demonstration of eggs or proglottids in the feces or cysticerci in tissues.

C. Nematodes are the **roundworms.**

  1. Nematodes have **round, unsegmented adult bodies covered by a tough cuticle.**

  2. They can be remembered by the following mnemonic: NEMA^{2}T^{3}ODES
    Necator (hookworm [United States])
    Enterobius (pinworm)
    Mosquito borne: *Wuchereria* and *Brugia*
    A^2: *Ascaris* and *Ancylostoma*
    T^3: *Trichuris, Trichinella,* and *Toxocara*
    Onchocerca (river blindness)
    Dracunculus (Guinea worm, nearly eradicated)
    Eye worm (Loa loa)
    Strongyloides (threadworm)

  3. Transmission can occur in several ways:

    a. Ingestion of eggs (*Enterobius, Ascaris, Trichuris,* and *Toxocara*)

    b. Ingestion of larvae in undercooked game or pork (*Trichinella*) (Ingestion mnemonic: EAT^3.)

    c. Direct invasion of skin by larval forms in soil contaminated with feces (*Necator, Ancylos-toma,* and *Strongyloides*)

    d. Larvae transmission via insect bite (*Wuchereria, Loa, Mansonella,* and *Onchocerca*)

Review Test

Please note that all parasite questions follow Chapter 10.

chapter 10 Parasitic Diseases

Although parasitic diseases still have a tremendous impact on world health, the level of sanitation, temperate climate in most areas, and reasonably good housing conditions in the United States limit their impact in this country. This review focuses on parasitic diseases common in the United States or commonly seen in travelers in the United States. The diseases are presented in a series of tables. Each table is organized to facilitate self-testing to check your preparedness for USMLE case-based questions. Symptoms are presented first. Your first task is to identify the causative agent based on the information presented. As you progress from the first left cell toward the right, your choices should narrow. Small images are incorporated into the tables; they are not to scale.

To use these tables for self-testing or later review, use two cover sheets, one to cover all subsequent rows and a second top sheet to move left to right on the row you are testing yourself on, starting with only the left cell revealed. On the top sheet, you may want to jot down the column headings, which are basically the most commonly asked USMLE questions, in order to make sure you can answer them for each of the organisms. See Tables 10.1, 10.2, and 10.3 (Figs. 10.1 and 10.2).

Signs/Symptoms/Case Details	Infective Form/Transmission	Diagnostic Form	Diseases/Treatment	Species/Type
Fever, auras (often odor), severe headache, rapid progression to coma and death; generally occurs during summer in the southern United States in healthy young children	Ameba acquired through cribriform plate from jumping or swimming in warm water swimming holes (environmental ameba)	Trophozoites (slug-like amebas) and smooth-walled cysts in CSF	Primary amebic meningoencephalitis Poor prognosis; amphotericin B	*Naegleria*/free-living ameba
Altered mental status with chronic onset in debilitated or immuno-compromised patients	Possibly transmitted in cyst-contaminated dust; probably enters through lungs or eyes (majority of infected individuals wear contact lenses); environmental organism	Trophozoites (below) and wrinkled cysts in CSF[1]	Granulomatous amebic encephalitis BSB (Beyond scope of book)	*Acanthamoeba*/free-living ameba
Neonate with fever, pneumonitis, and hepatosplenomegaly, or infant or young child with active chorioretinitis, encephalomyelitis, hydrocephaly, or microcephaly	Congenital transmission of tachyzoites across placenta if mother's primary infection occurs during pregnancy; maternal antibody from prior infection protects fetus	Clinical diagnosis Intracerebral calcifications PCR on amniotic fluid PCR on neonatal urine	Toxoplasmosis BSB	*Toxoplasma gondii*/protozoan parasite
Keratitis with severe ocular pain but a mild inflammatory response; corneal infection leading to ulceration may require both trauma (from contacts) and exposure (contaminated contact solution or dust); often a chronic onset; may lead to loss of eyesight	Cysts in environment; homemade contact saline solution has been implicated in some cases; almost all patients are contact wearers	Motile trophozoites (ameba) or cysts in corneal scraping; stain with calcofluor white and fluoresce	Keratitis BSB	*Acanthamoeba*/free-living ameba

(continued)

table 10.1 Central Nervous System, Eye, Blood, and Tissue (Including Skin) Parasites (*Continued*)

Signs/Symptoms/Case Details	Infective Form/Transmission	Diagnostic Form	Diseases/Treatment	Species/Type
Patient with posterior cervical lymph node enlargement, irregular fevers, rigors, headache, night sweats; patients eventually develop stupor; travel to Africa	Bite of tsetse fly carrying trypomastigotes	Flagellated trypomastigotes with undulating membrane in blood or CSF; hyper gamma-globulinemia[2]	African sleeping sickness; organisms are not cleared due to antigenic variation BSB	*Trypanosoma brucei*/ hemoflagellate noted for antigenic variation
Heart failure; autopsy reveals greatly enlarged heart; travel or residence in poor areas of South America	Defecating reduviid bug bites a person and deposits feces with trypomastigotes; bite itches; scratching inoculates organism into bite	Amastigotes (no undulating membrane nor flagella) in heart tissue; trypomastigotes in blood early	Chagas' disease[3] BSB	*Trypanosoma cruzi*/ hemoflagellates often C or U shaped
T-cell compromised patients; fever with lymphadenopathy and pneumonia; often changes in mental status (calcified lesions seen on CNS imaging); chorioretinitis (Symptoms in healthy adults resemble mononucleosis)	Ingestion of infective oocysts from cat feces or contaminated undercooked meat. Excreted form becomes an infective oocyst in approximately 2 days; may also be reactivated in AIDS	Serological diagnosis; the distinctive crescent-shaped replicating tachyzoites and cysts are seldom seen Immunofluorescent staining more sensitive	Toxoplasmosis Prophylaxis is TMP-SMT for *Pneumocystis* Treatment is BSB[4]	*Toxoplasma gondii*/ protozoan parasite Once infected, humans remain infected unless treated. *T. gondii* reactivates with immunosuppression but not pregnancy (see Fig. 10.1)

Influenza-like prodrome followed by recurring intense paroxysms[5] (chills [rigors for 10–15 minutes] followed by a hot phase for several hours ending with profuse sweating); patterns depend on species; anemia[6]	*Anopheles* mosquito bite bearing sporozoites; associated with travel to endemic area except in cases of rare "airport malaria," in which an individual who resides near an international airport is bitten by a mosquito	Hematocrit is low and urine often dark Merozoites in red blood cells	Malaria	*Plasmodium* sp./ apicomplexa (see life cycle in Fig. 10.2) See species features compared in Table 10.2
Subcutaneous nodules, dermatitis: wrinkled skin and eye infection Central America and Africa	Larvae-infected black fly bite (*Simulium*) near running water	Microfilariae are seen on skin exam (adults develop in nodules and migrate around)	Surgical removal of nodules and ivermectin	*Onchocerca volvulus*/river blindness
Fever, lymphangitis, and lymphadenitis; recurring fevers; limb or scrotal elephantiasis	Mosquitoes transmitting filarial worms	Often a clinical diagnosis in endemic areas; microfilaria in blood	Filarial worms BSB	*Wucheria* and *Brugia*
Calabar swellings with some pain and pruritis; migrating; may cross conjunctiva Western central Africa	Mango fly (*Chrysops*) transmit infective filariae	Eosinophilia and symptoms	Loiasis; little damage; surgical removal; ivermectin	*Loa loa*/african eye worms

[1]Trophozoites of *Acanthamoeba* spp. from culture. (Courtesy of Centers for Disease Control DPDx Parasite Image Library.)

[2]*Trypanosoma brucei* sp. in thin blood smears stained with Wright-Giemsa. (Courtesy of Centers for Disease Control DPDx Parasite Image Library.)

[3]*Trypanosoma cruzi* trypomastigote in a thin blood smear stained with Giemsa. (Courtesy of Centers for Disease Control DPDx Parasite Image Library.)

[4]Formalin-fixed *Toxoplasma gondii* tachyzoites stained by immunofluorescence (IFA). This is a positive reaction (tachyzoites + human antibodies to *Toxoplasma* + FITC-labeled antihuman IgG = fluorescence.) (Courtesy of Centers for Disease Control DPDx Parasite Image Library.)

[5]Paroxysms are caused by release of toxic hemoglobin metabolites when merozoites lyse red cells. Anemia is caused by loss of red blood cells. Cerebral malaria (*Plasmodium falciparum*) is due to adherence of infected erythrocytes in cerebral venules and effects of metabolic by-products in the CNS.

[6]A parasite called *Babesia microti* primarily causes disease in cattle and may cause anemia with malaria-like symptoms in humans (**babesiosis**). Because it is **transmitted by the *Ixodes* tick, coinfections with *Borrelia burgdorferi* or *Anaplasma*** may occur. Babesiosis is diagnosed by the presence of multiple ringlike forms in the red blood cells.

table	10.2	Malaria. All Plasmodia have two distinct hosts. A vertebrate (human or cattle) is the intermediate host where the asexual phase of the parasite's life cycle (schizogony) takes place in the liver and red blood cells. The *Anopheles* mosquito is the definitive host and is the site of the sexual phase of the parasite's life cycle (sporogony). (See Fig. 10.2 for the life cycle.)

Species[1]	Disease	Diagnosis (Giemsa stained)[4]	Treatment
Plasmodium vivax	Tertian malaria	Oval-shaped host cells with Schüffner's granules and ragged cell wall are seen on thick and thin blood examination	Chloroquine phosphate then primaquine
Plasmodium malariae[2]	Quartan malaria[2]	Bar and band forms; rosette schizonts	Chloroquine
Plasmodium falciparum	Malignant tertian malaria[3]	Multiple ring forms and crescents (gametocytes)→ schizonts rare in peripheral blood[5]	Chloroquine; chloroquine-resistant strains are treated with quinine sulfate with doxycycline; complicated falciparum malaria with quinidine sulfate[6]

[1]*Plasmodium ovale* (rare) causes benign tertian (ovale) malaria. Transmission, diagnosis, and treatment are similar to those for *P. vivax*. **Both *P. ovale* and *P. vivax* form hypnozoites (or sleeping forms) in the liver** that may not progress to merozoite production until months later (and like other liver forms are not sensitive to chloroquine). This recurrence of symptoms is called RELAPSE from LIVER forms.

[2]Recurrence of *P. malariae* symptoms, called RECRUDESCENCE, may result from a persistent low level of parasites in the RED blood cells.

[3]*P.* falciparum-infected red blood cells adhere to the endothelium of peripheral capillaries, resulting in "sludging." Severe anemia results from multiple infections of both immature and mature red blood cells. The severe disease that results constitutes a medical emergency.

[4]Immunofluorescent antibodies and agarose DNA gels and probes are now used in identification instead of morphology.

[5]Multiply-infected red blood cells with appliqué forms in thin blood smears. (Courtesy of Centers for Disease Control DPDx Parasite Image Library.)

[6]Left two are mature microgametocytes (female); Right two are mature macrogametocytes (male). (Courtesy of Centers for Disease Control DPDx Parasite Image Library.)

t a b l e 10.3 Gastrointestinal and Urogenital Parasitic Infections

Signs/Symptoms/Case Details	Infective Form/Transmission	Diagnostic Form	Diseases/Treatment	Species/Type
Dysentery; inverted flask-shaped ulcers of large intestine with extra-intestinal abscesses (particularly liver) common	Fecal-oral by water, fresh fruits, and vegetables; nonmotile cysts are infective stage	Cysts and motile trophozoites with wagon-wheel-like nuclei and ingested WBCs/RBCs are seen in stools; serologic testing	Amebic dysentery Metronidazole followed by paromomycin or iodoquinol	*Entamoeba histolytica*/amoeba[1] A B
Diarrhea with malabsorption; starts watery and then, as more and more trophozoites attach through their ventral sucking disk, the malabsorption gets worse and diarrhea more "fatty"; severe pain on ingestion of dairy is common	Quadrinucleate cysts Fecal (e.g., human, beaver, muskrat) by water, food, oral-anal intercourse, day care centers	Pyriform flagellated trophozoites with ventral sucking disk may not be seen; cysts found in stool Fecal antigen test is more sensitive	Giardiasis Tinidazole or nitazoxanide	*Giardia lamblia*/flagellate[2]
Transient diarrhea in healthy persons; severe diarrhea in immunocompromised persons	Chlorine-resistant cysts are found in up to 85% of United States surface water removed during water treatment by flocculation or filtration; AIDS patients should boil or filter water	Acid-fast oocysts in stool Biopsy: dots (cysts) in intestinal glands	Cryptosporidiosis No good treatment in AIDS except antiretroviral therapy	*Cryptosporidium* spp./apicomplexa protozoan
Vitamin B_{12} anemia in genetically predisposed; mild abdominal discomfort	Ingestion of late larvae (still viable) in smoked, pickled, undercooked, or raw fish from cold water lake regions such as Scandinavia or Canada[3]	Proglottids (*left*) and eggs in stool Proglottids wider than long ("broad" fish tapeworm); worm up to several meters long	Intestinal tapeworm: vitamin B_{12} anemia results if organism attaches in the proximal portion of the jejunum in genetically predisposed individuals	*Diphyllobothrium latum*/cestode (tapeworm)

(*continued*)

195

table 10.3	Gastrointestinal and Urogenital Parasitic Infections (*Continued*)			
Signs/Symptoms/Case Details	**Infective Form/Transmission**	**Diagnostic Form**	**Diseases/Treatment**	**Species/Type**
Perianal itching; sometimes with vaginitis; generally found in children[4] 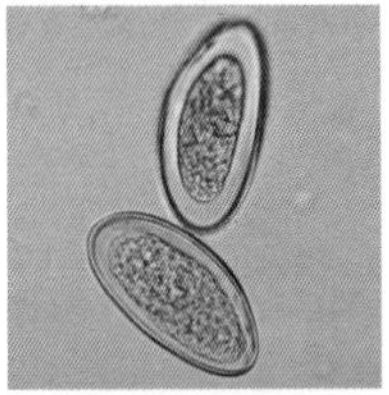	Eggs from bed linens and clothes are spread by air currents and stay viable for several days Reinfection by contaminated fingers is common	Scotch tape mount; eggs (*far left*) and 2- to 5-mm-long roundworms that are no more than 0.5 mm in diameter	Pinworms Albendazole or mebendazole	*Enterobius vermicularis*/(pinworm); the most common roundworm in the United States
Pneumonitis early, GI symptoms may be absent or a writhing sensation may be felt; anesthetics, fever, and drugs may induce adult worms to migrate to places such as the bile ducts or pancreas; intestinal blockage may occur in children with heavy worm burden	Ingestion of egg-contaminated feces; larvae exit GI tract into tissues and reach lymphatics and then lungs; larvae are coughed up and swallowed and then mature into adults in small intestines where they mate	Bile-stained knobby eggs (*right*) or 6- to 12-inch-long roundworms seen on radiograph or cholangiogram; serologic test shows some cross-reaction with *Trichuris*	Ascariasis Supportive therapy during pneumonitis; surgery for ectopic migrations Albendazole or mebendazole	*Ascaris lumbricoides*/(roundworm; egg shown below)[5] 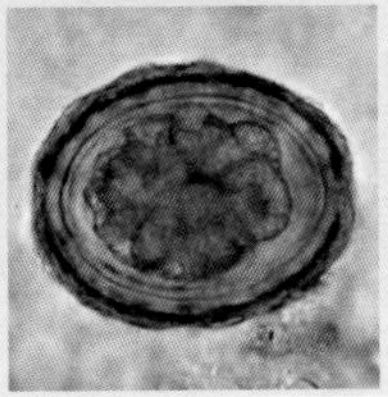
Generally asymptomatic but symptoms, when present, may be severe abdominal pain with bloody diarrhea, appendicitis, and rectal prolapse from strain to defecate	Ingestion of eggs (e.g., use of human feces as vegetable fertilizer; contaminated food and water)	Microscopic detection of barrel-shaped eggs with bipolar plugs (*right*)	Trichuriasis Albendazole[6] 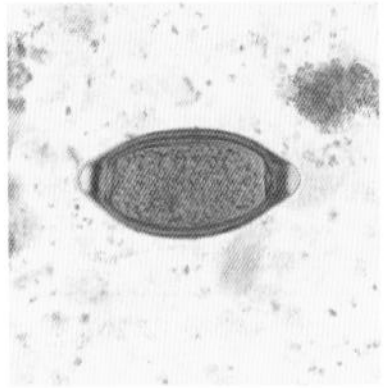	*Trichuris trichiura*/nematode (roundworm)

Symptoms/Signs	Transmission/Life Cycle	Diagnosis	Disease/Treatment	Organism
Diarrhea, vomiting, abdominal pain, iron deficiency anemia following ground itch at site of entry of parasite	Filariform larvae in soil penetrate intact skin of bare feet (shoes reduce transmission); larvae travel from skin to circulation to lungs, then ascend to epiglottis and are swallowed; adult worms attach to and mature in small intestine	Non-bile-staining segmented eggs in stool; possible occult blood in stools; no need to identify genus	Hookworm infection Albendazole or mebendazole	*Necator americanus* (New World hookworm); *Ancylostoma duodenale* (Old World hookworm)/nematodes
Skin pruritis, mild pneumonitis; asymptomatic to severe diarrhea with malabsorption	Filariform larvae penetrate intact **skin** of bare feet; free-living cycle occurs outside host; larvae migrate from skin to blood to lung to small intestine; adults lay eggs; larvae may hatch in GI tract, facilitating reinfection without exiting body (**autoinfection**)	Larvae in stool; serologic testing[7] 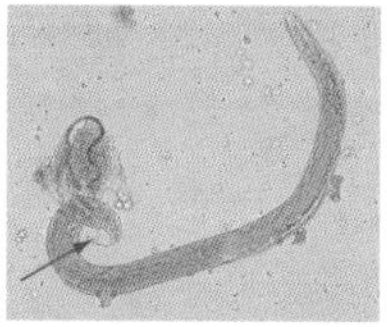	Strongyloidiasis Ivermectin	*Strongyloides stercoralis*/nematodes Because of auto- or reinfection, infections may last decades outside endemic area
Infections are commonly asymptomatic but may cause gastritis, fever, and muscle aches; high hemorrhages eosinophilia; splinter	Consumption of encysted larvae in **undercooked meat** (bear, pork, horse meat)	Eosinophilia with classic symptoms; serology; later, calcifications in muscle	Trichinosis	*Trichinella spiralis*/pork roundworm
Transient reaction and itching at skin site of infection; mild infections may be asymptomatic; may cause generalized malaise, fever, urticaria, abdominal pain with diarrhea or dysentery	Cercaria from infected snails enter water and penetrate intact skin of individuals swimming or standing in water. **Adults are shown here:**[8] 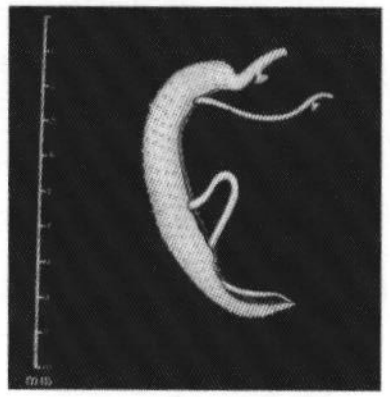	Eggs with lateral spine in feces[9] 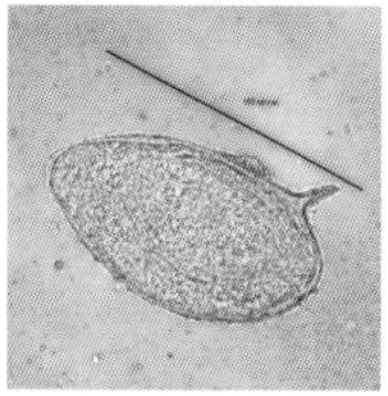	Intestinal schistosomiasis Praziquantel	*Schistosoma mansoni*/nematodes Mating pairs are found in vasculature; male is flat and fleshy and folds around the more cylindrical female in copulating pairs

(continued)

table 10.3 Gastrointestinal and Urogenital Parasitic Infections (*Continued*)

Signs/Symptoms/Case Details	Infective Form/Transmission	Diagnostic Form	Diseases/Treatment	Species/Type
Transient reaction and itching at skin site of infection; mild infections may be asymptomatic; may cause generalized malaise, fever, urticaria, abdominal pain with blood in urine at end of micturition, and dysuria	Cercaria from infected snails enter water and penetrate intact skin of individuals swimming or standing in water	Eggs with terminal spine in urine	Vesicular schistosomiasis Praziquantel	*Schistosoma haematobium*/mating pairs are found in vasculature; male is flat and fleshy but folded around the more cylindrical female in copulating pairs
Asymptomatic or may cause symptoms of vaginitis with discharge associated with burning or itching, or, in males, urethral discharge	Sexual contact; transmitted via trophozoites (below)[10]	Motile trophozoites with undulating membrane, tuft of four polar flagellae, and axostyle "tail"; excessive neutrophils in methylene blue wet mount; motility is jerky and nondirectional	Trichomoniasis Metronidazole or tinidazole (Good videos on YouTube.)	*Trichomonas vaginalis*/flagellates

[1](**A**) *Entamoeba coli* trophozoite stained with trichrome. Occasionally, the cytoplasm contains ingested bacteria (as seen in the photo), yeasts, or other materials. (**B**) Line drawing of an *Entamoeba histolytica/ Entamoeba dispar* trophozoite. (Courtesy of Centers for Disease Control DPDx Parasite Image Library.)

[2]*Giardia intestinalis* in in vitro culture, from a quality control slide. (Image contributed by the Oregon State Public Health Laboratory.)

[3]Carmine-stained proglottids of *Diphyllobothrium latum*, showing rosette-shaped ovaries. (Courtesy of Centers for Disease Control DPDx Parasite Image Library.)

[4]Eggs of *Enterobius vermicularis* in a wet mount. (Courtesy of Centers for Disease Control DPDx Parasite Image Library.)

[5]*Ascaris* fertilized egg in a wet mount with embryo in a more advanced stage of development. (Courtesy of Centers for Disease Control DPDx Parasite Image Library.)

[6]Egg of *Trichuris trichiura* in an iodine-stained wet mount. (Courtesy of Centers for Disease Control DPDx Parasite Image Library.)

[7]Free-living adult male *Strongyloides stercoralis*. Arrow points to spicule found in males. (Courtesy of Centers for Disease Control DPDx Parasite Image Library.)

[8]Adults of *Schistosoma mansoni*. The thin female resides in the gynecophoral canal of the thicker male. Note the tuberculate exterior of the male. (Courtesy of Centers for Disease Control DPDx Parasite Image Library.)

[9]Eggs of *S. mansoni* in unstained wet mounts. (Image contributed by the Wisconsin State Laboratory of Hygiene. Courtesy of Centers for Disease Control DPDx Parasite Image Library.)

[10]Two trophozoites of *Trichomonas vaginalis* obtained from in vitro culture stained with Giemsa. (Courtesy of Centers for Disease Control DPDx Parasite Image Library.)

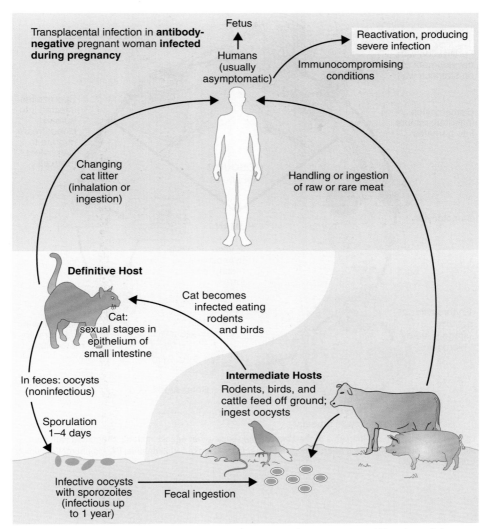

FIGURE 10.1. Toxoplasmosis Life Cycle. This illustration shows how widely distributed *Toxoplasma* is in nature and how humans can be infected and the populations which are impacted. (Modified from Engelberg NC, DiRita V, Dermody TS. *Schaechter's Mechanisms of Microbial Disease*. 5th ed. Philadelphia, PA: Wolters Kluwer Health/Lippincott Williams & Wilkins; 2013.)

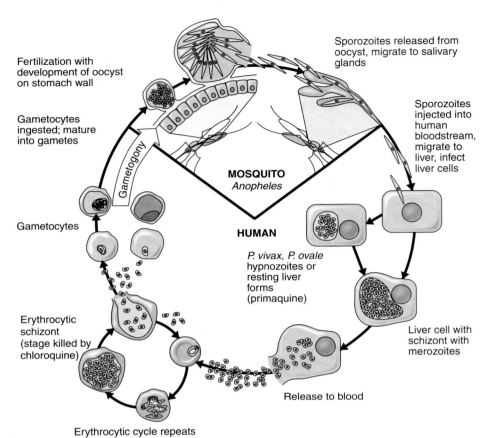

Fertilization with development of oocyst on stomach wall

Gametocytes ingested; mature into gametes

Sporozoites released from oocyst, migrate to salivary glands

Sporozoites injected into human bloodstream, migrate to liver, infect liver cells

Gametogony

MOSQUITO
Anopheles

HUMAN

P. vivax, P. ovale hypnozoites or resting liver forms (primaquine)

Gametocytes

Liver cell with schizont with merozoites

Erythrocytic schizont (stage killed by chloroquine)

Release to blood

Erythrocytic cycle repeats

FIGURE 10.2. The general life cycle of the *Plasmodium* species that causes malaria. (Reprinted with permission from Hawley L. *High-Yield Microbiology and Infectious Diseases.* Philadelphia, PA: Lippincott Williams & Wilkins; 2007:159.)

Review Test

Directions: *Each of the numbered items or incomplete statements in this section is followed by answers or completions of the statement. Select the ONE lettered answer that is BEST in each case.*

1. A biology graduate student who recently visited a tropical region of Africa presents with new visual impairment and the sensation that something is moving in her eye. She tells you that she is concerned because she had been warned about eye disease transmitted by black flies. When in Africa, she was in a river area, and despite her best efforts she received a lot of black fly bites. She also has some subcutaneous nodules. If her infection was acquired by black fly bite, what is the most likely causative agent?

(A) *Ancylostoma braziliense*
(B) *Dracunculus medinensis*
(C) *Loa loa*
(D) *Onchocerca volvulus*
(E) *Wuchereria bancrofti*

2. A woman who imports food from Mexico and spends several months per year in rural Mexico had to have a compound leg fracture pinned and set in Mexico and has returned 3 days later. She now has signs of acute appendicitis and is taken to surgery in Houston. When her appendix is removed, it is found to contain a light-colored, 20.5-cm-long roundworm as well as bile-stained, knobby eggs consistent with *Ascaris*. How did she acquire this infection?

(A) Ingestion of water containing filariform larvae
(B) Skin penetration by filariform larvae
(C) Skin penetration by rhabditiform larvae
(D) Ingestion of food contaminated with the eggs
(E) Inhalation of dust carrying the cysts

3. A patient whose major source of protein is smoked and cooked fish develops what appears to be pernicious anemia. What parasite is noted for causing a look-alike vitamin B_{12} anemia in certain genetically predisposed infected individuals?

(A) *Echinococcus granulosus*
(B) *Diphyllobothrium latum*

(C) *Hymenolepis nana*
(D) *Dipylidium caninum*
(E) *Taenia solium*

4. Which of the following protozoans is free living and is such that acquisition does not generally indicate fecal contamination?

(A) *Acanthamoeba*
(B) *Dientamoeba fragilis*
(C) *Entamoeba histolytica*
(D) *Entamoeba coli*
(E) *Giardia*

5. A 26-year-old woman with uncomplicated malaria who was treated initially with chloroquine now has relapsed. What is the reason for a chloroquine-treated case of *Plasmodium vivax* relapsing?

(A) *P. vivax* has a significant level of chloroquine resistance.
(B) *P. vivax* has a persistent erythrocytic stage.
(C) *P. vivax* has a persistent exoerythrocytic stage (hypnozoite).
(D) Chloroquine is not one of the drugs of choice.

6. How is *Leishmania donovani* transmitted?

(A) *Anopheles* mosquito bite
(B) Black fly bite
(C) *Culex* mosquito bite
(D) Sandfly bite
(E) Skin penetration by trauma

7. How is *Schistosoma haematobium* transmitted?

(A) Ingestion of raw or undercooked snail, frog, or snake
(B) Invasion of filariform larvae from soil
(C) Handling aquatic birds
(D) Standing or swimming in contaminated water
(E) Tsetse fly bite

8. An untreated AIDS patient (CD4$^+$ count of 180 cells/mm^3) from southern California has developed a progressively severe headache and mental confusion, along with ataxia and retinochoroiditis. Focal lesions are present on a computed tomography scan of his brain. No mucocutaneous lesions are found. He has been living under a bridge for the past 2 years. His level of immunoglobulin G (IgG) to the infectious agent is high. What is the most likely explanation for how this current infection started?

(A) Earlier exposure to pigeons
(B) Earlier exposure to desert sand
(C) Reactivation of bradyzoites in cysts from an earlier infection
(D) Recent exposure to cat feces
(E) Recent exposure to bats

9. Which of the following is the tapeworm acquired from eating undercooked pork?

(A) *Dipylidium* spp.
(B) *Echinococcus granulosus*
(C) *Taenia saginata*
(D) *Taenia solium*
(E) *Trichinella spiralis*

10. What roundworm is most likely to be transmitted by ingestion of food or water contaminated with feces?

(A) *Ascaris lumbricoides*
(B) *Enterobius vermicularis*
(C) *Necator americanus*
(D) *Taenia saginata*
(E) *Toxocara canis*

11. What roundworm is transmitted by filariform larvae that are found in the soil and penetrate the skin?

(A) *Dracunculus medinensis*
(B) *Enterobius vermicularis*
(C) *Strongyloides stercoralis*

(D) *Taenia saginata*
(E) *Toxocara canis*

12. How is *Clonorchis sinensis* (Chinese liver fluke) most likely transmitted to humans?

(A) Fish ingestion
(B) Mosquito bite
(C) Swimming or water contact
(D) Rare beef ingestion
(E) Mango fly (*Chrysops*)

13. A 48-year-old subsistence farmer from rural Brazil dies of heart failure. His autopsy shows a greatly enlarged heart. What was the vector for the most likely infectious agent that may have been responsible for his death?

(A) *Ixodes* tick
(B) Mosquito
(C) Reduviid bug
(D) Sandfly
(E) Tsetse fly

14. A 16-year-old man who recently returned from camping in Canada presents with fatty diarrhea and acute abdominal pain following many meals. How does the most likely agent cause the diarrhea?

(A) Coinfection with bacteria
(B) Enterotoxin production
(C) Suction disk attachment
(D) Tissue invasion leading to an inflammatory response and prostaglandin production

15. Which of the following protozoans is transmitted primarily by the motile trophozoite form?

(A) *Balantidium coli*
(B) *Entamoeba histolytica*
(C) *Giardia lamblia*
(D) *Taenia solium*
(E) *Trichomonas vaginalis*

Answers and Explanations

1. **The answer is D.** *Onchocerca volvulus* causes river blindness and is transmitted by the bite of a black fly. The patient may be able to detect movement of the parasite in the eye.

2. **The answer is D.** Fertilized *Ascaris* eggs released in feces may contaminate food or water, which is then consumed. *Ascaris* does not attach to the intestine but maintains its position by mobility. The worm may become hypermotile (e.g., during febrile periods, anesthetic use, or antibiotic use) and may migrate into the appendix or bile duct.

3. **The answer is B.** *Diphyllobothrium* is the tapeworm associated with anemia. It is transmitted in fish found in cool lake regions.

4. **The answer is A.** *Acanthamoeba* is a free-living organism with a sturdy cyst stage that is found in dust. A common way of acquiring *Acanthamoeba* infections in the United States is through homemade saline solutions for soft contact lenses. *Giardia* may be from animal contamination of water (rather than human) but is still not probably truly free living.

5. **The answer is C.** Both *Plasmodium ovale* and *Plasmodium vivax* may have resting liver forms, which are very slow to develop into schizonts with merozoites and proceed onto the chloroquine-sensitive erythrocytic stages after treatment is over. (It is not *over* with *P. ovale* or *P. vivax* unless you also treat with primaquine phosphate, which kills the liver stages.) (Papua, New Guinea, and Indonesia now have chloroquine-resistant *Plasmodium vivax*.)

6. **The answer is D.** All leishmaniae are transmitted by sandflies.

7. **The answer is D.** All schistosomes are transmitted by skin penetration from standing or swimming in contaminated water. Remember that snails are intermediate hosts.

8. **The answer is C.** The most likely disease in this case is encephalitis with focal lesions. Because the patient has high levels of immunoglobulin G, the current infection is likely a reactivation of an earlier infection; therefore, recent exposures (choices D and E) can be eliminated. Exposure to pigeons suggests cryptococcosis, which is often a reactivational infection. However, in cryptococcosis antibody levels are rarely monitored, and there is no mention of India ink stain or capsular polysaccharide in the cerebrospinal fluid, which are the major diagnostic methods. In addition, based on the patient's symptoms, the infection is more likely to be encephalitis rather than meningitis or meningoencephalitis; also, retinochoroiditis is usually not present in cryptococcosis. The retinochoroiditis and lack of mucocutaneous lesions makes infection with *Coccidioides* less likely. Reactivation of toxoplasmosis is most likely.

9. **The answer is D.** If you answered *Trichinella spiralis,* you fell for a typical testing "bait and switch." *T. spiralis* is the pork roundworm and *Taenia solium* is the pork tapeworm. *Dipylidium caninum* is the common tapeworm of both cats and dogs. It may be transmitted by ingestion of fleas harboring cysticercoid larvae. Transmission to humans usually occurs when crushed fleas harboring the disease are transmitted from a pet when it licks a child's mouth.

10. **The answer is A.** *Ascaris lumbricoides* is transmitted via the fecal-oral route. *Enterobius* is most likely transmitted via contaminated hands, clothing, or bedding. *Necator* enters by skin penetration. *Taenia* is not a roundworm. *Toxocara* is most commonly acquired from eating fecally contaminated dirt or soil.

11. **The answer is C.** *Strongyloides stercoralis* is a type of hookworm (also a roundworm). The filariform larvae of *S. stercoralis* are acquired when walking barefoot or sitting on the ground. *Dracunculus medinensis* (the guinea worm) is acquired by drinking water with copepods containing the larvae. Filtration of all drinking water through clean sari silk or T-shirt material has reduced the incidence of new cases dramatically and may allow its eradication. (For those

who are infected with *D. medinensis,* adults in subcutaneous nodules are slowly removed by rolling them out on a pencil.) *Toxocara canis* and *Toxocara cati* are acquired most commonly by pica, the ingestion of inert material; in this case, dirt or sand with animal feces. *Taenia saginata* is a flatworm. *Enterobius* (pinworm) eggs are ingested.

12. **The answer is A.** Raw, undercooked, smoked, or pickled freshwater fish are the most common route of transmission of *Clonorchis sinensis.* You should be able to answer this question from the general information in the preceding chapter without any specifics. The question told you it was a fluke, and so you know that water was involved in transmission; however, it is not a *Schistosoma* sp., so it has to be ingestion of aquatic plant or animal and in this case it is fish.

13. **The answer is C.** The case of the Brazilian farmer is a classic description of heart failure from chronic Chagas' disease, which is caused by *Trypanosoma cruzi. T. cruzi* is transmitted by reduviid bugs (cone-nose bugs or kissing bugs) that defecate as they bite. Scratching the bite spreads the trypanosome into the bite site, initiating the infection.

14. **The answer is C.** In this case, *Giardia lamblia* is the causative agent. *G. lamblia* is carried by muskrats and beavers, which is why it can be picked up in pristine northern lakes, such as those found in Canada. Attachment of numerous *Giardia* via their ventral sucking disks in the duodenal-jejunal area leads to malabsorption diarrhea and temporary lactose intolerance.

15. **The answer is E.** Protozoans transmitted by the fecal-oral route are transmitted in the cyst form, which survives stomach acid. Only the sexually transmitted *Trichomonas vaginalis* is transmitted in the motile form. *Taenia solium* is not a protozoan, but a flatworm.

chapter 11

Clues for Distinguishing Causative Infectious Agents (Systems Approach)

The infectious agents discussed in this chapter are not intended to be comprehensive lists of pathogens for the diseases, but rather the most common (or at least, with a few exceptions, the most likely to be encountered in the United States). They are the most likely to appear in the case-based questions on the USMLE step 1 examination. The clues listed relate to clinical symptoms, common laboratory data, and epidemiology. In the flowcharts, the **most common causes are in boldface.**

I. CONJUNCTIVITIS

Various types of infectious agents including viruses, bacteria, chlamydia, and protozoa can infect the eye and cause inflammation of the cornea. Viruses are the most common causative agents. Some of these infections occur in neonates (infants less than 2 weeks old) following passage through an infected birth canal. Red, irritated eyes are present in all cases. Diagnosis involves the presence or absence of pus, an examination of the conjunctiva for follicles or papillae, and Gram staining of discharge on conjunctival scrapings.

A. **Neonate (ophthalmia neonatorum).** Neonates can become infected during birth from infected mothers or by normal flora bacteria. Causative organism identification is important because of its potential for further systemic involvement (Fig. 11.1).

B. **Postnatal.** Postnatal infections are usually **self-limiting** except for those caused by *Staphylococcus aureus, Neisseria gonorhoeae, Chlamydia,* and herpes simplex virus, which penetrate into the deeper layers of the eye. Viral infections usually begin unilaterally. **Preauricular adenopathy is present on the involved side in adult viral and adult chlamydia infections and in ameba infections. Bacterial infections usually produce sticky eyelids.** *Staphylococcus aureus* and *Moraxella* may produce chronic conjunctivitis (Fig. 11.2).

II. PNEUMONIAS

Pneumonias may be classified in several different ways. One common classification is based on the time interval between infection and clinical symptoms (e.g., acute and chronic pneumonias). Acute pneumonias include community-acquired and nosocomial pneumonia, determined by where the infectious agents are acquired. Acute pneumonias may also be classified as typical or atypical, depending on their clinical symptoms. The following information combines important aspects of these classifications as well as other (e.g., geographic) considerations.

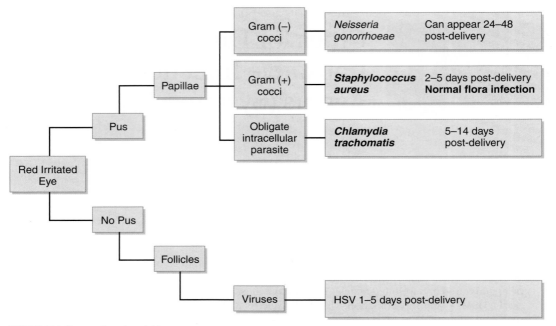

FIGURE 11.1. Neonatal conjunctivitis.

A. **Community-acquired pneumonia (CAP).** Considerable overlap and patient-dependent variability occurs, although some generalizations can be made. One important concept is that viruses are more common causes of acute disease in children under 2 years of age.

1. **Acute, typical.** Symptoms (abrupt onset, fever higher than 39°C/102°F, chills, productive cough, and chest pain) develop 1 to 2 days following infection (Fig. 11.3).

2. **Acute, atypical.** Symptoms (slower onset, fever less than 39°C, nonproductive cough, headache, sore throat, and gastrointestinal symptoms) develop 2 to 10 days following infection; **Gram staining is not helpful in diagnosis** (Fig. 11.4).

3. **Chronic pneumonia.** Symptoms are variable; primary infection may be asymptomatic; progresses or reactivates in some individuals to severe pneumonia; some fungal infections are associated with specific geological regions.

   a. **Cavitary lesions on x-ray:**
      (1) *Mycobacterium tuberculosis:*
         (a) **Primary infection** is mild but may cause **Ghon lesions** (areas of fibrosis on x-ray).
         (b) Reactivated or secondary tuberculosis occurs in 10% to 15% of those infected, particularly in middle-aged individuals. Findings include apical cavitary lesions and acid-fast bacilli in sputum.
      (2) *Histoplasma capsulatum* causes a progressive nodular to cavitary disease restricted to the Ohio and Mississippi River valleys and related to soil containing bird and bat droppings.

   b. **Variable x-ray patterns** are characteristic of *Nocardia asteroides* and several fungal infections where findings frequently depend on the stage of the **fungal disease.**
      (1) *Blastomyces dermatitidis* (central and eastern North America): large yeast cells are present in potassium hydroxide (KOH) preparations of sputum.
      (2) *Coccidioides immitis* ("**valley fever**") (Arizona, Nevada, New Mexico, western Texas, and parts of central and southern California): upper lobe nodules are frequently visible on x-ray; restricted to thick-walled "spherules" in KOH preparation of sputum; joint pain involved in disease process.

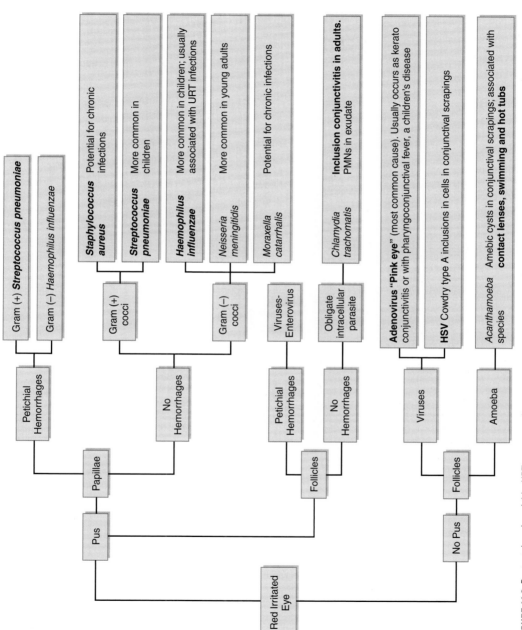

FIGURE 11.2. Postnatal conjunctivitis. URT, upper respiratory tract.

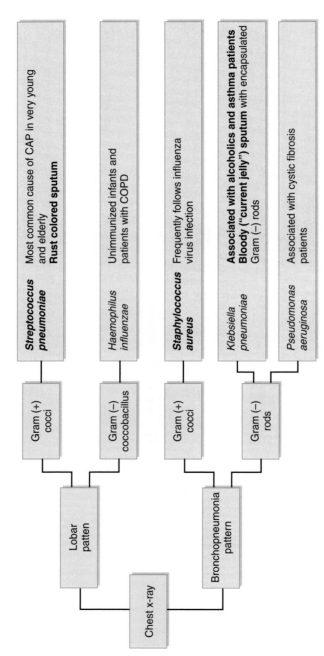

| | Gram (+)
cocci | **_Streptococcus
pneumoniae_** | Most common cause of CAP in very young
and elderly
Rust colored sputum |

Lobar
patten

| | Gram (−)
coccobacillus | _Haemophilus
influenzae_ | Unimmunized infants and
patients with COPD |

Chest x-ray

| | Gram (+)
cocci | **_Staphylococcus
aureus_** | Frequently follows influenza
virus infection |

Bronchopneumonia
pattern

| | Gram (−)
rods | _Klebsiella
pneumoniae_ | **Associated with alcoholics and asthma patients**
Bloody ("current jelly") sputum with encapsulated
Gram (−) rods |

| | | _Pseudomonas
aeruginosa_ | Associated with cystic fibrosis
patients |

FIGURE 11.3. Acute community-acquired typical pneumonias. COPD, chronic obstructive pulmonary disease.

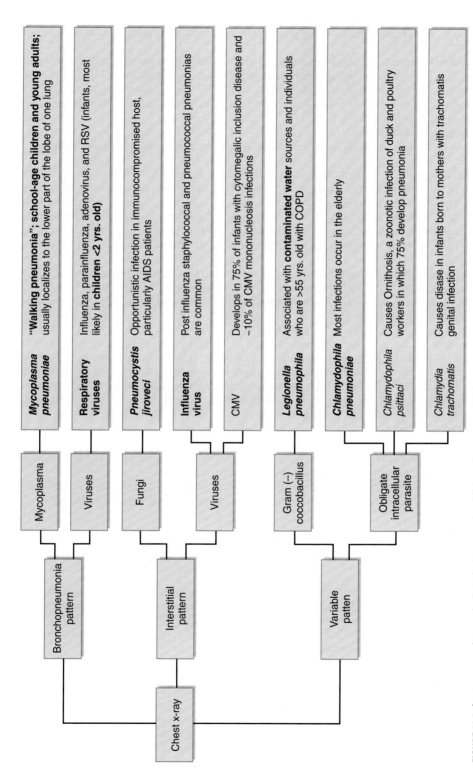

FIGURE 11.4. Acute community-acquired atypical pneumonias. RSV, respiratory syncytial virus.

(3) *Cryptococcus neoformans:* sometimes a single nodule on x-ray; organism is found in **pigeon and bird droppings.**

(4) *N. asteroides:* weakly Gram-positive rods are present in branching filaments in sputum.

B. **Nosocomial pneumonia.** These pneumonias are the leading cause of death from nosocomial infections. Risk factors include endotracheal intubation, malnutrition and underlying disease, metabolic acidosis, medications (particularly antibiotics and immunosuppressants), and advanced age (greater than 70 years of age). Clinical aids to identification of specific pathogens are found in the CAP information.

1. *Staphylococcus aureus.*

2. Gram-negative bacilli (*E. coli, Klebsiella pneumoniae,* and *Pseudomonas aeruginosa).*

C. **Aspiration pneumonia.** Aspiration pneumonia results in excessive aspiration of contaminated fluids or the loss of the reflexes utilized to protect the lungs from accumulating fluids or secretions. These situations occur in individuals who have a poor gag reflex or difficulty swallowing for various reasons or who have lost consciousness. They may result from aspiration of gastric contents or mouth flora during various conditions like endotracheal intubation, gastrointestinal (GI) endoscopy, general anesthesia, seizures, and so forth. Elderly stroke patients are particularly vulnerable.

1. **Anaerobic streptococci** infections are characterized by foul-smelling sputum containing no other leading CAP bacteria; frequently associated with periodontal disease.

2. *Staphylococcus aureus* **and Gram-negative bacilli** are the most frequent causes of nosocomial aspiration pneumonia.

D. **Pneumonia in an immunocompromised host.** In addition to being susceptible to the usual pneumonia-causing pathogens mentioned previously, immunocompromised individuals are also at risk for infection from several opportunistic pathogens. Pneumonia is a common infection in individuals infected with human immunodeficiency virus (HIV), patients undergoing cancer chemotherapy or with congenital immunodeficiencies, and individuals undergoing immunosuppressive treatment for organ transplants.

1. *Aspergillus fumigatus.* X-rays show fungus balls, nodules, and cavitation; aspirates or biopsy materials contain large, branching septate hyphae.

2. *Pneumocystis jiroveci.* X-rays indicate a bilateral defuse alveolar disease; silver staining of bronchoalveolar lavage material shows sporocytes (cysts).

3. **Cytomegalovirus (CMV).** This pathogen is an important consideration as the causative agent of pneumonias in organ transplant patients receiving immunosuppressive therapy.

III. DIARRHEAS AND DYSENTERY

Diarrheas are characterized by frequent and fluid stools that result from small intestine disease involving fluid and electrolyte loss. **Dysentery** is an inflammatory disease of the large intestine with blood or pus in the stool. However, clinicians frequently only apply the term "dysentery" to infections by a Shigella bacteria or an ameba. Thus, diarrhea can be classified on the basis of the nature of the diarrhea, which reflects the pathology and the site of infection.

The sources of infectious agents are food, water, zoonotic, or person-to-person transfer by the fecal-oral route. Toxins play a major role in the development of the symptoms observed with some bacteria and rotavirus infections, and the incubation times depend on whether a preformed toxin, colonization and toxin synthesis, or tissue invasion is involved. Many infections are self-limiting, but some, particularly in children without proper rehydration, can be fatal. Since it is impossible to clinically diagnose causative agents, recent food and travel history as well as examination of the stool is important. Specific diagnosis is dependent on laboratory analysis of the stool involving Gram staining for bacteria, staining for polymorphonuclear neutrophils (PMNs), and bacterial culture and immunologic-based tests for specific pathogens. Another important consideration related to diagnosis is whether the pathogen is associated with an epidemic; infection is frequently location-dependent, and in developed countries viral infections are the most common. An identification scheme initially based on the nature of the diarrhea and the presence or absence of vomiting is described.

A. **Watery diarrheas with vomiting.** Causative pathogens are the viruses and several bacteria, the majority of which synthesize **enterotoxins** involved in the pathogenesis of the disease. Some produce fever, but all have relatively **short incubation times, ranging from several hours to a few days,** due to the associated toxins or virus multiplication in the small intestine (Fig. 11.5).

B. **Watery diarrhea with no vomiting.** One bacterium and two protozoa are in this group. A variety of toxins contribute to the bacterial disease which has a short (less than 24 hours) incubation period. The protozoa have longer (1 to 4 weeks) incubation periods with disease that is usually moderate, but it can become chronic and serious in immunocompromised individuals. **No fever** is associated with these infections (Fig. 11.6).

C. **Bloody diarrhea with vomiting.** Two types of *E. coli* cause this form of diarrhea. Enterohemorrhagic *E. coli* (EHEC) strains release a verotoxin that is cytotoxic to intestinal villi and colon epithelial cells. Enteroinvasive *E. coli* (EIEC) strains invade and destroy colon epithelial cells. Both have incubation periods of 2 to 5 days (Fig. 11.7).

D. **Bloody diarrhea with no vomiting.** Both bacillary and amebic dysentery cause this form of diarrhea. Gram-positive and Gram-negative rods and a protozoan are involved. PMNs in the stool and fever occur with most infections. Tissue invasion is common (Fig. 11.8).

IV. ACUTE MENINGITIS

Meningitis is both an acute and chronic disease. Bacteria and viruses cause acute disease, while **Mycobacterium tuberculosis and fungi (Cryptococcus and Coccidioides) cause the chronic form.** Both types are preceded by infections that lead to meningeal invasion. Acute infections are usually preceded by a throat, ear, or lung infection. Clinical presentation and history, cerebral spinal fluid (CSF) characteristics, age of the patient, and time of the year are helpful in diagnosis.

A. **Bacterial meningitis.** Bacterial meningitis can either be acquired in the community or in the hospital. The symptoms (fever, severe headache, stiff neck, and **some cerebral dysfunction** like confusion or delirium) may develop in a few hours or a few days. Nausea, vomiting, and photophobia frequently occur. Specific pathogens need to be identified as quickly as possible so that appropriate intravenous administration of bacterial antibodies may be started (Fig. 11.9).

B. **Viral (aseptic) meningitis.** Acute viral meningitis is a milder disease than bacterial meningitis. There is usually **less neck stiffness and no cerebral dysfunction.** It is the **most common form of acute meningitis** and is frequently a component of common viral diseases like chickenpox. In temperate climates, the disease is usually observed in summer or early fall. The identification of the causative virus is rarely done (Fig. 11.10).

V. BACTERIAL AND VIRAL SKIN INFECTION AND RASHES

These infections may be localized and present with distinctive symptoms at the site of pathogen entry or attachment or they may result from their spread to subcutaneous tissues or the action of bacterial toxin upon the skin. Group A *Streptococci,* particularly *Streptococci pyogenes* and *Staphylococcus aureus,* are the most common pathogens in skin infections. Many systemic infectious diseases also produce rashes as part of their disease process.

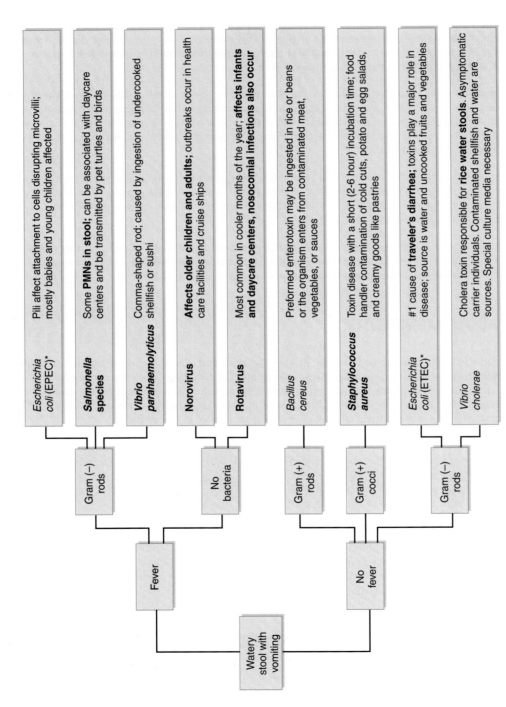

FIGURE 11.5. Watery stools with vomiting. EPEC, enteropathogenic *E. coli*; ETEC, enterotoxigenic *E. coli*.

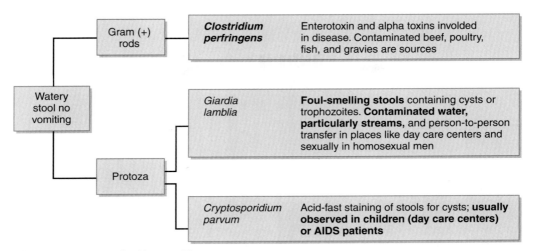

FIGURE 11.6. Watery stools with no vomiting.

A. **Localized infections of the skin.** Several viruses infect the epidermis, and some bacteria colonize the epidermis, sweat glands, sebaceous glands, and hair follicles. Diagnosis is usually accomplished by the nature of the skin lesion and perhaps recent patient history (Fig. 11.11).

B. **Spreading skin infections.** Two classes of these infections are recognized: cellulitis and necrotizing fasciitis. **Cellulitis** is a skin infection with an extension into subcutaneous fat. **Necrotizing fasciitis (NF)** is a serious infection of subcutaneous tissue that involves progressive destruction of fat and fascia. Both are accompanied by pain, fever, and chills, but NF may have delirium as well. A "hard feel" to the subcutaneous tissue distinguishes NF from cellulitis. It is a medical emergency that may involve surgical intervention (Fig. 11.12).

C. **Toxin-associated skin shedding.** Toxin-producing strains of **Staphylococcus aureus** can cause a "scalded skin" syndrome and **toxic shock syndrome** that includes desquamation of the epidermis as part of the disease process. "Scalded skin" syndrome occurs mainly in infants and children and may be associated with small epidemics. Toxic shock syndrome is a serious systemic disease frequently associated with a skin abscess or vaginal infection involving tampon use during menstruation. The rash observed with the disease resembles the scarlet fever rash.

D. **Rashes.** Many systemic bacterial, rickettsial, and viral infections, and some localized viral infections (cited previously), produce rashes as part of their disease process. They can be classified into four types: (1) maculopapular, (2) vesicular, (3) petechial-purpuric, and (4) diffuse erythroderma. They are helpful in identifying causative agents. Common pathogens found in the United States are listed in Tables 11.1 to 11.4.

VI. GENITOURINARY TRACT INFECTIONS

These infections are frequently classified according to the site of infection (i.e., urethritis, cervicitis, vaginitis, etc.). They produce some type of **exudate,** which usually contains the infectious agent; several form **genital lesions, which can be diagnostic.** Many cause sexually transmitted diseases (STDs).

A. **Urethritis.** Urethritis is characterized by dysuria and urethral exudate. Coinfections with *Neisseria* and *Chlamydia* are common (Fig. 11.13).

B. **Epididymitis.** Infection is painful with acute unilateral swelling of the testicle. Causative organism is found in urethral specimens or epididymal aspirates (Fig. 11.14).

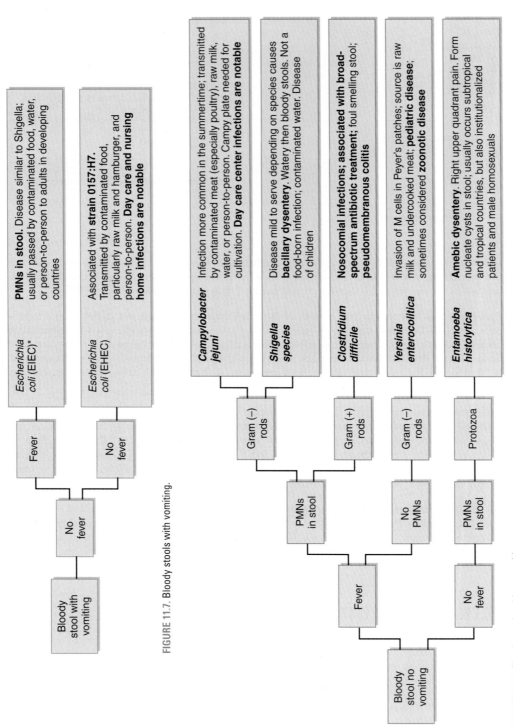

FIGURE 11.7. Bloody stools with vomiting.

Escherichia coli (EIEC)*	**PMNs in stool.** Disease similar to Shigella; usually passed by contaminated food, water, or person-to-person to adults in developing countries
Escherichia coli (EHEC)	Associated with **strain O157:H7.** Transmitted by contaminated food, particularly raw milk and hamburger, and person-to-person. **Day care and nursing home infections are notable**

Campylobacter jejuni	Infection more common in the summertime; transmitted by contaminated meat (especially poultry), raw milk, water, or person-to-person. Campy plate needed for cultivation. **Day care center infections are notable**
Shigella species	Disease mild to serve depending on species causes **bacillary dysentery.** Watery then bloody stools. Not a food-born infection; contaminated water. Disease of children
Clostridium difficile	**Nosocomial infections; associated with broad-spectrum antibiotic treatment;** foul smelling stool; **pseudomembranous colitis**
Yersinia enterocolitica	Invasion of M cells in Peyer's patches; source is raw milk and undercooked meat; **pediatric disease;** sometimes considered **zoonotic disease**
Entamoeba histolytica	**Amebic dysentery.** Right upper quadrant pain. Form nucleate cysts in stool; usually occurs subtropical and tropical countries, but also institutionalized patients and male homosexuals

FIGURE 11.8. Bloody stools with no vomiting.

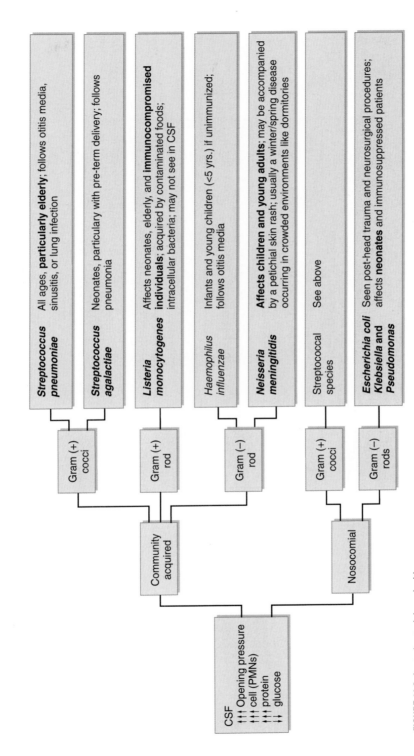

Streptococcus pneumoniae — All ages, **particularly elderly**; follows otitis media, sinusitis, or lung infection

Streptococcus agalactiae — Neonates, particularly with pre-term delivery; follows pneumonia

Listeria monocytogenes — Affects neonates, elderly, and **immunocompromised individuals**; acquired by contaminated foods; intracellular bacteria; may not see in CSF

Haemophilus influenzae — Infants and young children (<5 yrs.) if unimmunized; follows otitis media

Neisseria meningitidis — **Affects children and young adults**; may be accompanied by a petichial skin rash; usually a winter/spring disease occurring in crowded environments like dormitories

Streptococcal species — See above

***Escherichia coli* Klebsiella and Pseudomonas** — Seen post-head trauma and neurosurgical procedures; affects **neonates** and immunosuppressed patients

Gram (+) cocci

Gram (+) rod

Gram (−) rod

Gram (+) cocci

Gram (−) rods

Community acquired

Nosocomial

CSF
↑↑↑ Opening pressure
↑↑↑ cell (PMNs)
↑↑↑ protein
↓↓↓ glucose

FIGURE 11.9. Acute bacterial meningitis.

215

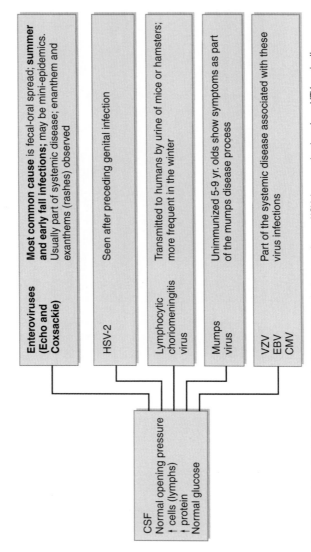

CSF
Normal opening pressure
↑ cells (lymphs)
↑ protein
Normal glucose

Enteroviruses (Echo and Coxsackie) — **Most common cause is fecal-oral spread; summer and early fall infections;** may be mini-epidemics. Usually part of systemic disease; enanthem and exanthems (rashes) observed

HSV-2 — Seen after preceding genital infection

Lymphocytic choriomeningitis virus — Transmitted to humans by urine of mice or hamsters; more frequent in the winter

Mumps virus — Unimmunized 5-9 yr. olds show symptoms as part of the mumps disease process

VZV EBV CMV — Part of the systemic disease associated with these virus infections

FIGURE 11.10. Acute viral (ascetic) meningitis. EBV, Epstein-Barr syndrome; HSV, herpes simplex virus; VZV, varicella zoster virus.

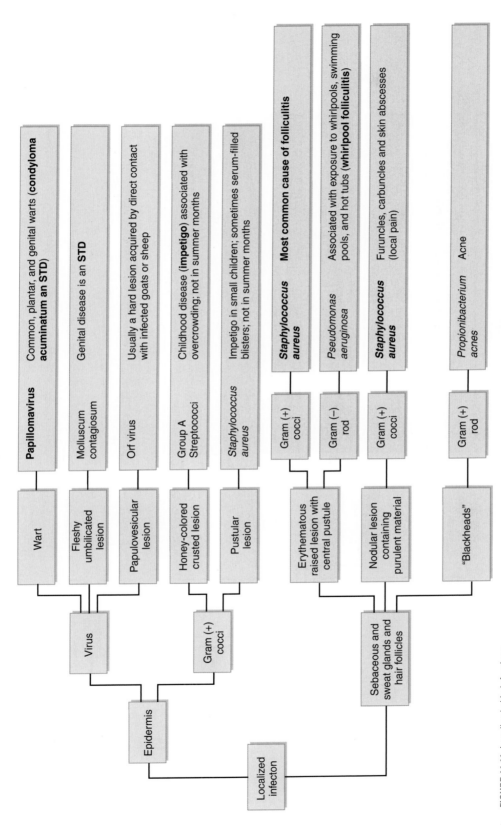

FIGURE 11.11. Localized skin infections.

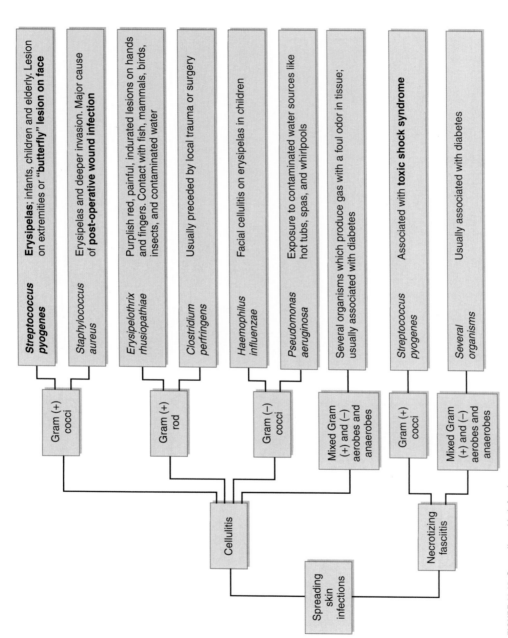

FIGURE 11.12. Spreading skin infections.

table 11.1 Maculopapular Rashes

Viral	Bacterial	Rickettsial
Colorado tick fever CMV mononucleosis Dengue Enterovirus infections EBV Erythema infectiosum (Parvovirus B19) Lymphocytic choriomeningitis Roseola (HHV-6) Rubella Rubeola	*Leptospirosis* Lyme disease (*Borrelia burgdorferi*) *Meningococcemia* *Pseudomonas* *aeruginosa bacteremia* Relapsing fever (*Borrelia recurrentis*) Rat bite fever (*Streptobacillus moniliformis*) Scarlet fever (*Streptococcus pyogenes*) Typhoid fever (*Salmonella typhi*)	Ehrlichia infections Rickettsial infections

table 11.2 Vesicular Rashes

Chickenpox (VZV)
Disseminated herpes simplex virus (HSV)
Disseminated herpes zoster
Hand-foot-mouth disease (Coxsackie H16)
Echovirus infections (enterovirus 11)
Smallpox

table 11.3 Petechial-Purpuric Rashes

Acute meningococcemia
Congenital cytomegalic inclusion disease
Congenital rubella
Echovirus 9 infections
Epidemic typhus
Infectious mononucleosis (EBV)
Rat bite fever (*Streptobacillus moniliformis*)
Relapsing fever (*Borrelia recurrentis*)
Rocky Mountain spotted fever (*Rickettsia rickettsii*)
Staphylococcus aureus *bacteremia*
Yellow fever

table 11.4 Diffuse Erythroderma Rashes

Scarlet fever (*Streptococcus pyogenes*)
Scalded skin syndrome (*Staphylococcus aureus*)
Toxic shock syndromes (*Staphylococcus aureus* and *Streptococcus pyogenes*)

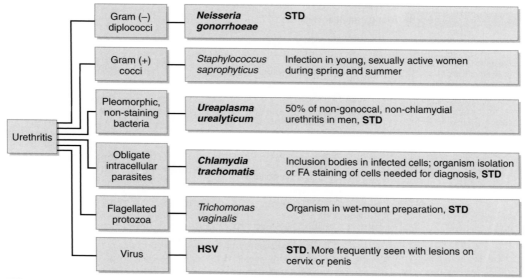

FIGURE 11.13. Urethritis. FA, fluorescent antibody; STD, sexually transmitted disease.

C. **Cervicitis.** Infection produces a mucopurulent discharge containing PMNs. The cervix is inflamed and friable. Causative agents are found in the exudate (Fig. 11.15).

D. **Vaginitis.** Certain invading organisms can cause infection, but overgrowth of the normal vaginal flora, including anaerobic bacteria and *Gardnerella vaginalis,* cause disease. Organisms in vaginal discharge are diagnostic (Fig. 11.16).

E. **Genital lesions.** Some infectious agents cause visible lesions (warts and ulcers) on the genitalia. The nature of these lesions is diagnostic (Fig. 11.17).

F. **Pelvic inflammatory disease (PID).** PID is **primarily an STD disease of young sexually active women.** Symptoms begin during or within a week of menstruation. They include lower abdominal pain, fever, and vaginal discharge in 50% of those infected. Causative organisms may be found in the discharge; however, since there is not always discharge, definitive diagnosis may be difficult. **Neisseria gonorhoeae** and **Chlamydophila trachomatis are the most common causes,** but a polymicrobial etiology involving normal vaginal flora is also possible. To prevent complications and sequelae, treatment is started even when a definitive diagnosis is not possible.

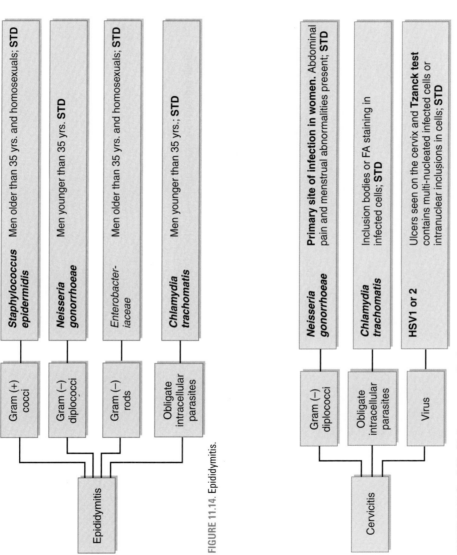

FIGURE 11.14. Epididymitis.

FIGURE 11.15. Cervicitis. FA, fluorescent antibody.

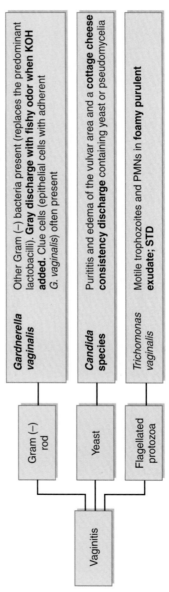

FIGURE 11.16. Vaginitis.

Vaginitis

Gram (–) rod → ***Gardnerella vaginalis***
Other Gram (–) bacteria present (replaces the predominant lactobacilli). **Gray discharge with fishy odor when KOH added.** Clue cells (epithelial cells with adherent *G. vaginalis*) often present

Yeast → ***Candida* species**
Puritis and edema of the vulvar area and a **cottage cheese consistency discharge** containing yeast or pseudomycelia

Flagellated protozoa → ***Trichomonas vaginalis***
Motile trophozoites and PMNs in **foamy purulent exudate; STD**

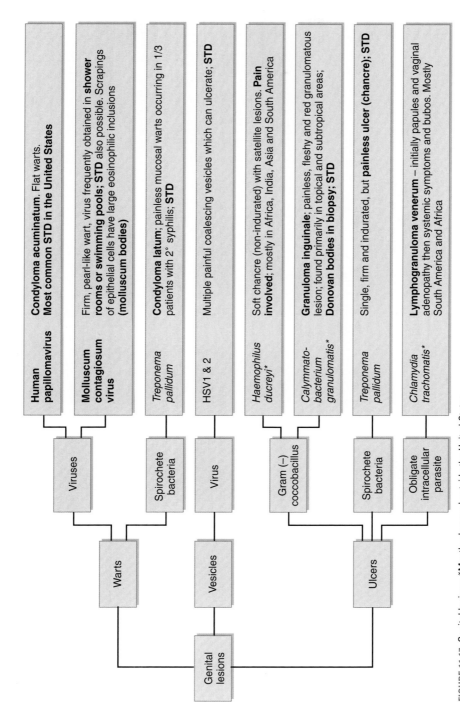

Human papillomavirus

Condyloma acuminatum. Flat warts. **Most common STD in the United States**

Molluscum contagiosum virus

Firm, pearl-like wart, virus frequently obtained in **shower rooms or swimming pools; STD** also possible. Scrapings of epithelial cells have large eosinophilic inclusions **(molluscum bodies)**

Treponema pallidum

Condyloma latum; painless mucosal warts occurring in 1/3 patients with 2° syphilis; **STD**

HSV1 & 2

Multiple painful coalescing vesicles which can ulcerate; **STD**

*Haemophilus ducreyi**

Soft chancre (non-indurated) with satellite lesions. **Pain involved**; mostly in Africa, India, Asia and South America

*Calymmato-bacterium granulomatis**

Granuloma inguinale: painless, fleshy and red granulomatous lesion; found primarily in topical and subtropical areas; **Donovan bodies in biopsy; STD**

Treponema pallidum

Single, firm and indurated, but **painless ulcer (chancre); STD**

*Chlamydia trachomatis**

Lymphogranuloma venerum – initially papules and vaginal adenopathy then systemic symptoms and bubos. Mostly South America and Africa

Viruses

Spirochete bacteria

Virus

Gram (−) coccobacillus

Spirochete bacteria

Obligate intracellular parasite

Warts

Vesicles

Ulcers

Genital lesions

FIGURE 11.17. Genital lesions. *Mostly observed outside the United States.

VII. SYSTEM SUMMARIES OF INFECTIOUS AGENTS

A. Characteristics of Important Causes of Encephalitis

Infection	Type of Microorganism	Microorganism	Virulence or Epidemiological Factors	Associated Disease	Prominent Groups	Diagnosis	Prevention/Treatment
ENCEPHALITIS	*Viruses*	Mosquito-borne Arboviruses (EEE & WEE viruses, LaCrosse virus, & St. Louis virus)	**Birds 1° reservoir for EEE, WEE viruses, & St. Louis viruses. Squirrels & chipmunks for LaCrosse virus**	**Flu-like illness**	**LaCrosse virus: children (mean age 7.5 yrs), St Louis virus: elderly people (>60 years)**	ELISA test for IgM in CSF for each virus	Supportive
		West Nile virus	**Birds, particularly jays, are 1° reservoir**, but breastfeeding, blood transfusion, & organ transplant transmission can occur	80% asymptomatic, 20% acute febrile illness, < 1% **encephalitis**	**Elderly persons (>60 years)**	ELISA for IgM in CSF	Supportive
		Tick-borne Arbovirus (Colorado Tick Fever)	**Small forest or field mammals are 1° reservoir**	GI symptoms & maculopapular or petechial rash can be present	**Children**	ELISA for IgM in serum	Supportive
		Poliovirus	**1% of those infected get paralytic disease**			RT-PCR of CSF for virus RNA	Salk trivalent inactivated vaccine/supportive
		Other enteroviruses	Summer months		Neonates (<7 days old)	PCR of CSF for virus RNA	Supportive
		HSV-1 and -2	**Most common cause of sporadic encephalitis in U.S.,** 90% of cases are HSV-1; 1° infections cause latent infections		½ cases <20 years ½ cases >50 years	PCR of CSF for virus DNA	Acyclovir
		Rabies virus	**G protein of envelope attaches to nicotinic acetylcholine receptor;** infection initiated by animal bite	Nonspecific prodromal period with fever, malaise, and fatigue	**Persons bitten by skunks, dogs, raccoons, cats, bats, and foxes**	Applied to possible rabid animals; negri bodies or FA tests of biopsy material	Active immunization with inactive rabies vaccine and passive immunization with human rabies immune globulin
	Protozoa	*Naegleria fowleri*	Secrete cysteine proteases, form cysts; **found in warm recreational fresh water like swimming holes;** nasal inoculation	Preceding changes in taste or smell	**Children and young adults**	PCR of CSF for amoeba DNA	Amphotericin B (intrathecal and IV miconazole and rifampin)
		Acanthamoeba	Mannose surface glycoproteins, IgA protease	Cutaneous lesions **and sinus infections**	Debilitated immunosuppressed individuals	Culture of brain biopsy, wet-mount exam of CSF	Sulfamethazine or trimethoprim/sulfamethoxazole
		Toxoplasma gondii	Forms cysts; **cyst transmission from cat feces and undercooked meat, particularly pork & lamb**	Toxoplasmosis; most **common focal CNS infection in AIDS patients**	**Congenitally infected fetuses and newborns;** immunosuppressed persons	PCR of CSF for organism DNA, ELISA of serum for IgA or IgG	Sulfadiazine plus pyrimethamine and leucovorin

B. Characteristics of Important Causes of Meningitis

Infection	Type of Microorganism	Microorganism	Epidemiological or Virulence Factors	Associated Disease	Prominent Groups	Diagnosis	Prevention/Treatment
ACUTE MENINGITIS	Bacteria	*Strep. pneumoniae*	**Polysaccharide capsule, IgA protease**	**Otitis media, respiratory infections,** neurologic sequence	**<2 years and elderly**	Gram stain and antigen latex agglutination test of CSF to be confirmed by culture	**13-valent vaccine (very young), 23-valent (Pneumovax 23) > 5 years**/ Penicillin G (drug susceptible) & ceftriaxone plus vancomycin (drug resistant)
		Neisseria meningitidis	**Polysaccharide capsule, IgA protease,** pili, outer membrane proteins, endotoxin	**Hemorrhagic skin rash,** neurologic sequelae	**Children and adolescents**	Same as strep pneumonia	**Tetravalent meningococcal polysaccharide vaccine**/ Penicillin G, if susceptible, ceftriaxone if not
		Haemophilus influenzae type b	**Polysaccharide capsule, IgA protease,** pili, outer membrane proteins, endotoxin	**Otitis,** neurologic sequelae	**Infants and young children (<5 years)**	Gram stain and culture	**Polysaccharide-protein conjugate vaccine**/ceftriaxone
		Streptococcus agalactiae	**A surface protein, pili, polysaccharide capsule**	Asymptomatic in pregnant females, generalized disease in neonates	**Neonates (<7days)**	Latex agglutination for antigen in serum or urine; culture or Gram stain of CSF	Ampicillin
		Borrelia burgdorferi	Spirochetal surface protein facilitates binding to host cells	**Preceding rash,** arthritis succeeds rash after a variable period of time	All bitten by infected tick	Clinical, but aided by serology and PCR of CSF or serum for bacterial DNA	Ceftriaxone
		Listeria monocytogenes	**Grows during refrigeration, food-borne;** mother-child transmission, iron, cell surface internalin, listeriolysin	Febrile gastroenteritis, neonatal bacteremia	**Neonates (<7 days),** Immuno-compromised persons including AIDS patients	CSF Gram stain and culture	Ampicillin
	Viruses	Enteroviruses, echoviruses, & coxsackie viruses	**Causes 80% of meningitis cases**	**Pharyngitis**	Infants, young children; also adults	RT-PCR of CSF for viral RNA	Supportive
		HSV-2 (rarely other herpesviruses)	Viral glycoprotein C, B, and D	**1° genital infection with HSV-2**	All with 1° HSV-2 infection	PCR of CSF for virus DNA	Acyclovir
		Mumps virus	Envelope glycoproteins	Mumps	Males 2 to 5 times greater than females; peak incidence in children 5–9 yrs	Clinical, also IgM serology possible	**Jeryl Lynn strain of attenuated virus vaccine**/supportive

(continued)

Infection	Type of Microorganism	Microorganism	Epidemiological or Virulence Factors	Associated Disease	Prominent Groups	Diagnosis	Prevention/Treatment
ACUTE MENINGITIS	Viruses	Lymphocytic choriomeningitis virus		Nonspecific febrile illness	**Contact with rodents or their excretia, esp. young adults**	IgM serology of serum aid CSF	Elimination of infected rodents/ supportive
CHRONIC MENINGITIS	Bacteria	Mycobacterium tuberculosis	**Waxy coat**	**Miliary TB**	HIV-infected individuals	PCR of CSF for bacterial DNA, lung lesions culture	**Four drug therapy: isoniazid, rifampin, pyrazinamide, and ethambutol;** adjunctive corticosteroids
		Treponema pallidum		2° syphilis, neurosyphilis	**2° syphilic individuals**	EIA tests for abs, microhemagglutination test	Penicillin G
		Borrelia burgdorferi (see Acute Meningitis)					
	Fungi	Cryptococcus neoformans	Polysaccharide capsule	Cryptococcosis	**Immunosuppressed individuals, particularly AIDS patients**	Cryptococcal latex agglutination on CSF	Amphotericin B plus flucytosine
		Coccidioides immitis	Formation of endospores	Coccidioidomycosis	**Persons living or traveling in southwest U.S.;** immunosuppressed individuals	Fungal immunodiffusion test on serum; complement fixation test on CSF; culture	Fluconazole
		Histoplasma capsulatum	**Bird or bat guano**	Histoplasmosis	Immunosuppressed individuals; **persons living/traveling in Ohio or Mississippi River valleys**	EIA for ag in CSF and culture of CSF	Liposomal amphotericin B (4–6 wks) followed by itraconazole for a year
	Protozoa	Acanthamoeba	Mannose surface glycoproteins, IgA protease	**Cutaneous lesions and sinus infections**	Debilitated or immunosuppressed individuals	Culture of brain biopsy, wet-mount exam of CSF	Sulfamethazine or trimethoprim/ sulfamethoxazole

C. Characteristics of Important Causes of Pneumonia

Infection	Sub-Type	Type of Microorganism	Microorganism	Epidemio- Logical or Virulence Factor	Associated Disease	Prominent Groups	Diagnosis	X-Ray Pattern	Prevention/Treatment
ACUTE COMMUNITY ACQUIRED PNEUMONIA	Typical (80%–90%)	Bacteria	*Streptococcus pneumoniae* (both drug sensitive and resistant strains)	**Estimates of 65% of CAP isolates resistant to penicillin due to alterations in PBPs;** polysaccharide capsule, pneumococcal surface protein A, pneumolysin, and neuraminidase	**Otitis media and meningitis**	**Newborns and infants (<2 yrs old) and elderly (>65 yrs old)**	Gram stain of sputum, urinary ag test, and PCR	**Single lobe lobar**	Three pneumococcal vaccines: 1) protein conjugate to 13 capsular polysaccharides (2–59 mo. children & 60–71 mo. children with under-lying medical conditions); 2) protein conjugate to 7 capsular polysaccharides (children <5 yrs); 3) 23-valent pneumococcal polysaccharide vaccine (>65 yrs old)/Empiric treatment (outpatients); amoxicillin & azithromycin; hospitalized adults; IV ceftriaxone and azithromycin
			Haemophilus influenzae (both drug sensitive & resistant strains)	Minor % of CAP except in older adults; **most common bacterial cause of COPD**	Otitis media and sinusitis	**Older adults**	Gram stain and culture of sputum	Patchy or lobar	**Hib polysaccharide protein conjugate vaccine.** Drug sensitive; amoxicillin, drug resistant ceftriaxone
			Staphylococcus aureus	**Minor % of CAP:** polysaccharide capsule; lipoteichoic acids, Protein A, hemolysins Panton-Valentine toxin, **pathogenicity islands, resistance to a variety of antibacterials (ex. penicillinase & active efflux) mechanism**	Soft tissue infections, endocarditis, and **20%–30% of nosocomial pneumonia**	**Hospitalized patients**	Gram stain of sputum and PCR	Patchy	MSSA: IV Nafcillin MRSA: Linezolid
			Moraxella catarrhalis	Minor % of CAP, outer membrane protein, pili, lipo-oligosaccharide, and penicillinase; second most common bacterial cause of COPD	Otitis media Sinusitis	**Elderly and hospitalized persons, COPD persons**	Gram stain of sputum	Diffuse	Azithromycin

(continued)

227

ACUTE COMMUNITY ACQUIRED PNEUMONIA

Infection	Sub-Type	Type of Microorganism	Microorganism	Epidemio-Logical or Virulence Factor	Associated Disease	Prominent Groups	Diagnosis	X-Ray Pattern	Prevention/Treatment
ACUTE COMMUNITY ACQUIRED PNEUMONIA	Typical (80%–90%)	Bacteria	*Pseudomonas aeruginosa*	**#1 cause of nosocomial pneumonia (associated with mechanical ventilation)**; pili, mucoid exopolysaccharide (MEP) endotoxin extracellular cytotoxins β-lactamases and efflux pumps	"Swimmer's ear"	Immunocompromised patients and **HIV and cystic fibrosis patients**	Gram stain and culture of sputum	Diffuse with some nodules	IV Piperacillin; Tazobactam plus Tobramycin (2–3 week treatment)
	Atypical	Bacteria	*Mycoplasma pneumoniae*	Largest number of atypicals (10%–15% of CAP); surface cytohesin protein (p1)	Bronchitis	**School-age children and young adults (5–20 years old)**	Serology for "**cold agglutinins**", PCR of lower respiratory tract specimens	Alveolar and inter-stitial	Doxycycline
			Chlamydophila-pneumoniae	**5%–10% of CAP: can cause persistent infections**; elementary and reticulate bodies	Pharyngitis and asthma	**School-age children and teenagers;** more severe in elderly	PCR on naso-pharyngeal swabs or sputum	Patchy sub-segmental	Azithromycin
			Legionella pneumophila	**1%–5% of CAP**, no person-to-person transmission, **transmission by aerosolized bacteria from aquatic habitats (ex. cooling towers, spas, potable water, etc.)** Also multiply in free-living amoebas; Mip protein, Hsp60 (heat shock protein), endotoxin, secreted degradative enzymes, & possible toxins	"**Pontiac Fever**"	Hospitalized individuals	RIA urine ag test	**Patchy, unilateral lower lobe**	Prevent aerosol formation; azithromycin

ACUTE COMMUNITY ACQUIRED PNEUMONIA

Atypical

	Organism						Treatment
Bacteria	*Coxiella burnetii*	Zoonotic disease, inhalation of small particle aerosols; reservoirs are cattle, sheep, and goats	Fever; chronic disease featuring endocarditis	**Occupational disease of farmers, veterinarians, and abattoir workers**	IFA serology on paired sera	Lobar or segmented rounded alveolar	Doxycycline
Virus	Lower respiratory tract viruses (mostly influenza, parainfluenza viruses, and RSV)	80% of infants and children, but only 10%–20% of adults; likely to occur during seasonal epidemics	**Predispose to 2° bacterial infection**	Infants (RSV) and children		Diffuse interstitial	See individual viruses in Upper and Lower Respiratory Tract Infections
	Hantavirus (Sin Nombre virus)	**Related to excreta of deer mice; most infections in SW U.S.**	Hantavirus pulmonary syndrome & cardio-pulmonary syndrome		Serology test for Sin Nombre virus IgM ab or RT-PCR of plasma	Diffuse interstitial	Fluid replacement and restoration of electrolytes and supportive measures
Fungi	*Pneumocystis jiroveci*	Transmission from other infected individuals, minor source of CAP except in **specific immunocompromised populations;** major surface glycoprotein, protease, antigenic variation		Malnourished and premature infants and **AIDS patients**	RT-PCR and PCR on oro-pharyngeal washes	Diffuse alveolar	Trimethoprim-sulfamethoxazole

(continued)

Infection	Type of Microorganism	Microorganism	Epidemiological or Virulence Factor	Associated Disease	Prominent Groups	Diagnosis	X-Ray Pattern	Prevention/Treatment
NOSOCOMIAL PNEUMONIAS	Bacteria	*Pseudomonas aeruginosa*	**Accounts for 50%–70% of these infections;** transmissible airborne pathogen; **found in moist microenvironments in hospitals (ex. sinks, inhalation equipment, etc.)**, pili, and extracellular poly-saccharides Pel, Psl, & mucoid exopolysaccharide (MEP) endotoxin & wide variety of antimicrobial resistance factors	Bacteremia; also causes both acute (small %) and chronic pneumonia	Hospitalized neutropenic patients and **CF patients**	Culture from sputum or bronchial-veolar lavage	Diffuse with some nodules	Piperacillin and Tazobactam
		Staphylococcus aureus (MRSA and MSSA)	**Accounts for 20%–30% of these infections;** capsular polysaccharide, variety of surface proteins including Protein A, several cytotoxins and secreted enzymes, **pathogenicity islands, & multiple antibiotic resistance mechanisms including penicillinase**	Bacteremia; endocarditis	**Lung abscess or thoracic surgery patients**	Sputum Gram stain and culture, also PCR of sputum	Patchy	MRSA: vancomycin or linezolid; MSSA: nafcillin
		Klebsiella pneumoniae	Minor % of infections, but usually associated with other nosocomial infections; polysaccharide capsule, pili, penicillinase, & other β-lactamases with extended spectrums (ex. cephalosporin)	**Insertion of intravascular and other invasive devices;** infections, meningitis, bacteremia	Debilitated patients	**"Currant jelly" sputum,** culture and Gram stain of sputum	Lobar	Susceptible organisms; IV ceftriaxone, resistant organisms; IV colistin
	Viruses	Influenza viruses, para-influenza viruses and RSV	**2%–10% of these infections**				See Listings in Upper and Lower Respiratory Tract Infections	
ASPIRATION PNEUMONIA	Bacteria	Anaerobic. Gram-negative bacilli (*Bacteroides, Prevotella,* and *Fusobacterium* species); some *Strep. pneumo* & *Staph. aureus*	**Cause 60%–80% of these infections (usually polymicrobial).** Capsular polysaccharides, extracellular enzymes, and a penicillinase	**Periodontal disease**	Patients with altered consciousness or dysphagia and elderly individuals (>65 years old)	Anaerobic culture of sputum and Gram stain	**Patchy, uni- or bilateral, right lung**	IV Metronidazole

CHRONIC PNEUMONIA

	Organism	Characteristics	Clinical	Patients	Diagnosis	Imaging	Treatment
Bacteria	*Mycobacterium tuberculosis*	Most chronic infections due to reactivation from sites of dormancy (macro-phages and lung); mycolic acid in cell wall and lipoarabinomannan on cell surface; also drug resistance	Previous TB infection which is usually asymptomatic; empyema	AIDS patients; elderly	Acid-fast stain, PCR and culture of sputum. Tuberculin skin test	Patchy or nodular in apical regions or subapical posterior; some cavitation	Prolonged combination therapy with isoniazid, rifampin, pyrazinamide, and ethambutol
	Mycobacterium avium-intracellulare	40% of AIDS patients get it within 2 years; naturally occurring in indoor water systems, pools, and hot tubs; virulence factors same as TB organism	Disseminated disease in AIDS patients	Older men who are heavy smokers or alcoholics; AIDS patients	Acid-fast stain and culture of sputum, but difficult to distinguish from TB organism	Fibronodular and cavitary in upper lobes	Same as for TB
	Nocardia asteroides	Found in soil and areas of plant decay; adhesins and mycolic acid polymers	CNS disease with granulomas or abscesses in the brain	Individuals with defective T-cell immunity or immuno-suppressed	Modified acid-fast stain of sputum and culture; PCR of sputum	Diffuse with irregular nodules	IV Trimethoprim and sulfamethoxazole plus imiperem
Fungi	*Aspergillus fumigatus*	Surface binding proteins and extracellular enzymes (proteases, elastase, and phospholipases)	Aspergillus colonization and allergic bronchopulmonary aspergillosis	Patients with granulopenia	Demonstrated tissue invasion in histopathologic specimens	Multiple diffuse nodules; cavitation late	Oral voriconazole
	Blastomyces dermatitidis	Endemic soil fungus in south central, central, and SE U.S.; glycoprotein adhesion (BAD1)	Skin lesions, acute pneumonia, high incidence of subclinical infections		Yeast cells in KOH smears of sputum, chemiluminescent DNA probes	Lobar or segmental alveolar, + or −	Lipid forms of Amphotericin B or itraconazole
	Coccidioides immitis	Exposure to soil dust in alkaline soil of semi-arid zones (AZ, NV, NM, and arid CA); secreted protease, and spherule outer cell wall	1° Valley Fever; chronic in alcoholics/poor health +/− meningitis; disseminates in IC patients or late pregnancy	Farm and construction workers; high mortality for women in third trimester of pregnancy	Spherules in KOH preps of sputum or in biopsy specimens. EIA tests for IgM or IgG antibodies	Diffuse unilateral; sometimes cavitation	Amphotericin B
	Histoplasma capsulatum	Inhalation of mold microconidia found in soil containing bird or bat droppings (found in Ohio and Mississippi River basins)	Preceding interstitial pneumonitis; disseminated disease with the RES organs and adrenal glands	Farmers, construction workers, and spelunkers, AIDS patients	EIA histoplasma ag test on urine bronchoalveolar lavage	Patchy upper lobes progress to cavitation	Itraconazole

D. Characteristics of Important Causes of Lower Respiratory Tract Infections

Infection	Type of Microorganism	Microorganism	Epidemiological or Virulence Factors	Associated Disease	Prominent Groups	Diagnosis	Prevention/Treatment
BRONCHITIS	Virus	Any of the cold and URT viruses can be involved	**Viruses cause 90% of infections**				
	Bacteria	*Bordetella pertussis*	Adults can get disease in spite of immunization as a child. Filamentous hemagglutinin facilitates attachment and **pertussis toxin and other cytotoxins**, including an adenylate cyclase, contribute to the disease	**Whooping cough**	Infants and young children	PCR on nasopharyngeal swabs	**Acellular pertussis vaccine is part of DPT vaccine and Tdap vaccine given as a booster to teens and initial adult vaccine** /erythromycin
		Chlamydophila pneumoniae	**Can cause persistent infections; elementary and reticulate bodies**	Pharyngitis and asthma	School-age children and teenagers	PCR on nasopharyngeal swabs	Azithromycin
		Mycoplasma pneumoniae	**Account for 75% of agent's infections;** surface cytohesin protein (P1)	"Walking pneumonia" (25% of infections)	5- to 20-year-olds	Definitive diagnosis not done unless a serious infection, then PCR of lower respiratory tract specimens	Erythromycin
BRONCHIOLITIS	Virus	Respiratory syncytial virus	**Causes 50%–80% of cases (usually occurs in winter) and is the leading cause of all infant hospitalizations;** F and G surface glycoproteins important for attachment and penetration and nonstructural proteins NS1 & NS2 inhibit type 1 interferon synthesis	**Croup (2%–10% of cases)**; otitis media (children 1–3 years old). Colds or bronchiolitis in adults	**Infants <1 year old**	**Dipstick immunoassay for RSV ags** in nasal washings or nasopharyngeal swabs	**Passive immunization with palivizumab monoclonal antibody for high risk infants**; supportive, but aerosolised ribivirin for hospitalized infants
		Human metapneumovirus (hMPV)	Causes 3%–19% of cases; membrane G glycoprotein needed for attachment	Exacerbations of childhood asthma	**Infants 3–24 mos. old**	PCR of respiratory specimens; immunofluorescence of indicator shell cultures inoculated with nasopharyngeal swab	Supportive
		Other upper respiratory viruses (see individual viruses)	Less common than RSV and hMPV				

E. Characteristics of Important Causes of Upper Respiratory Tract Infections

Infection	Type of Microorganism	Microorganism	Epidemiological or Virulence Factors	Associated Disease	Prominent Groups	Diagnosis	Prevention/Treatment
COMMON COLD	*Virus*	Rhinoviruses	Optimum growth temperature is 33°C and > **100 serotypes**; cellular receptor is ICAM-1	Often exacerbate asthma attack in school-age children and LRT infections	Adults	Clinical; but specific virus identification usually not done	Supportive
		Coronaviruses	**Infection mostly in winter and spring**; cellular receptor is aminopeptidase N	SARS with SARS CoV	Children	RT-PCR, but not usually done	Supportive
		Parainfluenza viruses	HN protein binds to cellular sialic acid surface molecules, but **cellular proteolytic activation of F protein needed for entry**	**Otitis media and croup**	Children	RT-PCR, but not usually done	Live attenuated strains of type 3 virus developed, but not licensed
PHARYNGOTONSILLITIS	*Bacteria*	*Streptococcus pyogenes*	**M protein**, capsule, hyaluronic acid, lipoteichoic acids, exotoxins, **streptolysin O, streptokinase**	Epiglottis, **pneumatic fever**, and acute glomerulonephritis	Children (5–15 years)	Rapid antigen detection tests (RADTs) for wall carbohydrate ag	Oral penicillin V or amoxicillin
		Corynebacterium diphtheriae	**Diphtheria toxin**	Diphtheritic myocarditis	Unimmunized children and adults	Clinical	Diphtheria toxoid vaccine part of DPT vaccine; penicillin G procaine or erythromycin antibacterials and diphtheria antitoxin (DAT) available for treatment
	Viruses	Cold and mouth viruses (Coxsackie A viruses, parainfluenza viruses, and HSV)	**See Mouth and Cold listings for details**				

(continued)

Infection	Type of Microorganism	Microorganism	Epidemiological or Virulence Factors	Associated Disease	Prominent Groups	Diagnosis	Prevention/Treatment
PHARYNGOTONSILLITIS	*Viruses*	Infectious mononucleosis viruses (CMV and EBV)	**Throat manifestations are part of systemic infectious mononucleosis**	Infectious mononucleosis	CMV childhood EBV:15- to 25-year-olds	CMV hybrid capture assay on WBC; EBV PCR on sputum	Valganciclovir for CMV; supportive for EBV
		Adenoviruses	**Most infections in late winter and early spring, many serotypes, latent in lymphoid tissue; pentons have toxic activity**	Multiple respiratory syndromes and pharyngoconjunctival fever	Children (<2 yrs) and military recruits	PCR of throat swabs or sputum	Supportive
EPIGLOTTITIS	*Bacteria*	*Haemophilus influenzae*	Polysaccharide capsule, IgA protease, pili, outer membrane proteins, endotoxin	**Otitis media**, neurologic sequelae	Unvaccinated children	Gram stain and culture	**Hib polysaccharide-protein conjugate vaccine**/ceftriaxone + airway
		Streptococcus pyogenes	See above	See above	Adults		See above
LARYNGITIS	*Viruses*	Cold, mouth, and upper respiratory tract viruses		See those listed above			
CROUP	*Virus*	Parainfluenza virus	**Type 3 virus is most involved**	See listing under Common Cold			
INFLUENZA	*Virus*	Influenza virus	**Hemagglutinin glycoprotein (H) is virus receptor, Neuraminidase protein (N) is important for virus release; genetic reassortment and genetic shift & drift** are important epidemiological processes	**1° viral pneumonia and 2° pneumonia caused by bacterial superinfection**	Children and adults	Dipstick test of respiratory secretions for viral ags	**Trivalent killed virus vaccines/influenza A only: amantadine and rimantadine; influenza A & B: zanamivir and oseltamivir,** but not all for young children (<1 yr old). Some use of amantadine, rimantadine, or oseltamivir for prophylaxis

Review Test

Directions: Each of the numbered items or incomplete statements in this section is followed by answers or completions of the statement. Select the ONE lettered answer that is BEST in each case.

1. One week postdelivery, an infant boy becomes extremely irritable and continuously rubs his right eye, which contains a mucopurulent exudate. An examination of the eye shows papillae on the conjunctiva. No bacteria are seen in the exudate. The most likely causative infectious agent is

(A) *Candida albicans*
(B) *Chlamydophila trachomatis*
(C) Cytomegalovirus
(D) Herpes simplex virus

2. A 58-year-old man presents at your office complaining of extreme pain in his right testicle. Physical examination shows considerable swelling. A small amount of urethral exudate could be aspirated. Microscopic examination and Gram staining showed the presence of bacteria. Those bacteria most likely are

(A) Gram-negative cocci
(B) Gram-negative diplococci
(C) Gram-positive cocci
(D) Gram-positive rods

3. A 22-year-old woman presents with symptoms of vaginitis, including a yellowish discharge. She claims to have not been sexually active for 18 months. When KOH is added to the discharge, a "fishy" odor appears. She is most likely infected with

(A) *Candida albicans*
(B) *Chlamydophila trachomatis*
(C) *Gardnerella vaginalis*
(D) Herpes simplex virus 2

4. A known alcoholic appears at the emergency department with chest pain, a 40°C/104°F fever, chills, and a productive cough. He has no history of chronic pulmonary disease. There are red blood cells and encapsulated Gram-negative rods in the sputum. The symptoms are most likely caused by

(A) *Haemophilus influenzae*
(B) *Klebsiella pneumoniae*

(C) *Nocardia asteroides*
(D) *Pseudomonas aeruginosa*

5. There is an outbreak of gastrointestinal disease involving six children at a day care center. The children all have symptoms of fever, watery stool, and vomiting. Recent activities at the center involved playing with animals including kittens, turtles, birds, and hamsters. What types of bacteria are most likely to be observed in the stool?

(A) Gram-positive cocci
(B) Gram-negative cocci
(C) Gram-positive rods
(D) Gram-negative rods

6. A 75-year-old man is brought by his daughter to the community health center. He appears confused and has a stiff neck and severe headache. She indicates that the previous week he had a runny nose and other symptoms consistent with sinusitis. What organism would you expect to find in his cerebrospinal fluid?

(A) Coxsackie virus
(B) *Haemophilus influenzae*
(C) *Neisseria meningitis*
(D) *Streptococcus pneumoniae*

7. While on winter semester break, a 21-year-old male college student appears at his family physician's office with several skin lesions on his right arm. They consist of a central pustule within a raised erythematous area. He reports that the only recent unusual activities that have involved skin exposure have been hot tub parties at his friend's cabin during the previous two weekends. What is the most likely causative infectious agent?

(A) *Pseudomonas aeruginosa*
(B) *Streptococcus pyogenes*
(C) *Staphylococcus aureus*
(D) Papillomavirus

8. In July, you are called to a rural nursing home where several of the residents have developed a gastrointestinal disease consisting of fever, vomiting, and bloody stool. Lab analysis of the stool shows the presence of PMNs and Gram-negative rods. Epidemiological discussions with the residents indicate they all shared the same raw milk brought to one resident by his farmer son. The most likely cause of the infection is

(A) *Campylobacter jejuni*
(B) *Clostridium perfringens*
(C) *Staphylococcus aureus*
(D) *Vibrio parahaemolyticus*

9. An 18-month-old female infant is brought to the emergency department by her mother. The mother reports an abrupt onset of symptoms consisting of continual crying, high fever (40°C/104°F), and a cough producing rusty colored sputum. What would you expect a chest x-ray and lab findings to show?

(A) Lobar pattern and Gram-positive cocci
(B) Lobar pattern and Gram-negative cocci
(C) Bronchopneumonia pattern and Gram-positive cocci
(D) Bronchopneumonia pattern and Gram-negative rods

Answers and Explanations

1. **The answer is B.** This case of neonatal conjunctivitis is most likely caused by *Chlamydophila trachomatis* since no bacteria are present and papillae rather than follicles are observed. The mother was probably the source of the infection.

2. **The answer is C.** Both *Staphylococcus epidermidis* and various Enterobacteriaceae can cause epididymitis in men over the age of 35 years, but Gram-negative rods is not a choice; therefore, Gram-positive cocci is correct.

3. **The answer is C.** *Gardnerella vaginalis* and *Candida albicans* are the non-STD choices. *Gardnerella vaginalis* is correct because it produces the fishy odor when KOH is added to the discharge.

4. **The answer is B.** *Klebsiella pneumoniae* is associated with pneumonia in alcoholics. The other Gram-negative rod (*Pseudomonas aeruginosa*) is associated with chronic pulmonary disease in the immunocompromised.

5. **The answer is D.** The most likely bacteria to cause gastrointestinal disease with the symptoms and circumstances provided is a species of *Salmonella,* which are Gram-negative rods.

6. **The answer is D.** The symptoms of confusion and severe headache point to a case of bacterial meningitis. With preceding sinusitis in an elderly man, *Streptococcus pneumoniae* is the most likely cause. The other two bacteria are more often observed in infants or young adults.

7. **The answer is A.** *Pseudomonas aeruginosa* is associated with an infection known as "whirlpool" or "hot tub" folliculitis. Inappropriate care of whirlpools, hot tubs, and swimming pools can allow this organism to grow and enter the skin through small breaks.

8. **The answer is A.** The symptoms and lab analysis of the stool are consistent with *Campylobacter jejuni* infection. The raw milk was most likely the source of the infection.

9. **The answer is A.** The most common cause of CAP in infants and elderly is *Streptococcus pneumoniae*. The symptoms in this case are consistent, and the rusty colored sputum is suggestive of this bacteria. It is a Gram-positive cocci with a lobar pneumonia on a chest x-ray.

chapter 12

Immunology

I. OVERVIEW

A. Host defense mechanisms (Fig. 12.1).

A collection of physiological strategies used to police tissues for parasites like bacteria and non-compliant self-tissue such as cancer. The immune system is responsible for identifying self- and non-self-tissue, and to discern between normal and non-compliant tissue. Strategies include the following:

1. Barriers

2. Inflammation

3. Innate immunity

4. Adaptive immunity

B. Concerns in medicine.

1. Autoimmunity

2. Hypersensitivity

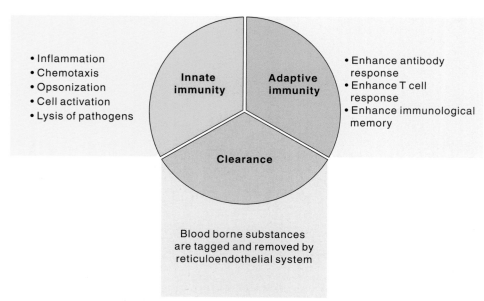

FIGURE 12.1. **Overview of host defenses.**

3. Cancer
4. Vulnerability to infection
5. Complications to tissue transplantation and blood transfusions

II. NON-SPECIFIC BARRIERS (FIG. 12.2)

These barriers are composed of epithelium and demarcated zones of immunity; for instance, inside vs. outside, mucosal vs. interstitial, exocrine (salivary and sebaceous glands), urogenital and kidney, respiratory region, synovia of articulating joints, blood-brain barrier, eye, germ line, and placenta.

A. Stratum corneum.
1. Demarcation of tissues from extracorporeal environment.
2. Effective protection; trauma and infections are rare events; examples are lacerations, punctures, bites or non-sterile needles, antigens, solvents, UV light, detergents, microorganism, toxins, nanoparticles.
3. Cornified epithelium produced as the terminally differentiated keratinocytes in the stratified squamous epithelium.
4. Composed of keratin filaments in the cells with a barrier of insoluble protein matrix and highly cross-linked.
5. Desquamation of skin, sloughs casting off carries bacteria.
6. Hair follicles, sebaceous glands, and sudoriferous glands flush the surface.
7. Common antigen-driven skin diseases include psoriasis and atopic dermatitis.
8. Skin surface area is 1.5 to 2.0 m^2.

B. Tight junctions.
1. Composed of epithelial proteins, occludins, claudins, and junctional adhesion molecules.
2. Provides a tight seal at the blood-brain barrier.
3. Provides a route for Langerhans cells to capture antigen.
4. Intraepithelial T lymphocytes release IFN-γ, IL-4, and IL-10 to disrupt the junction.

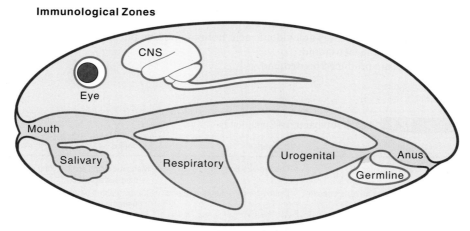

Immunological Zones

FIGURE 12.2. Zones for different immune responses. (1) Skin is the first line of defense, a rugged impermeable barrier shown as a blue solid line. **(2) The circulatory system** flushes the muscular and organelle tissue. **(3) Mucosal membranes** regulate material transfers into and out of the body. These barriers are specialized to separate physiological functions, and are continuously flushed clean with mucopolysaccharides; noted purple. **(4) Barrier membranes** incorporate tight junctions to rigorously regulate the select material transfers to provide tissue-specific protection, shown as green.

5. Antigen-driven tight junction diseases include:
   a. Skin: Pemphigus vulgaris, Pemphigus foliaceus
   b. GI/Mucosal: Inflammatory bowel disease, celiac disease, autoimmune bullous disease of oral mucosa, Crohn's disease and ulcerative colitis
C. **Mucous layer:**
   1. Demarcation between tissues and systemic environment.
   2. Dynamic protection using viscous fluid flow mixed with a highly enriched mat of micro flora; for example, oral or enteric bacteria.
   3. Mucosal surface area: intestine approximately 300 m^2, lung 70 m^2, and total 400 m^2.
   4. The acid mantle is a thin barrier to the penetration by bacteria and virus. Drastic pH alters the luminal environment from saliva pH of 6.2 to 7.4, Stomach pH of 1.5 to 3.5, small intestine at pH 6 for duodenum gradually increasing to pH 7.4 in the ileum, and large intestine ranging from 5.7 in caecum to pH 6.7 in the rectum.
   5. Intestinal mucosa is colonized by $<10^{14}$ luminal bacteria from more than 500 species.
   6. The largest pool of macrophages located in the intestinal wall accompanied by NKT cells to manage bacterial stasis to the intestinal lumina.
   7. Approximately 70% of all lymphocytes are located within the lamina propria.

III. INFLAMMATION AND SOLUBLE FACTORS

This is a rapid response system dependent on the circulatory system (cardiovascular and lymphatic systems). The system is based on a homeostatic equilibrium that rapidly responds to disturbances and utilizes complement and clotting to tag and trap foreign substances, vasodilation and extravasation to flush sites of infections, the **Reticuloendothelial system** to remove debris, and a chemical identification system of **pattern recognition receptors**. These receptors identify **PAMP**s (pathogen associated molecular patterns) and **DAMP**s (damage associated molecular patterns).

A. **Antimicrobial proteins (Table 12.1).**
   1. A collection of peptides between 12 to 50 amino acids.
   2. Net positive charge that disrupts membrane integrity.
   3. Many of the antimicrobial proteins are stored in neutrophils.

B. **Role of eicosanoids in inflammation (Fig. 12.3).**
   1. Prostaglandins, thromboxanes, leukotrienes, and lipoxins are membrane-derived lipids.
   2. Act as potent paracrine and autocrine signals.
   3. Phospholipase A2 releases arachidonic acid from membrane phospholipids, which are central to produce the eicosanoid.
   4. These lipids are produced on demand.

table 12.1   List of Antibacterial Compounds

Peptide	Site	Properties	Examples
Collectins	Extracellular	Collage-like domain	Mannin-binding protein, lung surfactant A, lung surfactant B
Defensins	Extracellular-vernix caseos, amniotic fluid Intracellular	Cysteine-rich cationic proteins	Neutrophils-α-defensin, release during phagocytosis Paneth cells-α-defensin Epithelial cells-constitutively release α- and β-defensin
Cathelicidins	Lysosomes of PMN and macrophage	Cationic peptide, release by elastase	LL-37
Saposin	CTL, NK cells	Acts on sphingolipids	Granulysin
Mucins	Saliva	Highly glycosidic proteins	MUC7

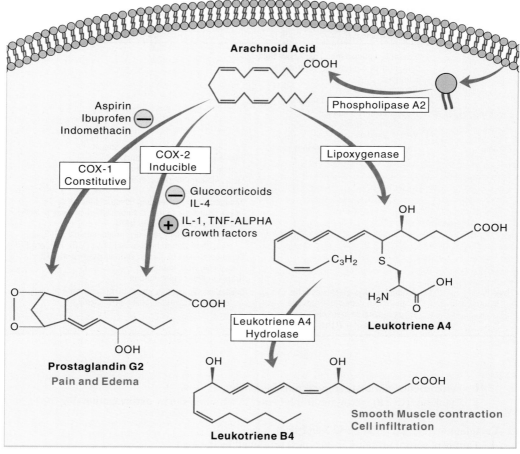

FIGURE 12.3. **Production of eicosanoids.**

5. These agents regulate vascular tone and smooth muscle contraction.
6. Eicosanoids are primarily responsible for the four signs of inflammation: *calor, rubor, dolor,* and *tumor.*
7. Eicosanoids play a significant role in anaphylaxis and asthma.

C. **Effects on vasculature (Table 12.2).**
    1. Conduit for fluid and nutrient exchange.
        a. Barrier to tissues built on endothelial cells interlocked together to form tubes.
        b. Blood passes through vascular channels lined with endothelium interlocked with tight junctions and wrapped with smooth muscle.
        c. Lymphatics are loosely connected endothelial cells that allow fluid entry driven by Starling pressure.
        d. **Vascular dilation** occurs immediately and rapidly when stimulated by histamine, bradykinin, and prostaglandins.
        e. Dilation leads to permeability and exudation.
        f. Vasoconstriction results from smooth muscle contraction.
        g. Restricted flow permits clotting and contains pathogen locally, thus preventing systemic dissemination.
        h. Mast cells regulate vascular tone by producing vasoactive substances.

t a b l e **12.2** Types of Inflammation		
Type	**Characteristic**	
Acute	Exudative inflammation– excessive fluid Suppurative or purulent–neutrophils Fibrinous Serous-clear fluid Hemorrhagic-vascular damage	
Lewis trip response	Flush: capillary dilatation Flare: arteriolar dilatation Wheal: exudation, edema	

Chronic	Persistent presence of noxious stimuli	Persistent presence of noxious stimuli
		Interferes with wound healing
		Normal wound healing process
		Mononuclear infiltration and elimination of pathogen
		Tissue destruction
		Resolution by regenerating tissue of fibrosis
		Tissue injury due to free radical oxygen, proteases, and
		    tissue plasmin activator (tPA)
		Fibrosis caused by cytokines, predominately TGFβ, but
		    also other growth factors including PDGF, FGF, or VEGF
		Common causes of chronic inflammation: Lyme, TB,
		    syphilis, viral hepatitis
		Granulomatous inflammation

Type IV
    hypersensitivity
	Attempt to physically isolate the
	    pathogen within macrophage
	Large nucleated foam cells form as a
	    syncytium of macrophage
		Examples: TB, leprosy, syphilitic gumma, foreign bodies,
		    fungal infections, silicosis, sarcoidosis

    i. Leukotrienes stimulate smooth muscle activity.

    j. Cytokines (CCL8) recruit neutrophil entry to a trauma site by **extravasation** (Fig. 12.4).

D. Complement (Fig. 12.5; Tables 12.3 and 12.4).

  1. Family of serum proteins ($>$30 types) produced by the liver.

  2. These proteins are functionally integrated; once triggered, they follow a cascade of reactions to instantaneously attack foreign substances.

  3. The complement proteins reside in the circulation in a homeostatic state.

  4. Any disturbance to this equilibrium causes a rapid and efficient shift in the local environment to the appearance of a series of highly reactive compounds.

  5. Recognition activates a sequence of caspases that generate **anaphylatoxin, opsonin,** and a **membrane attack complex (MAC)**. These three activities facilitate macrophage clearance of the foreign objects.

  6. Complement receptors on the follicular dendritic cell in draining lymph nodes collect debris for display and screening by mature B and T cells in germinal centers.

  7. Deficiencies lead to bacteral infections. Loss of C3 function leads to general bacterial infections. Loss of C5, C6, C7, C8, or C9 leads to succeptability to meningitis (i.e., *Neisseria meningitidis*). Loss of C1 inhibitor impacts complement fixation, clotting, and kinin pathways (i.e., Bradykinin), leading to edema.

E. Acute phase reaction.

  1. The liver will compensate for shifts in protein content in the plasma.

  2. A fast-acting, nonspecific response by hepatocytes during disturbances in homeostasis including trauma, infection, neoplastic growth, and immune hypersensitivities.

  3. Hepatocytes change protein secretion in response to the cytokines IL-1, IL-6, and TNFα release by macrophage located at the inflammatory site.

  4. Proteins such as C-reactive protein, serum amyloid, ceruloplasmin, complement factor-3, haptoglobin, fibrinogen, and α1-antitrypsin increase in secretion.

  5. Proteins such as albumin and transferrin decrease secretion.

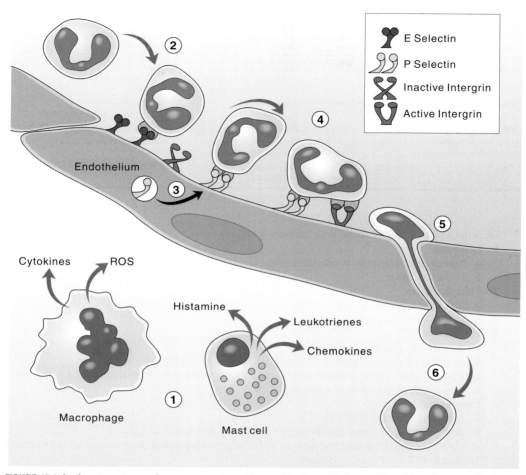

FIGURE 12.4. Leukocyte extravasation across post-capillary walls. Steps: (1) Recognition of PAMP, mast cell release of chemokines to recruit neutrophils, histamine, and leukotriene to promote inflammation; resident macrophage begins phagocytosis and cytolysis. (2) Neutrophil attaches to the endothelium using P-selectin; rolling action starts. (3) Weibel-Palade body exocytoses, presenting E-selectin to the surface. (4) Integrin activation and neutrophil stop moving. (5) Neutrophil crosses the endothelial barrier. (6) Neutrophil enters the site of inflammation.

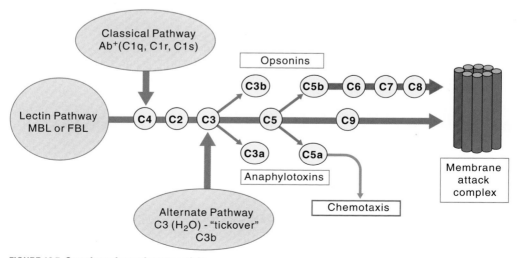

FIGURE 12.5. Overview of complement activity.

t a b l e **12.3**		List of Complement Receptors		
Receptor	CD	Complement Ligand	Function	Cell Type
CR1	CD35	C3b, C4b, iC3b	Phagocytosis Erythrocyte transport of immune complexes	Macrophage, monocytes PMN, erythrocytes, B cells, FDC
CR2	CD21	C3d, iC3b, C3dg	B-cell coreceptor	B cells, FDC
CR3	CD11b/CD18	iC3b	Phagocytosis	Macrophage, monocytes, PMN, FDC
CR4	CD11c/CD18	iC3b	Phagocytosis	Macrophage, monocytes, PMN, DC
C5a	CD88	C5a	Degranulation cellularity	Endothelial cells, phagocytes
C3a		C3a	Degranulation cellularity	Endothelial cells, mast cells, phagocytes

F. **Secreted enzymes and proteins with immune function.**
   1. **Lysozyme:**
      a. An enzyme of hydrolysis polysaccharide found on bacterial cell surfaces.
      b. Found in saliva.
   2. **Phospholipase:**
      a. An enzyme hydrolysis phospholipids into fatty acids and lipophilic substance.
      b. Initiates the release of **eicosanoids.**
   3. **Lactoferrin:**
      a. An iron-binding globular protein.
      b. Secreted by exocrine glands and specific granules in neutrophils.
      c. Upon degranulation, virtually all serum lactoferrin originates from neutrophils.
      d. Acts to deprive bacteria of a source of iron.
   4. **Lactoperoxidase:**
      a. A bactericidal oxidoreductase.
      b. Secreted from mucosal glands including salivary and mammary glands.
      c. Catalyzes oxidation and the production of water using hydrogen peroxide as the electron donor.

t a b l e **12.4**	Important Antibacterial Actions by Serum Complement
Function	Components

Recognition	Classical pathway
	    Natural antibodies to carbohydrate
	    Complement-fixing antibodies from adaptive immunity
	Lectin pathway
	    Sugar-binding proteins are ficolins and mannose-binding lectin
	    Bacterial surfaces have high density of mannose
	Spontaneous pathway
	    Nonspecific
	    Requires host proteins to prevent self-recognitions

Convertase	A serine endoprotease that converts the quiescent proprotein complement into a highly reactive form
	    C3 convertase
	    C5 convertase

Anaphylatoxin	Potent stimulator of phagocytosis
	    C3a
	    C4a
	    C5a

Opsonins	Coat targets for receptor-mediated phagocytosis
	    C3b-directs macrophage phagocytosis
	    C5b-directs formation of MAC

Permeabilization	Membranes attack complex C5b through C9

5. **Myeloperoxidase:**
   a. A bactericidal oxidoreductase.
   b. Expressed in neutrophils.
   c. Stored in azurophilic granules.
   d. Secreted following activation.
   e. Catalyzes chloride ion oxidation using hydrogen peroxide to form hypochlorous acid.
   f. The catalytic cofactor is a heme moiety that gives the green color to purulent pus.
6. **Xanthine oxidoreductase:**
   a. An oxidoreductase that produces hydrogen peroxide and water from the conversion of hypoxanthine to xanthine, which is further broken down to uric acid and an additional hydrogen peroxide.
   b. Converts aliphatic compounds to aliphatic alcohol and two superoxide radicals of oxygen.
   c. Xanthine oxidoreductase is widely expressed in tissues and is a major constituent of fat globules in breast milk.

IV. MEDIATORS OF INFLAMMATION AND IMMUNITY (TABLE 12.5)

A. **Chemokines:**
   1. Are defined as small peptides (8,000 to 16,000 Da) that are released by injury and are active at very low concentrations (10-8 to 10-11 M). They exhibit approximately 30% to 50% amino acid sequence homology.
   2. Function by transmitting signals through seven transmembrane, rhodopsin-like receptors, which activate and attract leukocytes to sites with tissue damage.
   3. Are classified into two subcategories based on the sequence of two pairs of the amino acid cysteine.
      a. C-X-C chemokines (alpha) have their first two cysteines separated by one amino acid. Most attract neutrophils; the most potent include IL-8, platelet factor 4, IFN-γ, inducible protein 10, and macrophage activation factors.
      b. C-C chemokines (beta) have two adjacent cysteine residues. Most attract monocytes and T lymphocytes, while a few attract eosinophils, basophils, and natural killer (NK) cells via MCPs, MIP, and RANTES (regulated on activation of normal T cells, expressed and secreted).

B. **Cytokines:**
   1. Are intracellular signaling proteins acting locally in a paracrine or autocrine manner by binding to high affinity receptors.
   2. Have frequently overlapping functions, as a single activity can be caused by multiple cytokines, and multiple activities can be caused by a single cytokine (pleiotropism).
   3. Lymphokines are cytokines that are produced by lymphocytes; monokines are cytokines that are produced by monocytes or macrophages.
   4. IL-1, IL-6, and TNF-α induce MCP and IL-8 and the acute phase response and are endogenous pyrogens.
   5. TGF-β is a potent wound healing and immunosuppressive agent inhibiting IL-2 effects and proliferation of many cell types. It also promotes the switching of B cells to immunoglobulin A (IgA) synthesis.
   6. Cytokine receptors on cells can have circulating forms, consisting of only the extra-cytoplasmic portion of the receptor, which can combine with and block the cytokine in serum before it reaches its cellular target.

table **12.5**   Cytokines and Their Actions

Cytokine	Major Cell Source	Major Immunologic Action
IL-1 (α, β)	Macrophages Endothelial cells Dendritic cells Langerhans cells	Stimulates IL-2 receptor emergence in T cells Enhances B-cell activation Induces fever, acute phase reactants, and IL-6 Increases nonspecific resistance Inhibited by an endogenous IL-1 receptor antagonist
IL-2	T_h1 cells	T-cell growth factor Activates NK and B cells
IL-3	T cells	Stimulates hematopoiesis
IL-4	T cells	Stimulates B-cell synthesis of IgE Down-regulation of IFN-γ
IL-5	T cells	Stimulates growth and differentiation of eosinophils B-cell growth factor Enhances IgA synthesis
IL-6	Monocytes T cells Endothelial cells	Induces acute phase reactants, fever, and late B-cell differentiation
IL-7	Bone marrow	Stimulates pre-B and pre-T cells
IL-8	Monocytes Endothelial cells Lymphocytes Fibroblasts	Chemotactic factor for neutrophils and T cells
IL-9	T_h cells	T-cell mitogen
IL-10	T_h2 cells	Inhibits IFN-γ synthesis by T_h1 cells Suppresses other cytokine synthesis
IL-11	Bone marrow	Stimulates hematopoiesis Enhances acute phase protein synthesis
IL-12	Macrophages B cells	Promotes T_h1 differentiation and IFN-γ synthesis Stimulates NK cells and CD8$^+$ T cells to cytolysis Acts synergistically with IL-2
IL-13	T_h2 cells	Inhibits inflammatory cytokines (IL-1, IL-6, IL-8, IL-10, MCP)
IL-15	T cells	T-cell mitogen Enhances growth of intestinal epithelium
IL-16	CD8$^+$ T cells Eosinophils	Increases Class II MHC, chemotaxis, and CD4$^+$ T-cell cytokines Decreases antigen-induced proliferation
IL-17	T cells	Increases the inflammatory response
IL-18	Activated macrophages	Increases IFN-γ production and NK cell action
TNF-α	Macrophages T cells B cells Large granular lymphocytes	Cytotoxic for tumors Causes cachexia Mediates bacterial shock
TNF-β	T cells	Cytotoxic for tumors
Transforming growth factor β	Almost all normal cell types	Inhibits proliferation of both T and B cells Reduces cytokine receptors Potent chemotactic agent for leukocytes Mediates inflammation and tissue repair

IFN, interferon; Ig, immunoglobulin; IL, interleukin; MCP, macrophage chemotactic protein; MHC, major histocompatibility complex; NK, natural killer; TNF, tumor necrosis factor.

V. INNATE IMMUNITY (FIG. 12.6)

A cellular response by leukocytes that targets pathogens decorated with chemical indicators (i.e., complement and antibody) derived from inflammation or adaptive immunity. Effector cells of innate immunity are often referred to as **granulocytes** due to their laden appearance with secretory vesicles, or **polymorphonuclear cells** due to their distinctively shaped nuclei. PMN cells attracted to the chemical indicators deliver a cytolytic attack or **cytolysis** using chemical warfare.

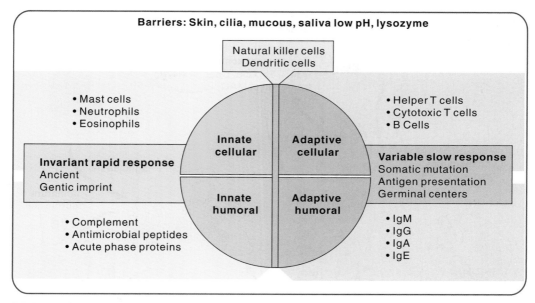

FIGURE 12.6. **Integrated immune system.**

1. Free radicals of oxygen (O_2^-, H_2O_2, OH^-, and $^1O_2$) and nitrogen (NO)
2. Antibacterial peptides (defensins and cathelicidins)
3. Apoptosis inducing peptides (granzymes)

A. **Innate immune response (Fig. 12.7):**
   1. A sequence of events beginning with recognition of infection by either PAMPs or DAMPs stimulating leukocytes such as mast cells and macrophage.
   2. Chemokines recruit additional leukocytes.
   3. Cytokines elicit specific physiological responses.
   4. Growth factors called colony-stimulating factors induce **hematopoiesis.**
   5. Bone marrow replenishes circulating leukocytes.
   6. Leukocytes extravasate into the site of inflammation or park in special niches such as draining lymph nodes.
   7. Leukocytes are generally short-lived and die by apoptosis as the inflammation resolves.

B. **Cell adhesion molecules:**
Immune cells interact with surface molecules on vascular epithelia to direct movement and to recruit cells to sites of trauma. Two systems provide cell recognition, selectins and integrins.
   1. **Selectins:**
      a. Initiate cell to cell contact
      b. Weak interaction, allows for rolling effect
      c. Must overcome shear force
      d. Structure, N terminus out, calcium-lectin, linked by complement-binding elements to a single membrane spanning domain-surface protease that down-regulates L-selectin binding or shedding
      e. Smallest family of adhesion molecules
      f. Three types:
         (1) **L-selectin:**
            (a) Found on most leukocytes
            (b) Necessary for lymphocyte entry into immune organs, steady-state process
            (c) Directs secondary tethering of neutrophils
            (d) Binding partners are E-selectin and cutaneous lymphocyte antigen (CLA)

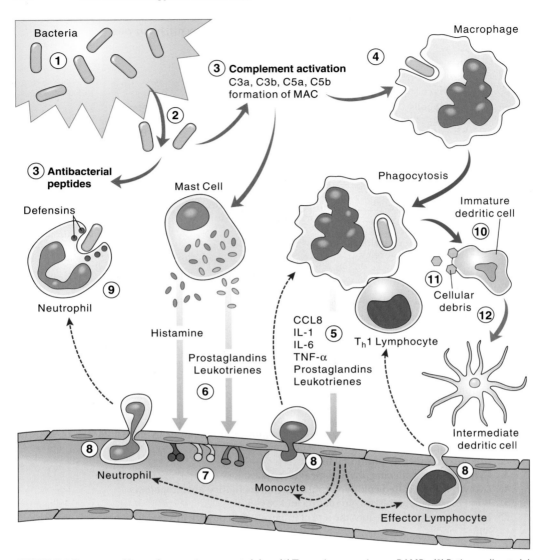

FIGURE 12.7. **Sequence of innate immune responses to injury.** (1) Tissue damage releases DAMPs. (2) Pathogen (bacterial or helminth) gains entry while presenting PAMPs. (3) Complement and antibacterial peptides begin immediate response. (4) Resident macrophage and mast cells are activated by C3a, C5a, PAMPs, and DAMPs. (5) Macrophage releases cytokines to recruit neutrophils, dendritic cells, and additional macrophage. (6) Mast cell initiates structural changes of the vasculature, vasodilatation/vasoconstriction, and relaxation of the tight junctions to facilitate extravasation. (7) Selectin expression is increased; Weibel-Palade bodies expel contents. (8) Cellular extravasation begins. (9) Neutrophils begin massive phagocytosis and cytolysis. (10) Dendritic cells scavenge debris from the wound site. (11) PAMPs stimulate dendritic cells to mature and egress the wound site by following lymphatic flow. (12) Mature antigen-expressing dendritic cells take residence in the paracortex of the lymph node to begin the adaptive immune response.

    (2) **E-selectin** found on endothelial cells:
       (a) Induced by IL-1β, TNFα, TNFβ, LPS
       (b) NF-κB regulation, a pro-inflammatory transcription factor
       (c) Down-regulated by internalization and routed to lysosome
    (3) **P-selectin** found on endothelial and platelets:
       (a) Prepackaged in **Weibel-Palade bodies**
       (b) Rapid surface expression induced by histamine, thrombin, and oxygen radicals

    (c) Rapid down-regulation by internalization but recycled from endosomes to secretory granules

    (d) Expression induced by TNFα and lipopolysaccharide (LPS)

2. Integrins:
    a. Chemokines emanating from inflammatory site induce tighter contact to stop leukocyte rolling.
    b. Chemokines are immobilized to proteoglycans.
    c. Other, platelet-activating factor.
    d. Chemokine induces allosteric effects to activate.

C. Pattern recognition receptors (*Commotus ingenio*) (Table 12.6).
    1. An invariant recognition mechanism that detects specific and unique molecular patterns associated with pathogens and inflammation.
    2. PPR are ancient and genetically imprinted into the host.
    3. Recognition molecules target molecular patterns that are also invariant and absolutely necessary for pathogen survival.
    4. Target signals emanating from a pathogen are called **PAMPs**; target signals emanating from inflammation and damaged host tissue are **DAMPs**.
    5. Pattern recognition receptors are cellular bound or soluble, and provide surveillance information to early responders for inflammation (mast cells, neutrophils, macrophage, and myeloid dendritic cells) and B cells.
    6. Two major receptor types screen for PAMPs/DAMPs.
        a. Toll-like receptors (TLR) are found on professional antigen-presenting cells (i.e., macrophage, dendritic cells, B cells).
        b. Intracellular pathogens are detected by **NBS-LRR proteins** (Nucleotide-binding site and leucine-rich repeat).

t a b l e 12.6 List of Selected Pattern Recognition Receptors

Pattern Recognition Receptor	Subcellular Location	Ligand	Cell Types
TLR-1	Cell surface	Lipoprotein	Monocytes, macrophages, dendritic cells, B cells
TLR-2	Cell surface	Glycolipid, lipoteichoic acid, HSP-70	Monocytes, macrophages, dendritic cells, mast cells
TLR-3	Intracellular compartment	dsRNA, polyI:C	Dendritic cells
TLR-4	Cell surface	Lipopolysaccharide, HSP, fibrinogen	Monocytes, macrophages, dendritic cells, mast cells, B cells
TLR-5	Cell surface	Flagellin	Monocytes, macrophages, and dendritic cells
TLR-6	Cell surface	Diacyl lipopeptides	Monocytes, macrophages, mast cells, B cells
TLR-7	Intracellular compartment	ssRNA	Monocytes, macrophages, plasmacytoid cells, B cells
TLR-8	Intracellular compartment	ssRNA	Monocytes, macrophages, dendritic cells, mast cells
TLR-9	Intracellular compartment	Unmethylated CpG DNA	Monocytes, macrophages, dendritic cells, B cells
TLR-10	Intracellular compartment	Unknown	
TLR-11	Intracellular compartment	Profilin	Monocytes, macrophages
TLR-12	Intracellular compartment	Unknown	
TLR-13	Intracellular compartment	Bacterial RNA	Monocytes, macrophages, dendritic cells
C-lectin receptor	Cell surface	Mannose, galactose	Macrophages, dendritic cells
NOD-like receptor	Cytoplasm	Peptidoglycan, Muramyl dipeptide	
RIG-I-like receptor	Cytoplasm	dsRNA	

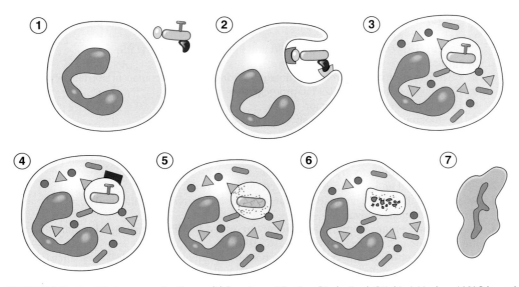

FIGURE 12.8. **Neutrophil clearance of pathogen.** (1) Complement fixation; C3a (yellow), C3b (dark blue), and MAC (green) are positioned on bacterium. (2) Fixed bacterium binds to complement receptors (C3a receptor, red; C3b receptor, yellow) and is phagocytosed. (3) Granules fuse to the phagosome (azurophilic granules, blue; specific granules, green; gelatinase granules, red). (4) NADPH oxidase (dark blue rectangle). Myeloperoxidase are activated. (5) Granules deliver antibacterial substances (i.e., defensins, lysosomes). (6) Bacteria is killed. (7) Neutrophil dies.

D. **Leukocytes.**

1. **Neutrophils** are the most abundant leukocytes in circulation having a multi-lobed nucleus and are "neutral" to staining. Neutrophils drive the active killing of invading bacteria by phagocytosis and cytolysis (Fig. 12.8).

   a. Most abundant leukocyte, 60% of circulating leukocytes.

   b. Cells in circulation have a short life span of hours to days:
      (1) Approximately 6 hours in circulation
      (2) Longer lived in spleen

   c. Occupy a temporary niche at the surface of vascular lumen:
      (1) Tethered by a transient interaction between CD62L on the neutrophil and CD34 on the vascular wall, which causes rolling along the surface (marginalization)
      (2) Released in the presence of glucocorticoids, causing a temporary spike in circulating neutrophils
      (3) Release is driven by a surface metalloprotease, ADAM-8

   d. First responders to inflammatory site.

   e. Neutrophils are recruited to the injury site by chemotaxis CCL8 (a.k.a., IL-8), C5a, and LTB_4.

   f. Principal function is phagocytosis:
      (1) Targets material labeled by C3b, IgG, or collectins.
      (2) Process is triggered by the anaphylatoxins C3a, C4a, and C5a.

   g. Kills internalized bacteria using antibacterial peptides, digestion by hydrolytic enzymes, and oxidation by free radicals (Fig. 12.9).

   h. The neutrophil has three types of secretory granules:
      (1) Azurophilic (defensins, myeloperoxidase, lysozyme)
      (2) Specifics (lactoferrin, lysozyme)
      (3) Gelatinase (acetyltransferase, gelatinase, lysozyme)

   i. Dies by apoptosis to release degraded materials.

   j. Accumulating debris constitutes pus; the greenish, purulent property comes from myeloperoxidase.

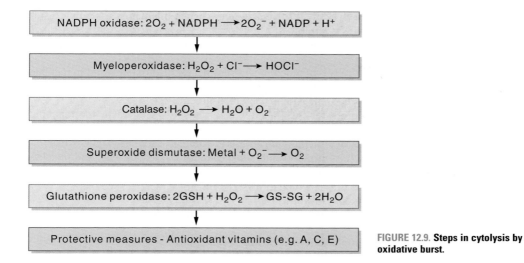

FIGURE 12.9. **Steps in cytolysis by oxidative burst.**

2. **Basophils** are an innate effector cell with a multi-lobe nucleus and stains a dark purplish blue to the presence of the basic dye methylene blue.
   a. Low abundance, 1% circulating leukocytes.
   b. Short-lived (hours to days) in circulation.
   c. Temporary residence in the lymph node.
   d. Directs T helper cell differentiation.
   e. Plays an active defense role toward allergens with protease activity.
   f. Basophils release histamine, leukotrienes, and prostaglandins and are a source for heparin, platelet-activating factor, and IL-4.
   g. Basophils express Fc receptors for IgE and MHC Class II for antigen presentation to T_h2 cells.
   h. Basophils complete their development in the bone marrow prior to entering the circulation.
   i. Enhance humoral memory.
3. **Eosinophils** are innate effector cells that stain red with the acidic dye eosin; they have a multi-lobed nucleus and numerous secretory vesicles.
   a. Bone marrow is induced by IL-5 to release eosinophils.
   b. 2% to 5% of circulating leukocytes.
   c. Secretory vesicles called granules contain destructive proteins including acid phosphatase, eosinophil peroxidase, major basic protein, eosinophil cationic protein, RNase, DNase, lipase, and plasminogen.
   d. Capable of phagocytosis or degranulation to release specific effector proteins.
   e. Perform cytolysis to flood the inflammatory site with high levels of effector proteins.
   f. Secrete leukotrienes and prostaglandins.
   g. Express Fc receptors for IgG and IgE, and MHC Class II, giving them the ability to activate $CD4^+$ T cells.
   h. Direct **cell-mediated cellular cytotoxicity** (CMCC):
      (1) Delivers toxic free radicals and proteases to the parasite.
      (2) Collateral host-tissue damage often results from the release of these cytotoxic agents.
   i. Defense to large extracellular parasite.
   j. Mediators of allergic inflammation.
4. **Mast cells** are a tissue resident myeloid cell.
   a. Ubiquitously placed in the body, including behind the blood-brain barrier.
   b. Do not ordinarily circulate.
   c. May proliferate, differentiate, and mature in the tissues.
   d. Long-lived and found throughout the body including the brain; they are particularly enriched at the boundaries to the environment where encounters with pathogens are likely.

e. Process trauma signals of trauma and release injury-specific mediators including histamine, serine proteases, and serotonin.

f. Perform similar functions compared to macrophage, including phagocytosis and antigen presentation.

g. Principal function of mast cells is to function as a sentinel for disturbances and to regulate inflammatory and adaptive immune responses.

h. Control vascular integrity and initiate neutrophil recruitment.

i. Express specialized receptors for IgE called Fcε; a sensory mechanism for **reagenic** molecules.

j. Source for histamine, heparin proteoglycan, and serine proteases tryptase and chymase.

k. Release reactive lipids such as thromboxane, prostaglandin D2, leukotriene, and platelet-activating factors to permit neutrophil and macrophage intrusion.

l. Function as sensors for trauma screening for DAMPs and PAMPs.

5. **Macrophages** are a tissue resident myeloid cell:
   a. Recruited to the inflammatory site to complete the clearance of debris and orchestrate wound healing.
   b. **Monocytes** in circulation replenish tissue resident macrophage.
   c. Monocytes constitute 5% of circulating leukocytes.
   d. Kill internalized bacteria using antibacterial peptides, digestion by hydrolytic enzymes, and oxidation by free radicals.
   e. Expression of microbial peptides using MHC Class II and phospholipids by CD1.
   f. Sequester bacteria by forming granulomas.
   g. Names for tissue resident macrophages are Kupffer cells (liver), histiocytes (dermis), alveolar macrophage (lung), microglia (brain), and osteoclasts (bone).
   h. Two functional states:
      (1) **M1** respond to bacteria and inhibit cancer growth.
      (2) **M2** support angiogenesis, suppress immunity, and promote cancer growth.

6. **Dendritic cells:**
Resident immature **myeloid-derived dendritic cells** (mDC) continuously collect samplings from the interstitial fluids and are responsible for recognition of non–self-antigen. Mature mDC take residence in secondary immune organs.
   a. **Immature mDC:**
      (1) Continuously process antigen for presentation to naive helper T cells.
      (2) Antigen is internalized by endocytosis and processed in lysosome and inserted into MHC Class II molecules.
      (3) Exposure to PAMP induces maturation of the mDC.
      (4) mDC migrates to lymph node.
   b. **Mature mDC:**
      (1) Reduces endocytosis activity.
      (2) Increases MHC Class II antigen expression.
      (3) Increases expression of coreceptors CD80/88.
      (4) Potential to release IL-12 depending on the identity of triggering PAMP.

VI. ANTIBODIES

A. **Definition.** Antibodies are mucoproteins that are found mainly in the gamma-globulin fraction of serum on electrophoresis. When injected into animals, human immunoglobulin, being foreign, becomes antigenic. The resulting antihuman antibodies are grouped into five classes: **IgG, IgA, IgM, IgE, IgD.**

B. **Structure:**
   1. The basic structural unit for each class is a four-chain protein with two heavy (H) and two light (L) chain polypeptides linked by disulphide bonds (Fig. 12.10).

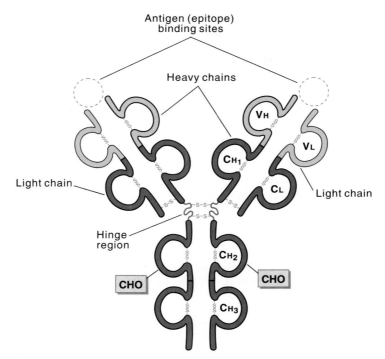

FIGURE 12.10. The basic four-peptide structure of immunoglobulins (Ig) is illustrated by this IgG pattern. Three heavy chain constant region domains (CH$_1$, CH$_2$, CH$_3$) and one light chain constant domain (CL) are shown in *dark blue*. The variable region of both the light and heavy chains (VL and Vh, respectively; in *orange*) associate to form the specific epitope-binding site. Several of the most critical disulfide bonds are shown (–*ss*–). CHO indicates where the carbohydrate is attached. (Redrawn with permission from Eisen HN. *General Immunology*. Philadelphia, PA: Lippincott-Raven;1990:48.)

    a. A differing, short amino acid sequence, specific for each of the H chains, permits differentiation into the five classes. These H-chain differences are called isotypes and are designated by the Greek letters gamma (γ), alpha (α), mu (μ), epsilon (ε), and delta (δ). Isotypes are genetic variations that all humans possess.

    b. All five classes have an amino acid sequence in common on the L chains. Thus, they can be classified together as immunoglobulins. In addition, two isotypes, designated kappa (κ) and lambda (λ), exist for all five classes.

C. Domains:

  1. Both H and L chains are divided into constant region domains, designated CH and CL, and variable region domains, designated VH and VL.

    a. The amino acid sequence in the constant regions of both the H and L chains is similar for all antibody molecules within each class.

    b. The amino acid sequence of the variable regions on both H and L chains varies with the epitope toward which the particular antibody is directed.

  2. Amino acids that show marked differences between antibodies of different specificities form a **hypervariable region** within each variable region.

  3. The hypervariable regions of both the H and L chains associate to form two epitope-binding regions known as the antibody **idiotype.**

  4. A **hinge region** also exists between the CH$_1$ and CH$_2$ domains, permitting flexibility in the movement of the two antigen-binding sites.

D. Monoclonal antibodies. Most antigenic preparations give rise to a mixture of antibodies. However, antibodies of a single specificity are highly desirable for many purposes, including specific diagnostic tests and immunotherapy.

  1. Monoclonal antibodies can be made routinely by fusing splenic B cells from an immunized animal with malignant (immortal) plasma cells, forming a hybridoma.

2. The B-cell hybridoma secreting the desired antibody can be isolated from the others by reactivity with the antigen of concern, then cloned and expanded in tissue culture, resulting in large amounts of antibody of a single specificity.

E. Immunotoxins.
1. Monoclonal antibodies can also be constructed using a murine antibody with the Fab domain specific for a cancer antigen; the Fc domain is removed and displaced by the toxin of choice.
2. Such antibodies bind specifically to the cancer cell antigen via the mouse Fab hypervariable region, thereby focusing the lethal toxin on only the designated target cell.

VII. PROPERTIES OF ANTIBODIES

A. Immunoglobulin G:
1. Structural properties (Table 12.7):
a. IgG is composed of two L chains (each with a molecular weight of 22,000 Da) and two H chains (each with a molecular weight of 53,000 Da). The total molecular weight is 150,000 Da.
b. The structural designation is ($\gamma 2\kappa 2$) or ($\gamma 2\lambda 2$), with the γ marker indicating the IgG H-chain isotype and the κ-marker or λ-marker indicating the L-chain isotype.
c. Four **subclasses** exist: $\lambda 1$, $\lambda 2$, $\lambda 3$, and $\lambda 4$. These subclasses are differentiated by slight changes in the amino acid sequences on the H chain.
d. Enzymatic cleavage (Fig. 12.11):
  (1) Papain splits IgG into three fragments:
    (a) Two of these fragments, **Fab** (fragment, antigen binding), are similar, with each containing only one of the reactive sites for the epitope. Because Fab is monovalent, it can bind to (but cannot enter into) lattice formation and precipitate or agglutinate antigen.
    (b) A third fragment (**Fc,** crystallizable) activates complement, controls catabolism of IgG, fixes IgG to tissues or cells via an Fc receptor, and mediates placental transfer of antibody.
  (2) Pepsin splits behind the disulfide bond, joining the two H chains, permitting the two Fab fragments to remain joined. Consequently, this fragment is termed **F(ab')2.**
    (a) Because F(ab')2 is bivalent, it is capable of lattice formation and thus facilitates removal of antigens.

table 12.7 Structural Properties of Human Immunoglobulins

Property	IgG	IgM	IgA	IgE	IgD
H-chain isotype	γ	μ	α	ε	Δ
H-chain subclass	$\gamma_1, \gamma_2, \gamma_3, \gamma_4$	—	α_1, α_2	—	—
L-chain isotype	κ or λ	κ or λ	κ or λ	κ or λ	κ or λ
Associated chains	—	J chain	J chain, SP	—	—
Structural designation	$\gamma_2\kappa_2$ or $\gamma_2\lambda_2$	$(\mu_2\lambda_2)_5$ or $(\mu_2\lambda_2)_5$	Serum: $\alpha\kappa_2$ or $\alpha\gamma_2$ Mucosa: $(\alpha_2\kappa_2)_2$ J, SP or $(\alpha_2\gamma_2)_2$ J, SP	$\varepsilon_2\kappa_2$ or $\varepsilon_2\lambda_2$	$\delta_2\kappa_2$ or $\delta_2\lambda_2$
Percentage carbohydrate	4	15	10	18	18
Molecular weight (Da)	150,000	Monomer: 180,000 Pentamer: 950,000	Monomer: 160,000 Dimer: 318,000 Dimer + SP: 380,000	188,000	184,000

J, J chain; SP, secretory piece
From Johnson A, Clarke B. *High-Yield Immunology.* 2nd ed. Philadelphia, PA: Lippincott Williams & Wilkins;2006:15.

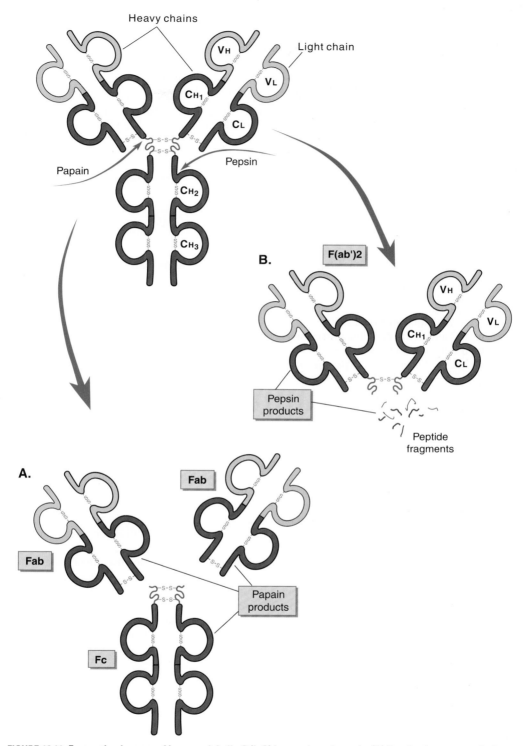

FIGURE 12.11. Enzymatic cleavage of immunoglobulin G (IgG) by pepsin and papain. (A) Papain cleavage results in two unlinked antigen-binding (Fab) fragments with the disulfide bonds (–*ss*–) remaining with the crystallizable (Fc) fragment. Because the fragments are univalent, they cannot precipitate or agglutinate antigens. **(B)** Pepsin cleavage results in retention of the disulfide bonds with the two Fab fragments linked as F(ab')2. The Fc portion is degraded. CH_1, CH_2, CH_3, and one light chain constant domain CL (blue), heavy chain constant region domains; VL, VH (*orange*), variable region of light and heavy chains, respectively. (Redrawn with permission from Abbas AK, Lichtman AH, Jober JS. *Cellular and Molecular Immunology.* 3rd ed. Philadelphia, PA: W.B. Saunders;1997:50.)

t a b l e **12.8**	Functional Properties of Human Immunoglobulins								
	IgG					*IgA*			
Property	γ1	γ2	γ3	γ4	IgM	α1	α2	IgE	IgD
Average serum concentration (mg%)	900	300	100	50	150	300	50	0.03	3
Serum half-life (days)	23	23	8	23	5	5	5	3	2.5
Activates complement	+	±	+ +	−	+ + +	−	−	−	−
Binds to Fc receptor	+	±	+ +	+	+	−	−	+	−
Crosses placenta	+	±	+	+	−	−	−	−	−

From Johnson A, Clarke B. *High-Yield Immunology*. 2nd ed. Philadelphia: Lippincott Williams & Wilkins, 2006, p. 17.

      (b) F(ab')2 is removed more rapidly from the circulation than the intact IgG.

      (c) The Fc fragment is extensively degraded.

  2. **Functional properties (Table 12.8):**

    a. IgG has the highest serum concentration of all immunoglobulins (700 to 1,500 mg%) and a serum half-life of 18 to 25 days.

    b. IgG adheres to cells that possess a receptor for the Fc fragment from IgG (Fcγ).

    c. IgG fixes complement, a series of enzymes resulting in cell lysis.

    d. IgG mediates placental passage of maternal antibody to the fetus.

B. Immunoglobulin M.

  1. **Structural properties (see Table 12.7):**

    a. IgM exists in two structural forms:

      (1) A monomer is synthesized by B cells, retained on its membrane, and is designated μ2κ2 or μ2λ2.

        (a) It serves as the B-cell receptor specific for a single antigenic epitope.

        (b) The hypervariable region of the monomer differs for each B-cell clone.

      (2) Secreted IgM exists as a pentamer (i.e., five monomeric IgM molecules joined together by a J chain; Fig. 12.12). The IgM pentamer is designated (μ2κ2)5 or (μ2λ2)5.

        (a) The pentamer is secreted following antigen and cytokine activation of B cells, with the hypervariable regions on the pentamer the same as those on the membrane-bound monomeric receptor.

        (b) Of the 10 possible epitope-binding sites on the pentamer, five are of high affinity and five are of low affinity.

    b. Molecular weight: IgM has four constant domains on the H and L chains (in contrast with the three found on IgG, IgA, and IgD); therefore, its pentamer form has the highest molecular weight of the immunoglobulins, approximately 1 million.

  2. **Functional properties (see Table 12.8):** IgM, the earliest antibody to appear after antigenic stimulus, fixes complement avidly.

C. Immunoglobulin A.

  1. **Structural properties (see Table 12.7):**

    a. IgA exists in three forms: a **monomer,** a **dimer** (in which a J chain joins two monomers (Fig. 12.13A), and a **dimer plus** a secretory piece.

      (1) The dimer is transported across respiratory and intestinal mucosal barriers into the lumen by the secretory piece, which is a receptor for the IgA Fc region (FcαR) on the mucosal epithelium.

      (2) The secretory piece also protects IgA from proteolysis.

    b. The structural designation is (α2κ2) or (α2λ2) as the monomer and (α2κ2) or (α2λ2) as the dimer.

    c. Two subclasses exist: α1 and α2.

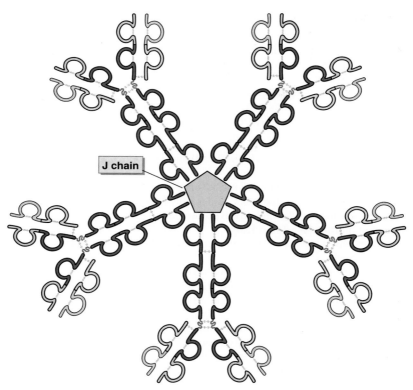

FIGURE 12.12. Immunoglobulin M pentamer. (Modified with permission from Abbas AK, Lichtman AH, Jober JS. *Cellular and Molecular Immunology.* 3rd ed. Philadelphia: W.B. Saunders;1997:48.)

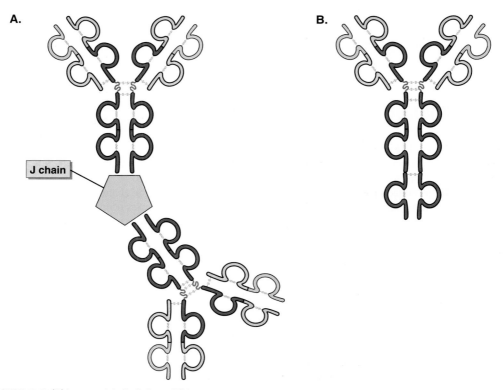

FIGURE 12.13. **(A)** Immunoglobulin A dimer. **(B)** Immunoglobulin E dimer. Note the four C domains. (Modified with permission from Abbas AK, Lichtman AH, Jober JS. *Cellular and Molecular Immunology.* 3rd ed. Philadelphia, PA: W.B. Saunders;1997:48.)

2. Functional properties (see Table 12.8):

a. IgA is found in high concentrations in secretions; in serum, IgA exists mainly as a dimer with a half-life of 5 days.

b. IgA is located in and protects mucosal tissues, saliva, tears, and colostrum by blocking bacteria, viruses, and toxins from binding to host cells.

D. Immunoglobulin E.

1. Structural properties (see Table 12.7):

a. IgE has four constant domains (Fig. 12.13B) and a carbohydrate content of 18%, resulting in a molecular weight of 188,000 Da.

b. The structural designation for IgE is $\epsilon 2\kappa 2$ or $\epsilon 2\lambda 2$.

c. The IgE molecule is unstable at 56C and is called reagin.

d. IL-4 mediates the B-cell switch to IgE production.

2. Functional properties (see Table 12.8):

a. IgE has an extremely low serum concentration and half-life because its Fc region binds avidly to mast cells and basophils.

b. IgE adheres to tissue-bound mast cells and circulating basophils via FCϵ receptors on these cells. The binding of antigen to these IgE-sensitized cells triggers the release of vasoactive amines (mainly histamine), resulting in atopic disease characterized by hives (a local reaction) and anaphylaxis (a systemic reaction).

c. IgE does not cross the placenta or fix complement by the conventional pathway.

d. The binding of IgE to IL-5 activated eosinophils results in elimination of parasitic Helminths.

e. Both total and allergen-specific IgE can be quantified.

E. Immunoglobulin D.

1. Structural properties (see Table 12.7). The structural formula for IgD is $\delta\kappa 2$ or $\delta\lambda 2$.

2. Functional properties (see Table 12.8):

a. IgD is found on the B-cell membranes of 15% of newborns and again on adult peripheral blood lymphocytes in conjunction with IgM; serum levels are very low. The serum half-life is 2 to 3 days.

b. IgD is a receptor on B-cell membranes for antigen.

VIII. IMMUNOGENETICS

A. Genetic control of immunoglobulin chain synthesis.

1. Genetic diversity: Human antibodies exhibit an enormous range (108) of specificities. The genetic basis for this remarkable diversity involves several factors.

a. Different genes code for the variable and constant region of the H and L chains.

b. Rearrangement of the variable region and constant region genes occurs during differentiation within the genome, such that any one of the many different variable region genes can be linked to a single constant region gene, thus conserving DNA.

c. An additional gene sequence, the **joining segment,** linking the VL gene to the CL region gene, is required during the formation of the L chain (Fig. 12.14).

d. During the formation of the H chain, an additional gene sequence, the **diversity segment,** also is required to link the VH gene to the J gene. These genes are then fused with the CH gene (Fig. 12.15).

e. A later rearrangement of **class genes** in the CH region dictates H-chain class switching from μ and δ to $\gamma 3$, $\gamma 1$, $\alpha 1$, $\gamma 2$, $\gamma 4$, ϵ, and $\alpha 2$, which is mediated by T-cell cytokines (IL-4, IL-13, INF-γ, TGF-β).

2. Random selection by each B cell from the variety of V, D, and J germ-line genes available results in a large number of structural possibilities for the VL and VH epitope-binding regions of the immunoglobulins. This random selection is primarily responsible for the vast diversity of antibodies.

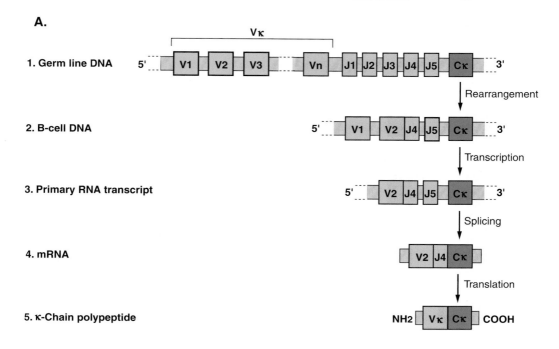

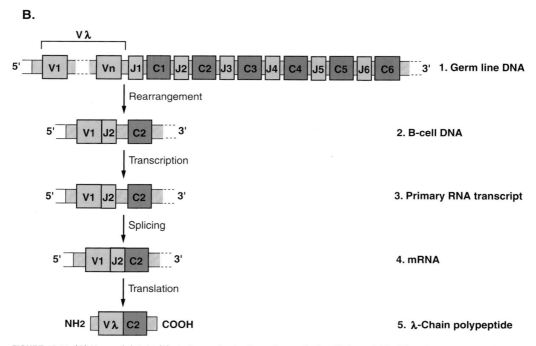

FIGURE 12.14. **(A)** Kappa (κ) light (L)-chain synthesis. From the pool of multiple variable (V) region genes on chromosome 2 in the germ line DNA (*1*), one V region is joined to a joining (J) region gene, resulting in B-cell DNA (*2*). Following removal of introns by recombinases, the primary RNA is transcribed (*3*), resulting in mRNA (*4*) results in the κ L-chain polypeptide (*5*). (Redrawn with permission from Benjamini E. *Immunology: A Short Course*. 4th ed. New York: Wiley-Liss, 2000, p. 121.) **(B)** Lambda (λ) L-chain synthesis. Rearrangement and synthesis of the λ, L-chain genes occurs in an identical manner on chromosome 22, except for the availability of up to six Cλ exons for union to the VJ combined region. This availability results in several subtypes.

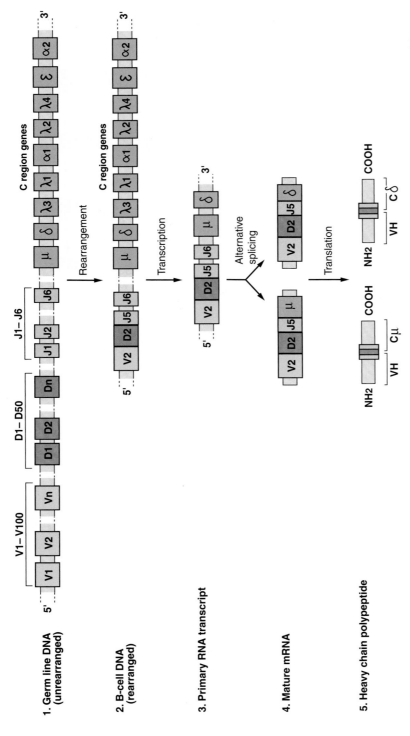

FIGURE 12.15. Heavy (H)-chain synthesis. (1) The variable region of the H chain is coded by three different gene complexes present on chromosome 14: variable (V) region genes, diversity (D) genes, and the joining (J) genes. The constant (C) region genes. The constant (C) region gene complex harbors the genes controlling all of the immunoglobulin (Ig) classes. (2) During rearrangement, a J region gene links to a D region gene, and then this complex links with a V region gene. The VDJ complex links to the μ or δ region genes. (3) A primary RNA transcript of the VDJ μδ complex is made; after splicing, mRNAs for a VDJ μ and a VDJ δ appear. (4) H chains of both IgM and IgD result after translation of the mRNAs (5). These H chains combine with light (L) chains and deposit on the B-cell membrane as the antigen receptors. Following antigen and cytokine stimulus, the IgM antibody is secreted (not illustrated). (Redrawn with permission from Benjamini E. *Immunology: A Short Course.* 4th ed. New York, NY: Wiley-Liss;2000:123.)

table 12.9   Association of Human Leukocyte Antigens with Disease

Disorder	HLA Type	Risk*
Ankylosing spondylitis	B 27	87
Dermatitis herpetiformis	DR 3	56
Reiter's syndrome	B 27	40
Insulin-dependent diabetes	DR 3/DR 4	33
Psoriasis vulgaris	C 6	13
Goodpasture's syndrome	DR 2	13
Rheumatoid arthritis	Dw 4/DR 4	10
Systemic lupus erythematosus	DR 3	5
Pernicious anemia	DR 5	5

*Times more likely to acquire the disorder than a person who does not have the specific HLA type.
From Johnson A, Clarke B. *High-Yield Immunology.* 2nd ed. Philadelphia, PA: Lippincott Williams & Wilkins;2006:23.

3. **Allelic exclusion** occurs since only one of the two parental alleles is expressed by a single B cell, resulting in a single H-chain isotype and L-chain subtype receptor capable of reacting with only one antigenic epitope.

B. Genetic control of HLAs.

1. HLAs control discrimination between self and non–self-antigen presentation to T cells, but only to the same HLA type since **self-MHC restriction** occurs.
2. HLAs determine individual susceptibility to immunologic disorders and infectious agents **(Table 12.9)**.

C. Classes of HLAs.

1. HLAs are organized into three MHC classes of molecules (Table 12 .10).
   a. **Class I HLAs** are glycoproteins that are found on the **membranes of most nucleated cells.**
      (1) They are encoded by three gene regions: A, B, and C.
      (2) They are linked to the **cytotoxic T (T_c) cell** through the **CD8** molecule and present peptidic epitopes to specific T_c receptors (Class I restriction). A single Class I molecule can bind several different epitopes.
      (3) Two chains form the Class I molecular structure; the α chain has three external domains, a transmembrane segment and a cytoplasmic tail, while the β_2-microglobulin is an invariant protein.
      (4) The peptide-binding site, found between domains α1 and α2, binds peptides containing 8 to 10 amino acids.
   b. **Class II HLAs** are glycoproteins that are found on the **membranes of dendritic cells, macrophages, activated T cells, and B cells.**
      (1) They are encoded by three gene regions: **DP, DQ,** and **DR.**
      (2) They are linked to the T_h cell through the **CD4** molecule and present peptidic epitopes to specific T_h-cell receptors (Class II restriction). A single Class II molecule can bind several different epitopes.

table 12.10   Human Leukocyte Antigen (HLA) Classes

	Complex			HLA				
MHC Class	I			II			III	
Region	B	C	A	DP	DQ	DR	C4, C2, BF	
Gene products	HLA-B	HLA-C	HLA-A	DP αβ	DQ αβ	DR αβ	C' proteins	TNF-α TNF-β

MHC, major histocompatibility complex; TNF, tumor necrosis factor
From Johnson A, Clarke B. *High-Yield Immunology.* 2nd ed. Philadelphia, PA: Lippincott Williams & Wilkins;2006:23.

A. Class I HLA molecule   **B.** Class II HLA molecule

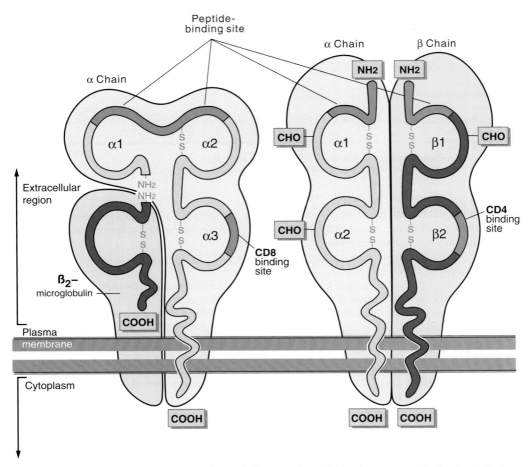

FIGURE 12.16. Structure of Class I and Class II human leukocyte antigen (HLA) molecules. −ss−, disulfide bond. (Redrawn with permission from Stites DP, Terr AI, Parslow TG. *Medical Immunology.* 9th ed. Stamford, CT: Appleton & Lange;1997:86.)

   (3) Two chains, α and β, form the Class II molecular structure. Each chain has two do-
        mains plus a transmembrane segment and a cytoplasmic tail (Fig. 12.16).
   (4) The peptide-binding site is formed by juxtaposition of the α1 and β1 domains, and
        binds peptides containing 13 to 18 amino acids.
   c. Class III HLAs control certain serum proteins, including several complement components
       and TNFs. Class III molecules are encoded by three gene regions: C4, C2, and BF.
   d. Polymorphism:
      (1) Many **alleles** of Class I and II are present at each locus on chromosome 6 and are the
            major obstacles to organ transplantation.
      (2) **Haplotypes** from both parents are inherited and expressed codominantly.

D. Genetic control of the T-cell antigenic receptor (TCR).
   1. The TCR is a dimer of either α and β chains (approximately 95%) or γ and δ chains
        (approximately 5%).
   2. TCRs do not respond to soluble antigens, in contrast to the monomeric IgM antigen receptor
        on the B cell membrane.
   3. TCRs recognize antigenic epitopes only as peptidic fragments bound to either Class I or
        Class II HLA molecules on an antigen-presenting cell (APC).

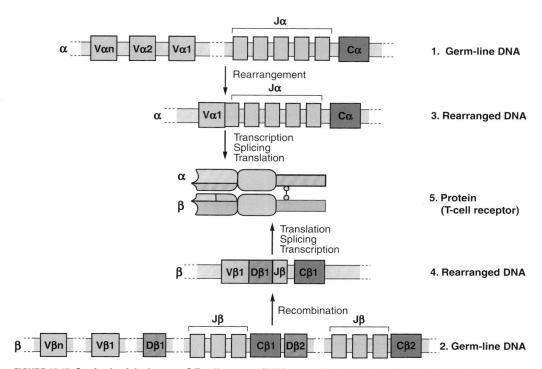

FIGURE 12.17. Synthesis of the human αβ T-cell receptor (TCR) genes. Synthesis of the γδ chains is thought to follow a similar pattern. (*1*) Multiple variable (V) region genes and joining (J) region genes occur at the TCRα locus on chromosome 14. (*2*) Similarly, multiple (V) region, diversity (D) segment, and J region genes occur at the TCRβ locus on chromosome 7. (*3*) During the rearrangement of α-chain genes, a randomly selected V gene is joined to a J gene and the exon is transcribed, combined with a constant (Cα) region gene, and translated. (*4*) Similarly, the β-chain exon is formed by the random linkage of a V region gene, first to a D region gene and a J region gene, and then to a Cβ gene. (Redrawn with permission from Janeway CA, Travers Jr. *Immunobiology: The Immune System in Health and Disease.* New York, NY: Garland Publishing;1997:4.35.)

4. **The coreceptors, CD4 or CD8, determine whether humoral or cell-mediated immunity occurs.**
    a. Binding of CD4 to a Class II HLA molecule on an APC results in HI.
    b. Binding of CD8 to a Class I HLA molecule on an APC results in CMI.
5. Union of the specific TCR and coreceptor with the peptide-HLA membrane complex is associated with signal transduction into the cytoplasm by a complex of proteins, collectively designated **CD3**.

E. **Genetic diversity.** Achieved among the TCRs through gene rearrangements similar to those of immunoglobulins (Fig. 12.17).
    1. Recombinase enzymes RAG-1 and RAG-2 are required for both heavy and light chain rearrangements in both early B-cell and T-cell antigen-receptor expression, which mediates the somatic recombination of V and J or V, D, and J genes.
    2. The phenomenon of allelic exclusion controls the genetic expression of TCRs.

IX. ADAPTIVE IMMUNITY (FIGS. 12.18, 12.19, 12.20)

The **adaptive immune system** is a collection of specialized leukocytes called **lymphocytes**. Each cell expresses multiple copies of the same antigen receptors. These receptors are highly specific to a single target referred to as an **antigen**. Lymphocytes are generally long-lived and itinerant, continuously trafficking between specialized niches (immune organs) and peripheral tissues while patrolling for non-self substances.

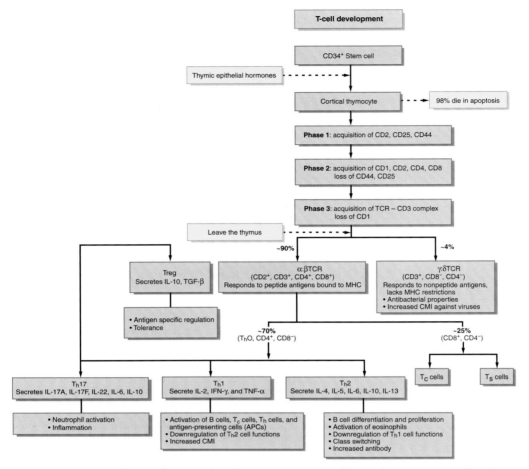

FIGURE 12.18. T-cell development. Stem cells from bone marrow bearing a CD34 marker migrate to the fetal thymus, where they become cortical thymocytes under the influence of epithelial hormones. Most of the cortical thymocytes die; the surviving 1% to 2% pass through three phases of development, during which they acquire and lose specific membrane markers (clusters of differentiation [CD]). During the final phase, which takes place in the medulla, the thymocytes acquire the T-cell antigenic receptor (TCR) and the CD3 signaling complex, and they lose the CD1 marker and leave the thymus. The T cells can have one of two types of TCR (α:βTCR or γ:δTCR); the types are differentiated according to the amino acids in the two peptide chains that form the receptor. The α:βTCR T cells respond to peptide antigens bound to the major histocompatibility complex (MHC), while the γ:δTCR cells respond to nonpeptide antigens. There are two populations of α:βTCR T cells: T_h1 cells and T_h2 cells. These cells secrete different cytokines and therefore have different functions. CMI, cell-mediated immunity; IFN, interferon; IL, interleukin; T_c, cytotoxic T (cell); T_h, T helper (cell); T_s, T suppressor (cell).

A. **Primary immune organs** are sites for the development of lymphocytes and provide a development of the lymphocyte antigen receptor.
  1. **Bone marrow** is the site for progenitor stem cell development for both T and B cells.
     a. Progenitor T cell stem cells are produced during adolescence and transferred to the thymus.
     b. Progenitor B cell stem cells differentiate into **mature B cells** (express functional surface IgM antigen receptor and IgD).
     c. Mature B cells enter the circulation and traffic between different secondary immune tissues.
  2. **Thymus** is the site for progenitor T cell stem cell differentiation into mature T cells.
     a. **Helper T cells** (T_h) express the coreceptor CD4 and recognize the antigen displayed on MHC Class II molecules.
     b. **Cytotoxic T cells** (T_c) express the coreceptor CD8 and recognize the antigen displays on MHC Class I molecules.
     c. **Regulatory T cells** (Treg) express the coreceptor CD4, high affinity IL-2 cytokine receptor subunit CD25, and recognize the antigen displayed on MHC Class II molecules.

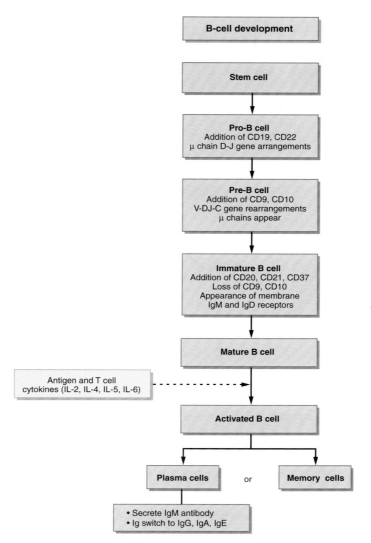

FIGURE 12.19. B-cell development. Stem cells differentiate in the bone marrow and pass through several stages of development before becoming mature B cells. Random selection by each B cell from a variety of germ line genes results in a large number of possible structures for the epitope-binding regions of the immunoglobulins. At the pro-B-cell stage, a joining (J) region gene links with a diversity (D) segment gene, and then the VDJ complex links to the IA constant (C) region gene. At the immature B-cell stage, the appearance of membrane IgM and IgD receptors defines B-cell clones. Activation of the mature B cells by antigen and T-cell cytokines leads to differentiation and division of the B cells and synthesis of antibody. CD, cluster of differentiation; Ig, immunoglobulin; IL, interleukin.

3. Development of the antigen receptor:
   a. Immature lymphocytes rearrange genes within the immunoglobulin gene loci (B cells) or the TCR loci (T cells) to assemble a unique antigen receptor.
   b. **Recombination activating genes** (RAG) direct the reassortment of immunoglobulin genes to produce an enormous variety of possible antigen receptors.
   c. **Positive selection** screens for functional antigen receptors.
   d. The final rearrangements must pass **negative selection**, to eliminate receptors that recognize host-specific antigens
   e. Failures to eliminate self-reactive antigen receptors result in autoreactive cells, a basis for **autoimmunity.**
   f. Mature, antigen naïve lymphocytes emerge and circulate.

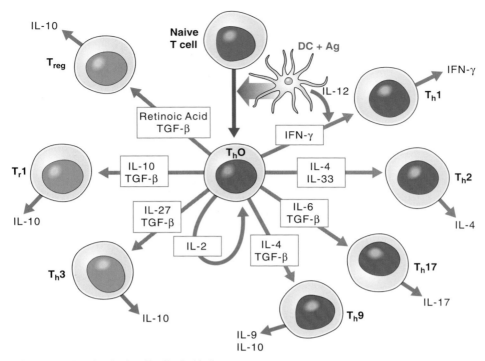

FIGURE 12.20. **Family of helper T cells.** Red indicates agents that stimulate activation and differentiation.

4. An **anticipatory response** provides antigen receptors for a large variety of encounters.
  a. An enormous number of cells are produced, each with an antigen receptor capable of recognizing a separate and unique antigen.
  b. The immune system attempts to produce a repertoire of lymphocytes capable of recognizing new and novel antigens that the host may encounter during a lifetime.

B. Secondary immune tissue.
Secondary immune organs provide a niche for mature B and T cells to be educated to respond to a specific antigen.
  1. A crossroads for itinerate naïve mature T cells to enter a compartment and screen for cognate antigen recognized by the T-cell receptor.
  2. Naïve lymphocytes, never exposed to antigen, enter secondary immune organs.
    a. Entry to lymph node occurs at the **high endothelial venule.**
    b. Naïve T cells express CD62L that recognizes CD34 on the endothelial wall.
    c. T cell enters by **extravasation.**
    d. Naïve T cells express CD62L, antigen-educated lymphocytes express CD44.
    e. Niche provides space for antigen-presenting cells (mDC) to display antigen recovered from inflammatory sites.
  3. Selected T cells proceed through a phase of proliferation and differentiation to specialize for an adaptive response.
  4. Differentiated T cells then guide responses as humoral (antibody) or cell mediated (cell-mediated cytotoxicity).
  5. **Germinal center** establishes niches for B cells to expand antibody diversity and specificity (Fig. 12.21).
    a. **Somatic hypermutation** provides a means to produce an enormous diversity of antibodies.
      (1) Series of point mutations that randomly alters the amino acid sequence in the **paratope** of immunoglobulins.
      (2) Deamination of cytosine to uracil driven **by activation induced (cytidine) deaminase** (AID).

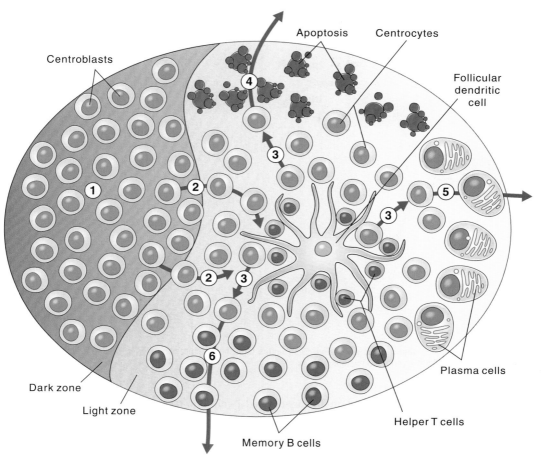

FIGURE 12.21. Germinal center. Centroblasts (light blue) are reconstructing immunoglobulin specificity by somatic hypermutation within the dark zone. The **centroblasts** then migrate toward **follicular dendritic cells** to become **centrocytes** (light purple) and begin immunoglobulin class under the guidance of T cell (orange) cytokines. Cells that fail to maintain a high affinity for antigen are removed by apoptosis. Cells retaining high affinity progress on to become **plasma cells** (light red) or **memory B cells** (dark purple).

   (3) Uracil is removed by **Uracil-DNA glycosylase.**
   (4) Error-prone DNA polymerase repairs the gap.
   b. The B cell is capable of editing the immunoglobulin to make higher affinity interactions with antigen.
   c. **Germinal center** forms, consisting of an outer mantle composed of transient lymphocytes; dark zone contains centrocytes; and light zone contains centroblasts.
   d. The dark zone is a site of active proliferation and somatic hypermutation.
   e. Epithelial-derived **follicular dendritic cells** bind complement-bound antigen.
   f. FDC collects antigen originating from the inflammatory site.
   g. B and T cells collect around the FDC screening for antigen.
   h. The B cell (centrocyte) and T cells remain associated with the antigen on the FDC.
   i. The B cell shifts antigen recognition by somatic hypermutation until the association with the FDC is lost or the T cell intervenes.
   j. Centrocytes proceed through **affinity maturation** while somatic hypermutation is sustained by T-cell intervention.
   k. The B cell can also change isotype to enhance antibody function within different tissues; for example, IgG in the circulation and IgA in mucosal tissues.
   l. Isotype switching is driven by neighboring T cells (Fig. 12.22).

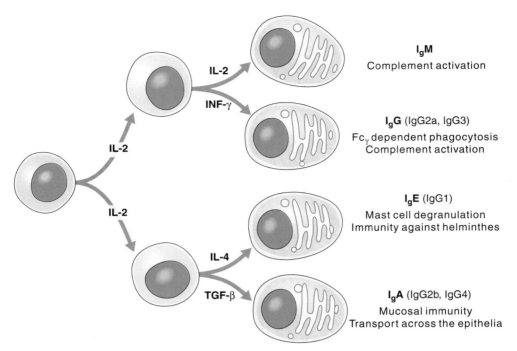

FIGURE 12.22. Immunoglobulin class switching. Centrocytes (light blue) expressing IgM can switch immunoglobulin secretion based on T-cell intervention with cytokines.

C. **Lymphocytes (Table 12.11).**

1. **αβ T-cell receptor** is found on thymus-derived T cells and recognizes peptides presented by MHC Class II molecules.

2. **γδ T-cell receptor** is found on mucosal epithelial T cells and can recognize free peptides; it does not need antigen presentation.

t a b l e 12.11 List of T-Cell Subsets

Cell	Symbol	Function	Secretory Cytokines
Naïve T Cell CD4$^+$ or CD8$^+$	T_h0	Quiescent, progenitor, must be activated by DC	None
Activated Helper T Cell	T_h0^*	Activated progenitor, receptive to cytokine control	IL-2
Helper T1	T_h1	Intracellular bacteria and virus	IFN-γ, LTα
Helper T2	T_h2	Extracellular parasites	IL-4, IL-5, IL-13, IL-25
Helper T9	T_h9	Immunity to helminthes	IL-9, IL-10
Helper T17	T_h17	Extracellular bacteria and fungi, mucosay	IL-21, IL-17a, IL-17f, IL-22
Natural Regulatory T CD4$^+$CD25$^+$	T_{reg}	Tolerance, regulation, and homeostasis	TGF-β
Regulatory 1 T CD4$^+$CD25$^-$	T_r1	Suppress naïve and memory T cells, inducible	IL-10
Anergic T CD4$^+$CD25$^-$	T_h3	Mucosal immunity, inducible	TGF-β
Suppressor T CD8$^+$CD28$^-$	T_s	Regulation, mucosal immunity	IL-10, TGF-β up-regulates ILT3 on monocytes
Cytotoxic T Cell CD8$^+$	T_c	Cell-mediated immunity	Perforin granzyme
(γδ)T	(γδ)T	Mucosal, respiratory tract	IFN-γ, TNF-α, IL-4
Natural Killer T Cell	NKT	Detect glycolipid antigen presented by CD1	IFN-γ, TGF-α, IL-4
Natural Killer Cell	NK	Cytotoxic T cell screens for missing MHC Class I, antiviral activity	Perforin, granzyme

3. Antibodies are produced by B cells.
   a. **B-1 cells** are found in mucosal areas and produce antibodies to polysaccharides. B-1 cell immunoglobulins have a limited repertoire to different antigens.
   b. **B-2 cells** are produced in germinal centers and have the ability of immunoglobulin gene rearrangements, somatic hypermutation, and class switching. B-2 cell immunoglobulins have a virtual limitless repertoire of antigen recognition ability. B-2 cells differentiate into plasma cells to produce large quantities of antibody.

4. mDC activate T cells.
   a. **Immature dendritic cells** accumulate and identify antigen as foreign substances at a site of inflammation; exposure to PAMP induces maturation and directs migration to the draining lymph node.
   b. **Mature dendritic cells** present antigen to **helper T cells (T_h)** using the major histocompatibility complex II in specialized niches, such as lymph nodes.
   c. Mature dendritic cells take residence in the lymph node adjacent to mature naive T cells in the paracortex.
   d. mDC present antigens and interrogate naïve T cells, express costimulatory molecule CD 80/86, and increase surface display of MHC Class II bound antigen.
   e. Antigen-specific T cells begin development and clonal expansion.
   f. Naïve B cells bind antigen percolating in draining lymph fluids; antigen is internalized and expressed on MHC Class II.
   g. Specific T cells recognize presented antigens and stimulate B cell activation.

5. Specialized lymphocyte:
   a. Generally localized to mucosal boundaries and express a low copy number of antigen receptors.
   b. **B-1 cells** secrete antibody specific for bacterial carbohydrates and lipopolysaccharides.
   c. **Marginal zone B** cells are located in the spleen to produce antibody to polysaccharides.
   d. **($\gamma\delta$) T cells** expressing an alternative T-cell receptor are located in the boundary areas of gut mucosa and epithelia.
   e. **NK cells** search for host cells with aberrant expression of **MHC Class I** surface molecules and execute target cells by cell-mediated cytotoxicity.
      (1) NK cells recognize target cells based on antibody labeling, complement labeling, and screening for low MHC Class I expression.
      (2) NK cells express receptors for complement (C3b, C3a, and C5a) and imunoglobulins IgG and IgA.
      (3) NK cells engage a target cell through lectin activity or recognition of labeling with antibody or complement.
      (4) NK cell engagement activates a cytolytic mechanism.
      (5) NK killer receptor screens for the absence of MHC Class I using an inhibitory receptor. MHC engagement to the killer inhibitory receptor (KIR) deactivates the NK cell.
      (6) The NK cell kills target cells by inducing apoptosis if the KIR is not triggered.
      (7) Target cell death by apoptosis is driven by granule exocytosis or TNF pathway.
   f. **Natural killer T cells** share properties with NK and T cells:
      (1) Displays a ($\alpha\beta$) TCR.
      (2) Recognizes glycolipids displayed by CD1.
      (3) Displays a killer cell lectin receptor NK1.1.
      (4) Produces IFN-γ.
   g. **Plasmacytoid cells:**
      (1) Low abundant leukocyte (less than 1% circulating leukocytes).
      (2) Lymphocyte derived.
      (3) Do not express complement receptor (CD110).
      (4) Do not express CD14, as it is not responsive to lipopolysaccharide.
      (5) Expresses toll-like receptor 7 to detect ssRNA.
      (6) Expresses toll-like receptor 9 to detect CpG.
      (7) Produces large amounts of interferon α and β.
      (8) Important to viral infections.

X. RESPONSE TO ANTIGEN (FIG. 12.23)

A. **Fate of antigen (or vaccine).**
   1. If antigen entry is intravenous, it is phagocytized or pinocytosed in the spleen; if entry is other than intravenous, it traffics to the lymph node draining the site of entry. They are processed at these sites by APC, monocytes, macrophages, and dendritic cells.
   2. Exogenous protein antigens enter the APC from the extracellular environment by pinocytosis and are processed in acidic endosomal vacuoles. The resulting peptides bind to the cleft in MHC **Class II** molecules and are transported to the cell membrane where they can be presented to **CD4$^+$ T cells** to activate B cells for antibody synthesis.
   3. Viruses and intracellular parasitic antigens are synthesized endogenously within the APC cytoplasm and endoplasmic reticulum and processed to peptides by proteasomes. The peptides bind to the cleft in **MHC Class I** molecules and migrate to the APC membrane, where they are presented to **CD8$^+$ T cells** to initiate CMI (Fig. 12.24).
      a. CMI is directed mainly against intracellular-dwelling microorganisms and aberrant, endogenous cells (e.g., cancer cells) (see Fig. 12.23).
      b. Antibody is not involved except in antibody-dependent cellular cytotoxic reactions (ADCC). In the latter, the effector cell is linked to the target cell by an antibody bridge, with the Fab portion binding to the specific membrane antigen on the target cell, and the Fc portion binding to the Fc receptor on an activated effector cell.

B. **Activation of T cells** is initiated when the specific CD4 or CD8$^+$ T-cell receptor binds to the appropriate APC peptide-HLA complex (Fig. 12.25).
   1. T-cell adhesion molecules CD28, CD2, and LFA-1 strengthen the binding.
      a. CD28 binds to B7.1 on the APC and increases IL-2 synthesis.
      b. CD2 binds to leukocyte functional antigen (LFA-3).
      c. CTLA4 binds to B7.2, which serves to down-regulate IL-2 synthesis following activation.
   2. An activation signal is transduced by the CD3 complex composed of three polypeptides—γ, δ, and ε—and two zeta chains.

C. **T$_h$ cell response pathways.** T$_h$ cells are classified into two compartments (T$_h$1 and T$_h$2) based on the cytokines they secrete, which determine the functions they effect.
   1. The **T$_h$1 cell** induces CMI following binding to the peptide-**Class I** MHC by transforming, differentiating, and dividing logarithmically and secretes:
      a. IL-2, which is necessary for T-cell and B-cell transformation.
      b. IFN-γ, which enhances CMI by activating macrophages and NK cells. It also triggers HLA antigen presentation by endothelial cells and can suppress antibody formation by down-regulating IL-4 synthesis.
      c. TNF-α, which activates macrophages and synergizes with IL-1 in inducing and stimulating the acute phase response.
      d. IL-12 and IL-18 from dendritic cells and macrophages aid the transition of macrophages, T$_c$ cells, and NK cells to CMI.
   2. The **T$_h$2 cell** induces activation of B cells and HI following binding to the peptide-**Class II** MHC and stimulation by IL-2. It transforms, differentiates, and divides logarithmically while secreting IL-4, IL-5, IL-10, and IL-13.
      a. IL-4 is essential for the development of antibody synthesis by stimulating B-cell differentiation. It is necessary for IgE production and down-regulates IFN-γ by T$_h$1 cells and thus can suppress CMI.
      b. IL-5 functions synergistically with IL-4 and IL-2 to aid B-cell differentiation. It stimulates growth and differentiation of eosinophils and facilitates IgA synthesis.
      c. IL-10, like IL-4, inhibits T$_h$1 release of IFN-γ and IL-2, thus reducing macrophage activation by IFN-γ.
      d. IL-13 mimics IL-4 actions, inhibiting T$_h$1 cytokine release.

D. **B-cell response** is initiated by antigen selecting the clone of B cells with the membrane-bound IgM antigen receptor that is specific for the antigen epitope.

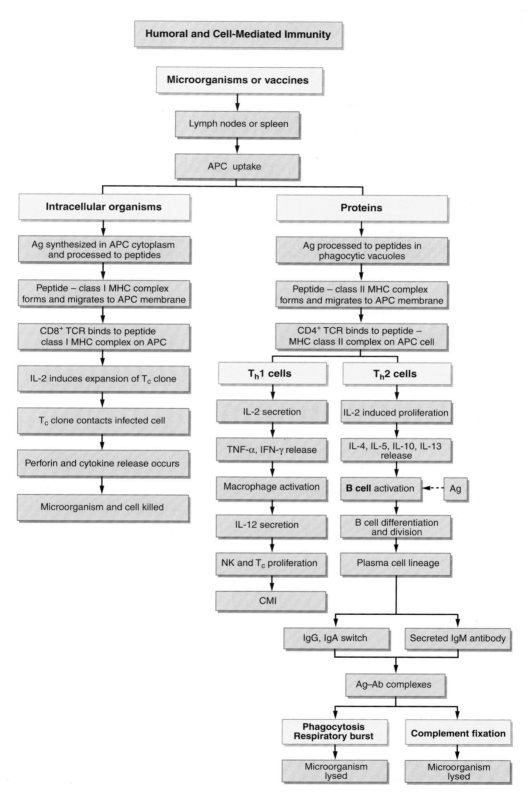

FIGURE 12.23. Humoral and cell-mediated immunity. ag -ab, antigen–antibody; APC, antigen-presenting cell; CD, cluster of differentiation; CMI, cell-mediated immunity; IFN, interferon; Ig, immunoglobulin; IL, interleukin; MHC, major histocompatibility complex; NK, natural killer; T_c, cytotoxic T cells; TCR, T-cell receptor; T_h, helper T cells; TNF, tumor necrosis factor.

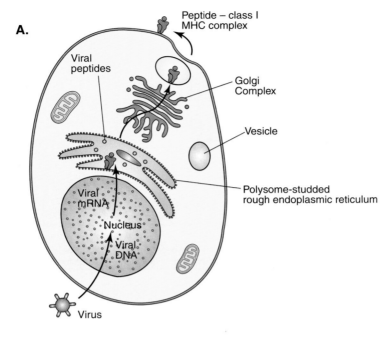

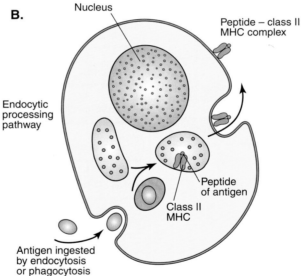

FIGURE 12.24. Antigen processing (A) of intracellular organisms and (B) of exogenous proteins. MHC, major histocompatibility complex. (Redrawn from Kuby J. *Immunology*. 3rd ed. New York, NY: W.H. Freeman; 1997.)

1. Binding of antigen, along with stimuli from the T-cell cytokines IL-2 and IL-4, triggers differentiation of that B-cell clone into a large blast cell, and logarithmic division occurs.

2. IL-5 continues this process, during which the B cell acquires the cytoplasmic "machinery" necessary for antibody synthesis.

   a. H and L chains are synthesized and assembled; under IL-6 influence, terminal differentiation into a plasma cell and secretion of IgM occurs.

   b. Subsequent gene rearrangements result in a switch to IgG, IgA, and IgE synthesis and secretion.

      (1) IL-4 and IFN-γ influence the switch to IgG; TGF-β influences the switch to IgA; and IL-4 influences the switch to IgE.

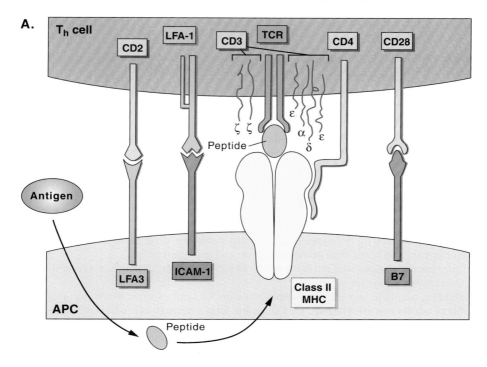

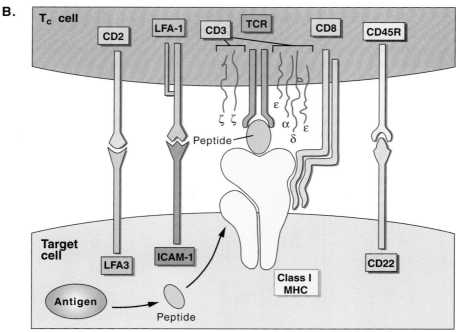

FIGURE 12.25. **(A)** Activation of CD4$^+$ helper (T$_h$) cells. The specific T-cell antigenic receptor (α:βTCR or γ:δTCR) binds to the peptide-Class II major histocompatibility complex (MHC) by the antigen-presenting cell (APC). The CD4 molecule links to the MHC. An activation signal is transduced by the TCR–CD3 complex, which is composed of three polypeptides (α, δ, ε) and two ζ chains. Accessory T-cell adhesion molecules (e.g., CD2, leukocyte function-associated antigen-1 [ILFA-1], and CD28) facilitate adherence of the T$_h$ cell to the APC and influence interleukin-2 synthesis. **(B)** Activation of CD8$^+$ cytotoxic T (T$_c$) cells. CD, clusters of differentiation; ICAM, intracellular adhesion molecule. (Redrawn from Kuby J. *Immunology.* 3rd ed. New York, NY: W.H. Freeman; 1997.)

(2) The binding of CD40 on the B cell to its ligand on the T_h cell (CD40L) is necessary for switching to occur.

E. **Memory cells** of all classes are generated independently of the plasma cell lineage. They migrate to various lymphoid tissues, where they have an extended survival.

F. **A secondary response** to the same antigen can result in the following:
   1. A shorter induction period to antibody synthesis
   2. More rapid class switching from IgM to IgG
   3. Increased IgG with antibodies of higher affinity
   4. Predominant IgA synthesis in mucosal tissues

XI. IMMUNOLOGIC ASSAYS

A. Antigens, antibodies, antigen-antibody reactivity, cytokines, drugs, and cells can be detected in vitro or in vivo, and some even in the nanogram and picogram range.
   1. The union of antigen with antibody is very sensitive, specific, and firm, but reversible; multiple short-range forces are involved.
   2. Binding occurs in seconds but is not visible until a lattice forms, which occurs more slowly. Since antibodies are bivalent, they form the lattice through cross-linkages (Fig. 12.26). The composition of the lattice depends on the ratio of antigen to antibody.
   3. **Affinity** measures the binding energy between an antibody and a univalent epitope; **avidity** is the total binding energy between an antibody and a multivalent antigen.
   4. Changing the position of atoms, double bonds, structural conformation, or the composition of amino acids or sugars of the epitope changes specificity.

B. **Protection tests** are used to determine the potency of vaccines.
   1. Active. Following immunization with the vaccine that is being tested, groups of animals are challenged with increasing numbers of microorganisms. The lowest number of microorganisms lethal for 50% of the animals (i.e., LD50) is determined and compared to the LD50 in nonvaccinated animals in order to measure the protective power of the vaccine.
   2. Passive. Graded amounts of serum from immunized individuals are transferred to normal animals, which are then challenged with the infectious agent. The highest dilution of serum effective at protecting 50% of the animals (i.e., ED50) is determined as a measure of the efficacy of the vaccine.

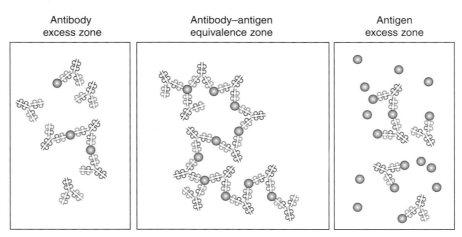

| Antibody excess zone | Antibody–antigen equivalence zone | Antigen excess zone |

FIGURE 12.26. The size of antigen–antibody (ag-ab) complexes is determined by the ratio of antigen to antibody. In vivo, larger complexes (in antibody excess and at equivalence) are phagocytosed; smaller complexes (in antigen excess) escape and lodge in blood vessels and behind the renal basement membrane, causing vasculitis and glomerulonephritis. Antigen is depicted in pink color.

C. **Agglutination tests** are used to detect antibody union with large, particulate antigens.
1. Rapid, slide **identification of bacteria** can occur by mixing a loopful of bacteria from the patient's culture with a battery of specific antibacterial antisera and noting which antiserum causes agglutination.
2. Semiquantitative **diagnostic test for bacterial diseases** involves addition of the suspect bacterium (killed) to dilutions of the patient's serum. The highest dilution that results in visible agglutination is called the **titer.** A fourfold increase in titer is necessary for diagnosis due to low levels of "natural" antibodies occurring in the serum of most normal human beings.
3. **Slide agglutination** is used in blood grouping to determine qualitatively whether the donor's cells or serum possess antigens or antibodies that are reactive with the recipient's serum or cells.
   a. **Major crossmatch** uses the donor's cells plus the recipient's serum to determine whether anti-red blood cell (RBC) antibodies are present in the recipient's serum. Rapid clumping of the donor's cells will occur in vivo if antidonor RBCs are present.
   b. **Minor crossmatch** uses the donor's serum plus the recipient's cells. Agglutination of the recipient's cells occurs if anti-RBC antibodies are present in the donor's serum. However, a transfusion reaction under these conditions would be much less severe than one associated with a major crossmatch because the amount of antibodies transfused in the donor's serum is minimal relative to the number of RBCs in the recipient.
4. **Coombs direct test** involves the detection of **weak or nonagglutinating anti-Rh antibody** by adding antihuman immunoglobulin **directly to the infant's RBCs,** to which the Rh antibody has been attached in utero, and noting any agglutination. An **indirect test** involves measuring these same weak antibodies in the **maternal circulation** by adding the mother's serum to Rh+ RBCs in vitro. The addition of antihuman immunoglobulin results in agglutination of the sensitized RBCs.
5. IgM complement-fixing antibodies, which agglutinate RBCs at temperatures below 37°C, can be detected by incubation at lower temperatures. These **cold agglutinins** are frequently autoimmune in nature and occur commonly in patients with **primary atypical pneumonia** caused by *Mycoplasma pneumonia.*
6. A diagnostic test for myxoviruses (e.g., influenza, mumps, some pox viruses, and arborviruses) involves neutralization of their ability to spontaneously agglutinate RBCs by the infected patient's serum. The patient's serum titer is determined by the highest dilution blocking the agglutination.

D. **Precipitation reactions** are used to detect soluble proteins, polysaccharides, and antigen-antibody complexes.
1. Either antigen or antibody in serum can be measured **quantitatively** with analytical precision.
   a. Increasing amounts of antigen are added in separate tubes containing a constant amount of the patient's serum.
   b. The resulting precipitate in each tube is washed and analyzed by micromethods, and the precipitated antibody is plotted as a function of antigen added. Three zones result: antibody excess, equivalence, and antigen excess (see Fig. 12.26).
2. **Immunoelectrophoresis** may be used to identify a specific antigen in a mixture and in immunologic disorders. Components of an antigen mixture are separated in agar, first by migration in an electric field, followed by their diffusion and subsequent precipitation with specific antibody diffusing from an overhead trough.
3. **Radioimmunoassay (RIA)** is based on the displacement of a known, radiolabeled antigen from an ag-ab complex by an unknown, unlabeled antigen (e.g., hormone) in a patient's body fluids. The extent of loss of the labeled antigen from the ag-ab complex can be measured and is a function of the concentration of the unknown antigen in the patient's fluid. Sensitivity is less than 1 ng.
4. **Radioimmunosorbent test (RIST)** is used to measure **total** (nonspecific) IgE in allergic patients' serum.
   a. The patients' serum is added to rabbit antihuman IgE, which has been adsorbed onto particulate (agarose) beads, and the complex is washed.
   b. Iodine-125-labeled rabbit antihuman IgE is added, again washed, and the amount of radioactivity is quantified, which reflects the total concentration of IgE in the patient's serum.

5. Radioallergosorbent test (RAST) is used to measure IgE in patients' serum **specific** for a given allergen.

   a. The suspected allergen is coupled to an insoluble matrix and the patient's serum is added and washed.

   b. Iodine-125-labeled rabbit antihuman IgE is added, the complex is washed, and the bound radioactivity is quantified, reflecting the serum level of IgE specific for that allergen.

6. Enzyme-linked immunosorbent assay (ELISA) is a sensitive, practical assay useful in detecting either antigens or antibodies in low concentrations in a patient's body fluids.

   a. To measure low (nanogram) concentrations of **antigen** (e.g., hormones, drugs, serum proteins, etc.), dilutions of the fluid containing antigen are added to its antibody, which is adsorbed onto plastic wells. The resulting complex is washed, and an enzyme-conjugated antibody specific for a different epitope on the test antigen is added.

   b. After washing, the enzyme substrate is added, and the color reaction is measured using a spectrophotometer. The titer is recorded as the highest dilution of antigen giving a color above the background.

   c. **Specific antibodies** in low concentrations in a patient's serum (e.g., HIV) can also be measured by adding dilutions of the test antibody to its antigen adsorbed onto plastic wells; the complex is washed and an enzyme-conjugated anti-isotype antibody is added. After washing, the enzyme substrate is added, the color is measured, and the titer is determined, as above.

   d. The use of an enzyme label eliminates problems associated with radioisotope disposal in radioimmunoassays.

E. The complement complex (C) is an important component of both innate and adaptive immunity.

   1. It is comprised of nine major factors (C1 to C9), most of which are pro-enzymes present in normal serum and not increased by antigenic stimulation. It is effective via three pathways:

   a. The **classical pathway** results in lysis of microbial or mammalian cells to which IgM or a doublet of IgG1, IgG2, or IgG3 antibody has been bound to the membrane, followed by sequential "fixation" of C to the antigen–antibody complex.

   (1) C1qrs is bound initially via C1q, resulting in enzymatic cleavage and fragmentation of C4 and C2.

   (2) C4b and C2a bind to the cell surface as C4b2a, becoming a C3 convertase that cleaves C3 into fragments C3a and C3b.

   (3) C3b complexes with C4b2a to become a C5 convertase, which cleaves C5 into C5a and C5b.

   (4) C5b combines with C6 and C7 and inserts into the cell membrane.

   (5) C8 and C9 combine with the C5b,6,7 complex to form the **MAC,** resulting in increased permeability, changes in osmotic pressure, and cell lysis.

   b. The **alternate pathway** is activated by cell walls of certain Gram-negative and Gram-positive bacteria, viruses, yeasts, and aggregated IgA.

   (1) It acts independent of antibody or C1, C4, or C2.

   (2) It is initiated by cell wall absorption of small amounts of C3b existing in normal serum.

   (3) Binding of a serum protein, factor B, follows, which serves as a substrate for an enzyme, factor D. The resulting complex, C3bBb, is stabilized by properdin and has C3 convertase activity, which generates additional C3b.

   (4) A complex, C3bBbC3b, forms, which becomes a C5 convertase, leading to the further reactions resulting in the MAC.

   c. The **mannan-binding lectin pathway** follows the binding by an acute phase protein, mannose-binding lectin (MBL), onto mannose residues on the cell walls of certain bacteria, fungi, and viruses.

   (1) This complex acts similar to C1 and thus follows the classical pathway, forming C3 and C5 convertases that result in cell lysis via MAC.

   (2) It is an adjunct to innate immunity, independent of antibody.

   2. Complement-induced chemotaxis and opsonization:

   a. Fragments C3a and C5a are potent vasodilating and chemotactic adjuncts, adding cells and cytokines to the inflammatory response.

   b. The binding of fragment C3b to microorganisms promotes their opsonization via a C3b receptor on phagocytic cells.

F. **Fluorescent antibody** permits the visualization of either antigen or antibody in cells or tissues.
   1. In the **direct technique** fluorescinated (or another appropriate label) antibody to the antigen is added directly to the specimen (e.g., tissue) containing antigen and visualized under ultraviolet light.
   2. The more sensitive **sandwich technique** is used to:
      a. Detect antigen: its antibody is added first to the specimen, followed by fluorescinated anti-immunoglobulin, and the specimen is visualized under ultraviolet light.
      b. Detect antibody: the antigen is added to the specimen followed by fluorescinated antibody against the antigen, and the specimen is visualized under ultraviolet light.

G. **The Western Blot technique** is valuable in identifying an antigen or antibody within a mixture.
   1. The components of the mixture are separated by electrophoresis on a sodium dodecyl sulfate-polyacrylamide gel and "blotted" onto a nitrocellulose matrix. It is labeled, and a known antibody is added to locate and identify the antigen of interest.
   2. As a confirmatory test for acquired immunodeficiency syndrome (AIDS), the patient's serum suspected of containing anti-AIDS antibody is added to known HIV antigens bound to a nitrocellulose matrix. Binding of a labeled, antihuman immunoglobulin antibody to the HIV-anti-HIV complex confirms exposure.

XII. CLINICAL IMMUNOLOGICAL DISORDERS

Although the immune system functions efficiently in protecting the vast majority of the population, a small percentage of individuals react in an aberrant manner or lack some of the basic elements necessary for an adequate response. These disorders encompass individuals who exhibit (1) hypersensitivity to certain antigens, (2) inadequate or unresponsiveness to microbial or other antigenic exposure, or (3) loss of mechanisms regulating the immune system from reaction against self. The role of the immune system in transplantation, cancer, and vaccination is included in this section.

A. **Hypersensitivity diseases (Table 12.12).**
   1. **Anaphylaxis (type I)** reactions occur in genetically susceptible individuals who respond rapidly and excessively to the release of mediators following complexing of an allergen to mast cell-bound IgE. During the initial sensitization phase, IgE is formed in excess and binds avidly via its Fc domain to its receptor (FcFRɛ, CD23) on the surface of mast cells and basophils. The F(ab')2 domains containing the antigen-binding sites remain free to bind the allergen. When an allergen is **re**introduced, it aggregates several cell-bound IgE molecules, causing membrane perturbations and degranulation of mast cells and basophils, releasing pharmacologically active agents systemically or locally (**atopy**).
      a. **Anaphylactic shock** is a rapid, severe, generalized reaction that occurs when the allergen IgE-complex-induced mediators are released systemically (e.g., histamine, leukotrienes, TNF-α, IL-1, IL-6, serotonin and bradykinin, and platelet-activating factor [PAM]).
         (1) These agents rapidly contract smooth muscle, increase vascular permeability and secretions, change coagulability, and induce hypotension, leading to multiple organ failure and death.
         (2) Common inducers of IgE and subsequent triggers include *Hymenoptera* venom, foods, drugs, and antibiotics (e.g., penicillin).
      b. **Urticaria** (hives) is an IgE-mediated, cutaneous form of immediate hypersensitivity characterized by vasodilation and increased vascular permeability of the skin. Histamine release following the allergen-IgE union is mainly responsible for the wheal and flare lesion and pruritis.
      c. **Asthma** is characterized by airway obstruction and acute respiratory distress caused by mucus secretion and mediator-induced constriction of the smooth muscle surrounding the bronchioles following allergen-IgE complexing. Symptoms include wheezing, dyspnea, chest tightness, and cough.

t a b l e **12.12**	Hypersensitivity Classifications	
Type	Conditions	Distinguishing Characteristics
I: Anaphylaxis	Atopy (Local reactions) Urticaria Asthma Allergic rhinitis Anaphylactic shock (systemic reactions)	IgE Fc adherence to mast cells and basophils Degranulation and histamine release Smooth muscle contraction
II: Cell surface Ag-Ab Cytotoxicity	Hemolytic disease of the newborn Transfusion reactions Goodpasture's syndrome Glomerulonephritis	Exogenous cell antigens Complement-induced target cell lysis Phagocytosis ABO, Rh blood loss Endogenous cell antigens Autoimmunity Neutrophil influx & damage
III: Ag-ab complex Disease	Arthus reaction Serum sickness Polyarteritis nodosa Glomerulonephritis Systemic lupus erythematosus Rheumatoid arthritis	Precipitating antibody Vasculitis Complement-mediated neutrophil influx and damage dsDNA-anti-dsDNA complexes Rheumatoid factor
IV: Delayed-type hypersensitivity	Tuberculosis Granulomatous reactions Contact dermatitis	Cell-mediated immunity Activated macrophages Epithelioid cells TDTH, T_h1, $CD8^+$ cells Haptens

Ag-ab, antigen-antibody; CD, cluster of differentiation; dsDNA, double-stranded DNA; T_{DTH}, delayed-type hypersensitivity effector cells; T_h1, T helper cell type 1
From Johnson A, Clarke B. *High-Yield Immunology.* 2nd ed. Philadelphia, PA: Lippincott Williams &Wilkins;2006:60.

(1) An influx of mast cells, $CD4^+$ cells, T_h2 cells, basophils, and eosinophils results in cytokine release and inflammation.

(2) Important mediators are the leukotrienes, platelet-activating factor, eosinophil chemotactic factor (ECF), and histamine; important triggers are respiratory infections, environmental pollutants, aspirin, and nonsteroidal anti-inflammatory drugs.

(3) Chronic exposure to occupational, environmental, and food allergens results in extrinsic asthma, whereas intrinsic asthma can be induced by nonimmunologic means (cold, exercise).

d. Allergic rhinitis is the most common clinical expression of atopy. Inflammation of the mucous membranes of the nose occurs, leading to profuse rhinorrhea, paroxysmal sneezing, nasal obstruction, itching, and conjunctivitis (e.g., hay fever).

(1) Common allergens involved are pollens, fungal spores, house dust, and animal dander.

(2) Binding of the allergen to cell-bound IgE releases cytokine mediators, including histamine, leukotrienes, prostaglandin D2, and ECF.

(3) With certain allergens a **hyposensitive state** can be achieved by repeated parental injection of the agent in subliminal doses. Desensitization is associated with an increase in **IgG** antibody, which combines avidly with the allergen in the circulation, thus blocking union with cell-associated IgE and mediator release.

2. Cellular antigen–antibody cytotoxicity (type II) occurs when antibody is directed against epitopes that occur on the cellular surface membranes of organs and tissues. Subsequent damage results from: (a) the osmotic, lytic action of activated complement; (b) opsonization by phagocytic cells or killing by ADCC; and (c) killing of the target cell by T_c lymphocytes, NK cells, or both. Destruction of the target cell results mainly from the release of perforins and serine proteases (granzymes), which cause pore formation and osmotic lysis. Examples include the following:

a. Transfusion reactions occur mainly following the transfusion of blood containing RBC antigens foreign to the recipient (Table 12.13). ABO incompatibility reactions are the most common; Rh reactions are the most severe.

t a b l e **12.13**	Blood Grouping				
ABO System			*Rh*	*Genotype*	
RBC Genotype	**Phenotype**	**Serum Antibody**	**Terminal Epitope**	**Rh+**	**Rh-**
OO	O	Anti-A and anti-B	Fucose, galactose	DCe	dce
AA or AO	A	Anti-B	*N*-acetylgalactosamine	DcE	dCe
BB or BO	B	Anti-A	Galactose	DCE	dcE
AB	AB	Neither	—	Dce	dCE

RBC, red blood cell
From Johnson A, Clarke B. *High-Yield Immunology.* 2nd ed. Philadelphia, PA: Lippincott Williams & Wilkins;2006:62.

(1) Preformed antibodies in the recipient clump or agglutinate the donor's blood cells, resulting in complement-mediated RBC lysis or rapid phagocytosis.

(2) Fever is the most common reaction; in severe reactions chest pain, hypotension, and disseminated intravascular coagulation (DIC) may occur.

b. Hemolytic disease of the newborn (*erythroblastosis fetalis*) can occur following placental transfer of a nonsaline agglutinating, maternal, anti-Rh IgG antibody (usually anti-RhD), which binds to RhD+ fetal erythrocytes. The presence of this antibody in either the mother's circulation or on the infant's cells can be detected by the Coombs test.

(1) Complement-mediated lysis or rapid phagocytosis follows, resulting in hemolysis and hemoglobinuria, which convert to toxic indirect bilirubin.

(2) Accumulation of the latter causes **kernicterus** (jaundice) with respiratory and brain damage.

(3) Injection of the Rh– mother with anti-Rh antibody (Rhogam) within 1 to 2 days following delivery prevents this disease. Anti-RhD antibody neutralizes the fetal Rh+ antigens entering the mother's circulation following spillage during removal of the placenta and prevents stimulation of the maternal immune system and injury to future Rh+ newborns.

c. Autoimmune reactions occur in genetically susceptible individuals who produce antibodies against their own cellular membrane antigens by unknown mechanisms. Exemplary is **Goodpasture's syndrome,** which is characterized by glomerulonephritis (GLN) and pulmonary hemorrhage (also termed Masugi type GLN).

(1) The inciting antigen is a glycoprotein dispersed uniformly on the glomerular basement membrane (GBM).

(2) Susceptible hosts produce an IgG antibody, which binds to the membrane antigen and activates complement, releasing the potent chemotactic factor C5a.

(3) Neutrophils are attracted to the antibody-GBM complex where they release lysosomal enzymes, causing severe necrosis of the glomeruli and a loss of filtration capacity.

3. Antigen-antibody complex reactions (type III) occur when circulating ag-ab complexes of small size, with antigen in slight excess, escape phagocytosis and deposit in tissues or on the surface of blood vessels. These complexes cause damage by activating complement and releasing the chemotactic factor C5a, anaphylatoxins, and clotting factors. Neutrophils are attracted to the area of deposition, releasing lysosomal enzymes that destroy tissue. Examples include the following:

a. Arthus reaction is a rare inflammatory response to gross, intravascular ag-ab precipitates of intermediate size, occurring when highly sensitized humans or animals are injected with antigen. Complement-activated chemotactic factors, PMN infiltration, and platelets result in thrombi and hemorrhagic, necrotic lesions.

b. Serum sickness occurs following injection of foreign serum or its products. It is characterized by a complement-dependent, systemic reaction with fever, pruritic rash, lymphadenopathy, and joint pains.

(1) The incidence of this condition is rare since use of such products is restricted to several toxic diseases and immunosuppression.

(2) A similar but milder allergic vasculitis can be elicited by drugs (e.g., sulfonamides, penicillin, cephalosporins, dilantin, and thiourea).

c. Polyarteritis nodosa (PAN) is characterized by continuous insult of arteriolar walls by deposition of circulating ag-ab complexes, causing thrombosis and interruption of blood flow. Hepatitis B antibody complexes are involved frequently.

d. Glomerulonephritis is characterized by soluble ag-ab complexes depositing on and behind the basement membrane of the kidney, causing an inflammatory response.

   (1) Complexes can be detected with fluorescent antibody against either the antigen, antibody, or complement as a lumpy-bumpy pattern of fluorescence due to the random deposition of the complexes.

   (2) Antigens implicated most often are: DNA, insulin, thyroglobulin, and group A nephritogenic streptococci.

   (3) Damage is due to the release of lysosomal enzymes by PMNs attracted by chemotactic agents that destroy the glomeruli, resulting in loss of filtration.

e. Systemic lupus erythematosus (SLE) is a chronic, exacerbating inflammatory disease usually presenting in women ages 20 to 45. Its cause is unknown, but it may be initiated by an antibody response against bacterial or viral DNA followed by loss of regulatory control of self-tolerance. The clinical pattern is associated mainly with polyarthralgia or arthritis. An ultraviolet light-induced skin rash, facial "butterfly rash," pleurisy, pericarditis, vasculitis, and rheumatoid factor can also be present.

   (1) SLE is characterized by the formation of autoantibodies to many **endogenous** antigens: RBC, white blood cells, platelets, dsRNA, and various nuclear antigens (antinuclear antibodies), with anti-dsDNA predominating.

   (2) dsDNA, anti-dsRNA, and other circulating complexes in slight antigen excess lodge at random in the kidney, giving rise to the **cardinal lesion of GLN.**

   (3) A lumpy-bumpy pattern of fluorescence distinguishes lupus GLN from the smooth pattern seen in the **Masugi** type of GLN, where the kidney antigen is dispersed uniformly.

f. Rheumatoid arthritis is a chronic, recurrent inflammatory disease thought to be initiated by an unknown antigen that stimulates local antibody formation in the synovium. Approximately 70% of patients possess the HLA-DR4 haplotype. Inflammation of the pannus and loss of cartilage characterize the joint lesions.

   (1) Union of the antigen with the local antibody alters the tertiary structure of the latter, revealing "buried" amino acid sequences now recognized as foreign by the immune system.

   (2) These newly available epitopes stimulate production of an antibody, usually IgM, termed **rheumatoid factor,** which reacts with the Fc domain of IgG molecules (i.e., an antibody against a now "foreign" antibody). As a consequence, IgM-IgG complexes form in synovial fluid, activate complement, and release chemokines. PMNs are attracted, which, while attempting to phagocytize the complexes, release lysosomal enzymes that destroy articular cartilage.

   (3) TDTH cells predominate and contribute to the damage, as do macrophages, which release IL-1, IL-6, and TNF. Osteoclasts emerge, which injure bone.

   (4) Rheumatoid factor, as one diagnostic sign, can be detected by latex agglutination tests employing IgG-coated latex particles added to the patient's serum.

   (5) Rheumatoid arthritis is also classified as an autoimmune disease.

4. Delayed-type hypersensitivity (type IV) reactions are effected by sensitized T cells, macrophages, and NK cells on direct contact with the target cell. Antibody is not involved. The basic lesion is an inflammatory response induced by activated macrophages, cytotoxic T lymphocytes, and NK cells to intracellular-dwelling microorganisms as well as reactivity to small molecular chemical irritants.

   a. The tuberculin skin test is exemplary of delayed-type hypersensitivity reactions in internal organs (e.g., lungs). It identifies human beings exposed to, or actively infected with, *Mycobacterium tuberculosis* and epitomizes delayed-type hypersensitivity activity to other intracellular dwelling organisms.

   (1) The patient suspected of having been exposed to the organism is injected intradermally with an antigenic extract of *M. tuberculosis* (called purified protein derivative [PPD]).

(2) A contained lesion of induration and erythema, peaking in 1 to 2 days, results from the inflammatory response induced by sensitized T-cell action at the site of PPD deposition.

(3) The skin lesion is initiated by Langerhans cell presentation of antigen to **previously sensitized TDTH** cells that have been recruited to the site of antigen deposition by chemokines.

(4) Subsequent APC and T-cell secreted cytokines and chemokines attract PMNs followed by CD4$^+$ T cells. A nonspecific perivascular accumulation of monocytic or macrophage cells results in destruction of the organisms, tissue, or both.

b. **Granulomatous reactions** occur if the microbial antigens persist in the tissues and continue to stimulate host reactivity.

(1) IL-1 and IL-8 are released in response and attract an inflammatory cell influx.

(2) IL-4 and IFN-γ promote the retention of macrophages and cause the fusion of monocytes at the site, leading to an **epithelioid cell granuloma** derived from macrophages, histiocytes, and epithelioid cells.

c. **Contact dermatitis** can occur following deposition of small molecular weight chemicals (haptens) or other irritants into the skin of a previously sensitized individual, causing a CMI reaction.

(1) The haptenic agent becomes antigenic by combining with intradermal host proteins as carriers via NH3 or S groupings. Langerhans cells and endothelial cells serve as APCs.

(2) Subsequent reexposure to the agent results in chemokine and cytokine release, monocytic or macrophage infiltration, and a **vesiculating lesion** with erythema and induration.

(3) Common eliciting agents include nickel, dinitrochlorobenzene, rubber, poison ivy, and poison sumac.

B. **Immunodeficiency diseases** occur mainly during the prenatal period or early childhood. A depressed immune response is also associated with the aging process. The child presents with a history of **recurrent infections** verified by below normal level values for IgG, IgM, or IgA, or abnormal T cell:B cell or CD4:CD8 ratios, as well as diminished response to standard vaccines in vivo. Since both T and B cells possess specific membrane markers (CD3 on T cells and membrane-bound IgM or CD19 or CD20 on B cells), they can be counted with a fluorescent microscope following addition of the respective fluorescent-labeled, monoclonal antibody to a blood smear. Monoclonal antibodies against CD4 and CD8 differentiate T-helper and suppressor subtypes, respectively.

1. **Transient physiologic hypogammaglobulinemia** occurs **normally** in infants between the ages of approximately 3 and 6 months. Although infants are born with adult levels of placentally transferred IgG, this level is diminished due to:

a. The slow disappearance of maternal antibody, which has a half-life of 22 to 28 days.

b. The infant's early low rate of synthesis of secretable immunoglobulins.

2. **X-linked agammaglobulinemia (Bruton's disease)** is a sex-linked (male) disorder that affects infants around the ages of 5 and 6 months. These patients present with recurrent pyogenic infections (e.g., *Streptococci* and *Hemophilus*) and digestive tract disorders. The thymus, CMI, and reactivity to viral infections appear normal, yet very few mature B cells are found.

a. The defect has been found to occur in the transition from pre-B to B cells in the bone marrow and involves the loss of a tyrosine kinase gene.

b. The absence of tonsils and germinal centers, as well as B cells and antibody, is diagnostic.

c. Treatment involves prophylactic transfer of adult serum immunoglobulin to diminish infections.

3. **Dysgammaglobulinemia** describes an immunoglobulin deficiency where the patient has decreased levels of a selective immunoglobulin class (usually IgA, with 1 in 600 to 800 individuals affected). Mucosal surface protection is diminished or lost.

a. Although the number of IgA-bearing cells is normal, they fail to differentiate into secreting plasma cells.

b. An increased susceptibility to autoimmune diseases is seen.

4. **Congenital thymic aplasia (DiGeorge syndrome)** patients exhibit poorly developed or absent thymus and parathyroid glands resulting in depressed CMI. Infections caused by opportunistic organisms (e.g., *Candida, Pneumocystis,* viruses) occur in the absence of T cells.

The disorder is not hereditary but is caused by an unknown intrauterine injury to the third and fourth pharyngeal pouches that occurs around the 12th week of gestation.

   a. The germinal centers, plasma cells, and serum immunoglobulins appear normal.

   b. The absence of parathyroid glands results in hypocalcemia and tetany.

   c. Vaccination with live vaccines (e.g., measles) is contraindicated.

5. Chronic mucocutaneous candidiasis is a highly specific T-cell disorder that is characterized by an absence of immunity to *Candida*. Patients have apparently normal T-cell and B-cell absolute numbers and functions. Approximately 50% of patients also have endocrine dysfunctions (e.g., hypothyroidism).

6. Wiskott-Aldrich syndrome is a sex-linked (male) disorder occurring mainly in children. It features thrombocytopenia (bleeding), eczema, and recurrent infections. A poor response to bacterial capsular polysaccharide antigens is seen. An increased incidence of lymphoreticular malignancies or lymphomas may occur.

   a. Depressed CMI and a low serum IgM level are seen, but IgG and IgA levels appear normal.

   b. The primary defect is on the short arm of the X chromosome and may result in an absence of specific glycoprotein receptors on cells and platelets.

7. Severe combined immunodeficiency disease (SCID) is a rare disorder characterized by a genetic defect in stem cells that results in the absence of the thymus gland and T and B cells. Affected children are extremely susceptible to infections and have a very short life span.

   a. A deficiency in the enzyme adenosine deaminase (ADA) occurs in 50% of patients. This deficiency results in the accumulation of toxic deoxyadenosine triphosphate (DATP), which inhibits ribonucleotide reductase and prevents DNA synthesis.

   b. A mutation in the γ chain of the IL-2 receptor gene is found in other patients with SCID.

8. Chronic granulomatous disease (CGD) results from a genetic defect in the nicotinamide adenine dinucleotide phosphate (NADPH) oxidase system in neutrophils. Patients are inordinately susceptible to infections by age 2 years, especially to organisms of low virulence.

   a. Neutrophil bactericidal activity (i.e., respiratory burst) is defective due to depressed NADPH oxidase, superoxide dismutase activity, and decreased hydrogen peroxide levels.

   b. Diagnosis is based on failure of neutrophils and macrophages to reduce a nitroblue tetrazolium dye.

   c. Treatment with IFN-γ has been successful.

9. AIDS is caused by human immunodeficiency virus (HIV) (see Chapter 5) whose major target cell is the $CD4^+$ T_h cell and its lysis. Macrophages, astrocytes, and dendritic cells with much lower membrane levels of CD4 also can be infected. Depletion of the T_h cell population results in a loss of cytokines and the capacity to activate other immunocompetent cells. Consequently, infections by endogenous and nosocomial agents predominate.

   a. Common organisms include *Pneumocystis,* cytomegalovirus (CMV), *Toxoplasma, Candida, Mycobacterium,* herpesvirus, and *Cryptococcus.*

   b. HIV binds to the CD4 receptor and an obligate chemokine coreceptor (CXCR4) via gp120. Membrane fusion and entry of the virus through the cell membrane is mediated by gp41 (Fig. 12.27).

   c. A viral reverse transcriptase transcribes the viral RNA into DNA, and its integration into the target cell genome is facilitated by an integrase.

   d. Following activation of the infected T cell by other viruses or antigens, the now provirus is transcribed, translated into viral proteins, assembled, and replicated, leading to lysis of the host cell.

   e. The indirect ELISA test detects the antibody to HIV in a patient's serum, which is confirmed by Western blot testing.

10. Functional deficiencies in any of the many cytokines and chemokines or their receptors could contribute to an immunodeficient state.

C. Autoimmune disorders occur as a result of a breakdown in regulation of the self-tolerant state characteristic of normal human beings. HI or CMI against their own tissues results. Tolerance to self-antigens is specific for the inducing epitope and is more readily induced and lasts longer in T cells than in B cells. Suppression of autoreactive T lymphocytes has recently been ascribed to

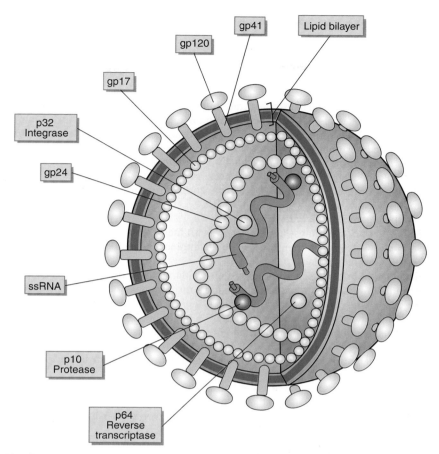

FIGURE 12.27. Components of the human immunodeficiency virus (HIV). The virus consists of an envelope formed from glycoproteins (e.g., gp120 and gp41) that houses several core proteins. The virus has several genes that code for enzymes (e.g., integrase, reverse transcriptase, protease) that play a role in integrating viral DNA into the host genome and degrading polyprotein precursors into smaller proteins and peptides. (Redrawn from Johnson A, Clarke B. *High-Yield Immunology.* 2nd ed. Philadelphia, PA: Lippincott Williams & Willkins; 2006.)

the convergence of CD4$^+$ T lymphocytes into Tregs by Fox P3, a suppressive protein. Their impact on prevention of certain autoimmune disorders is being assessed.

1. Self-tolerance is hypothesized to be caused by clonal deletion, clonal anergy, or peripheral suppression.

   a. **Clonal deletion** is postulated to result when immature CD4$^+$ T cells, which bear receptors for endogenous molecules, are deleted after contact with self-antigens in the neonatal thymus gland. Immature B cells with self-reactive receptors likewise are eliminated after contact with potential self-antigens in the bone marrow.

   b. **Clonal anergy** describes the loss of T-cell and B-cell functions after exposure to antigens in the absence of mandatory costimulatory signals or following exposure to cells lacking major histocompatibility complex Class II molecules.

   c. **Peripheral suppression** can occur if CD8$^+$ T cells or macrophages secrete cytokines (e.g., TGF-β), which down-regulate the immune response, or if high-dose or low-dose antigen produces an anergic state.

2. Occurrence of an autoimmune disorder in a previously normal individual can be reasoned to occur in several different ways varying with the disorder.

   a. **Microbial antigens** that cross-react with human tissue antigens have been demonstrated in *Streptococci,* which cross-react with sarcolemmal heart muscle and the kidney. Antimicrobial DNA antibodies react with cells from patients with SLE. Although an "autoimmune" reaction against the patient's tissues is induced, the antigenic stimulus is of exogenous origin.

   b. **"Hidden" antigenic determinants** that were unavailable when fetal clonal deletion was occurring can become available following damage by surgery. Illustrative also are patients with rheumatoid arthritis who form rheumatoid factors, which are mainly IgM antibodies, against the Fc fragment of IgG.

   c. **Adsorption of a foreign hapten** (e.g., quinidine, sulfathiazole) onto an endogenous molecule or cell (e.g., platelets) leads to the formation of an antigenic hapten-carrier complex. Antibody to the drug is formed and reacts with the drug on the platelet membrane. Complement is activated, resulting in platelet lysis.

   d. If the normally occurring **suppression by T regulatory cells** of B-cell clones that arises with idiotype specificity for self-antigens is lost or diminished, autoantibodies may result. An inordinate switch from T_h1 to T_h2 cell activation during antigenic stimulus may favor autoantibody synthesis.

3. **Systemic autoimmune disorders:**

   a. **SLE** is an episodic multisystemic disease with major lesions being an erythematous rash, vasculitis, arthritis, and nephritis. Multiple autoreactive antibodies against diverse cellular constituents are formed.

   b. **Rheumatoid arthritis** is a chronic, systemic inflammatory disease that is characterized by granulation tissue (pannus) formation and subcutaneous nodules in joints. IgG-IgM complexes activate complement, resulting in lesions.

   c. **Sjogren's syndrome** is characterized by autoantibodies formed against salivary duct antigens, lymphocytic infiltration, and immune complex formation in the salivary glands. Clinical features occur primarily in postmenopausal women, including dryness of the mouth, trachea, bronchi, eyes, nose, vagina, and skin. It may occur secondary to rheumatoid arthritis and SLE.

   d. **Polyarteritis nodosa** is one of several human vasculitides of varying causes. The condition often involves hepatitis B ag-ab complexes, which are found in the vessel walls of 30% to 40% of patients. Similar lesions can be reproduced in animals using other ag-ab complexes.

4. **Organ-specific autoimmune disorders:**

   a. **Blood disorders:**

      (1) **Anemia, leucopenia, and thrombocytopenia** disorders possess antibodies that react with RBCs, white blood cells, and platelets, respectively.

      (2) **Multiple myeloma** is characterized by the malignant transformation of a single plasma cell clone, resulting in an excess of IgG or another immunoglobulin class (termed paraproteins). Patients secrete Bence Jones proteins (monoclonal light chains) in their urine.

   b. **Central nervous system (CNS) disorders:**

      (1) **Allergic encephalomyelitis** is a demyelinating disease that can occur after infection or immunization. A nonapeptide isolated from an extract of brain has been implicated as the antigen since the disorder can be mimicked in animals by injection of the peptide in adjuvant.

      (2) **Multiple sclerosis** is a chronic, relapsing disease of unknown etiology that is characterized immunologically by mononuclear cell infiltrates and demyelinating lesions (plaques) in the white matter of the CNS. A decrease in suppressor cell function and elevated titers to measles and other viruses appear in the cerebrospinal fluid, suggesting a virus etiology.

      (3) **Myasthenia gravis** patients often exhibit thymic hyperplasia or a thymoma along with muscle weakness and fatigue. A defect in neuromuscular transmission is indicated by the presence of an **antiacetylcholine receptor antibody,** which binds to the receptor at the postsynaptic membrane of the neuromuscular junction. An inability to transmit the acetylcholine-induced signal to muscle fibers results and causes the clinical signs.

   c. **Endocrine disorders:**

      (1) **Chronic thyroiditis (Hashimoto's disease, hypothyroidism)** is a self-limiting disease with a probable genetic basis that affects mainly women. It is characterized by autoantibodies and CMI to thyroglobulin or thyroid peroxidase, causing progressive

destruction of the thyroid gland. Antibody-dependent cell-mediated cytotoxicity may be responsible for the tissue damage.

(2) Graves disease (hyperthyroidism) is characterized by a diffuse goiter and thyrotoxicosis. T and B cells infiltrate the thyroid gland, leading to the formation of autoantibodies to the thyroid-stimulating hormone (TSH) receptor. The autoantibodies compete with TSH, bind to the TSH receptor site, and induce uncontrolled TSH-like activity.

(3) Diabetes mellitus (insulin-dependent diabetes, juvenile onset, type 1 diabetes) is characterized by the destruction of insulin-producing cells in the pancreas. Either HI or CMI anti-islet cell activity can be operative. There is no evidence for an autoimmune pathogenesis for non–insulin-dependent (maturity onset, type 2) diabetes.

d. Gastrointestinal tract disorders:

(1) Pernicious anemia is caused by impaired gastrointestinal absorption of vitamin B_{12}, resulting in weakness and chronic fatigue. It occurs secondary to T-cell damage in the gastric parietal cell. The latter normally synthesizes intrinsic factor, the agent responsible for the transport of vitamin B_{12} into the blood. Antiparietal cell and anti-intrinsic factor antibodies, which block the transport function of intrinsic factor, are found in most patients. Injection of vitamin B_{12} bypasses the need for gastric absorption and corrects the deficiency.

(2) Ulcerative colitis is characterized by chronic inflammatory lesions that are confined to the rectum and colon and are accompanied by infiltration of monocytes, lymphocytes, and plasma cells. Patients' lymphocytes exert cytotoxicity against colonic epithelial cells in culture, and they may have antibodies that cross-react with *Escherichia coli,* but the disease is of unknown etiology.

(3) Crohn's disease is a chronic inflammatory granulomatous disease that involves T and B cells, macrophages, and neutrophils. The disease usually occurs in the submucosal area of the terminal ileum. It has often been suspected, but has not been established as being of microbial etiology.

D. Transplantation immunology is governed mainly by allogeneic differences in histocompatibility antigens (i.e., HLAs) between donor and recipient. The genes for the HLAs are located in the MHC on chromosome 6.

1. HLAs have two major functions:

a. To bind and present processed, foreign antigenic peptides to T cells, thus initiating the immune response.

b. To identify and distinguish the MHC membrane antigens on a transplanted donor organ from those of the recipient.

2. Class I and Class II HLA genes, which encode the histocompatibility antigens, exhibit enormous polymorphism since multiple alleles exist at each locus.

a. Class I antigens are found on all nucleated cells. They have three gene loci—HLA-A, HLA-B, and HLA-C—identified serologically with anti-HLA antibodies. Their function is to present foreign antigenic peptides to **CD8$^+$ cells.**

b. Class II antigens are found on immunologic effector cells (e.g., macrophages, dendritic cells, B cells, activated epithelial cells). They have three gene loci within the D region—HLA-DP, HLA-DQ, and HLA-DR—defined by cellular reactions. Their function is to present foreign antigenic peptides to **CD4$^+$ cells.**

3. Matching the donor and recipient at the HLA locus improves graft acceptance.

a. Both donor and recipient are typed for HLA profiles with anti-HLA antisera and for ABO and Rh antigens with their respective antisera.

b. The donor must be tested for preexisting anti-HLA antibodies and CMI since sensitization to HLA antigens can occur as a result of prior blood transfusions, pregnancy, or other organ grafts.

4. The degree of genetic disparity between donor and recipient governs the vigor and speed of rejection of the graft. CD8$^+$ cytotoxic T cells and macrophages (activated by CD4$^+$ T cells) mediate most rejections.

a. Acute rejection is characterized by swelling and tenderness over the allograft. It is initiated by HLA antigens on allografts stimulating recipient CD4$^+$ T cells, which respond by secreting cytokines and inducing adhesion molecules and inflammation. Injury to the renal vasculature by the T_c cells and their products follows, with resulting ischemia of the renal parenchyma.

b. A **second allograft** from the same donor as the initial allograft (second set rejection) is rejected more quickly than the initial allograft (the memory response).

c. **Chronic rejection** is characterized by episodic bouts of rejection occurring months to years after transplantation. Both cellular and humoral mechanisms are active, eventually resulting in interstitial fibrosis, vascular occlusion, and loss of function.

d. **Hyperacute rejection** occurs when a graft never takes because of preexisting sensitivity (**white graft**). Rejection occurs within minutes.

5. Graft-versus-host reactions can occur when **immunocompetent** tissues (e.g., bone marrow, thymus, spleen, organs harboring passenger leukocytes) are allografted. If they recognize the recipient as foreign, CMI damage results. If the recipient is immuno**in**competent, a host-versus-graft reaction does not take place.

6. Immunosuppression is used to prolong graft acceptance; however, it predisposes the individual to infection. Consequently, appropriate killed (but not live) vaccines should be administered before transplantation. **Major organisms** that cause infections are:

a. CMV, present in more than 50% of donors.

b. *Candida,* present in more than 90% of donors.

c. Epstein-Barr virus, present in more than 90% of donors.

d. Aspergillus.

e. Respiratory syncytial virus.

7. Immunosuppressive agents include cyclosporine A, tacrolimus (FK 606), mycophenolate mofetil, azathioprine, corticosteroids, and antilymphocyte globulin (ALG).

E. Immunologic aspects of cancer.

1. Oncogenes. Cancers arise from cells in which growth-regulating and repair genes (**proto-oncogenes**) have become ineffective as a result of random mutation or following viral infection or chemical damage. When proto-oncogenes become altered or damaged, they are termed **oncogenes,** and their actions are capable of causing neoplastic growth. Examples of oncogenes and their actions include the following:

a. p53 gene: As a proto-oncogene, p53 encodes a nuclear phosphoprotein that inhibits cell division, thus suppressing tumor growth. Mutations in p53 result in uncontrolled growth.

b. *ras*: As a proto-oncogene, *ras* controls a guanosine triphosphate (GTP)-binding protein involved in signal transduction. Mutation results in failure of guanosine triphosphatase (GTPase) inactivation of *ras* and continuous *ras* activity.

c. *c-myc*: When this proto-oncogene is translocated onto a different chromosome (e.g., as in Burkitt's lymphoma), it becomes oncogenic, resulting in loss of regulation of B-cell growth and a B-cell lymphoma.

d. Bcl-2 gene: The cellular protein produced by this gene inhibits apoptosis at normal concentrations. At high concentrations in B cells, Bcl-2 promotes cell expansion and follicular lymphoma.

e. bcr/abl gene fusion results in a protein with increased tyrosine kinase activity, which is involved in chronic myeloid leukemia.

2. Cancer cells arise from normal cells. In order for the immune system to attack cancer cells, they need to be distinguished from normal cells (i.e., they need to possess antigens).

a. Tumor-associated antigens exist, but are not found exclusively on cancer cells; however, they are generally present in higher amounts in cancer patients and aid in diagnosis. Examples are:

(1) Carcinoembryonic antigen (CEA), which is present on fetal gastrointestinal and liver cells, but normally disappears at birth. It reappears in the serum of most patients with colorectal cancer.

(2) β-fetoprotein attains high levels in patients with hepatomas and testicular teratocarcinomas. Levels are lower in normal adults.

b. Tumor-specific antigens (TSAs) are unique to cancer cells. They can be induced by viruses (e.g., papovaviruses, herpesviruses, adenoviruses) or chemical or physical carcinogens.

(1) **Virus-induced TSA are cross-reactive** (i.e., the genome of a particular virus synthesizes the same viral antigens in whatever cell that virus infects). Consequently, immunotherapy should be applicable to all individuals infected by the same virus.

(2) **Carcinogen-induced TSA induce random mutations** in the genome of affected cells. Consequently, each mutated gene product (antigen) differs depending on which gene has been affected by the carcinogen, and immunologic cross-protection is not feasible.

3. **Immune response to cancer antigens:**

   a. **Immunocompromised hosts** with diminished CD4 and CD8 **T-cell functions** have a higher incidence of lymphoproliferative cancers, implicating a T-cell protective function.

   b. **Macrophages** are found frequently in the bed of regressing tumors. They must be activated by macrophage-activating factor (MAF) (e.g., IFN-γ) in order to eradicate tumor cells via the respiratory burst, nitric oxide, and TNF-α.

   c. **NK cells** kill cancer cells through ADCC and lysis following contact. Their cytolytic activity is increased by IL-2, IL-12, and IFN-γ.

   d. **Monoclonal antibodies** directed to tumor-associated and tumor-specific antigens can be infused into a patient either directly or conjugated with a toxin, drug, or radioisotope to kill the tumor (e.g., humanized anti-CD20 for B-cell lymphomas).

F. **Immunization** is the most cost-effective weapon available against infectious diseases, as shown in the current (2008) recommended Department of Health and Human Services, Centers for Disease Control and Prevention schedules for children and adolescents (Fig. 12.28).

1. Four types of vaccines are currently in use or undergoing testing:

   a. **Live attenuated vaccines** permit replication of the organism in the host, increasing antigenic stimulation. Attenuation occurs mainly by passages in cell culture, growth in embryonic tissue or at low temperatures, or by selective deletion of genes involved in pathogenesis.

   b. **Killed vaccines** contain organisms that have been inactivated by chemical or physical means. Multiple doses must be given and adjuvants might be required for a protective response.

   c. **Recombinant vaccines** (e.g., hepatitis B vaccine): Formulation requires identification of an epitope involved in the organism's pathogenicity. Synthesis of the vaccine antigen follows isolation and expression of the gene coding for the epitope in an appropriate host cell.

   d. **Plasmid DNA vaccines** are under development based on the isolation of microbial DNA containing the genes coding for an antigen involved in pathogenicity. Potential advantages of DNA vaccines include stability, low cost, ease of production, and long-lasting protection.

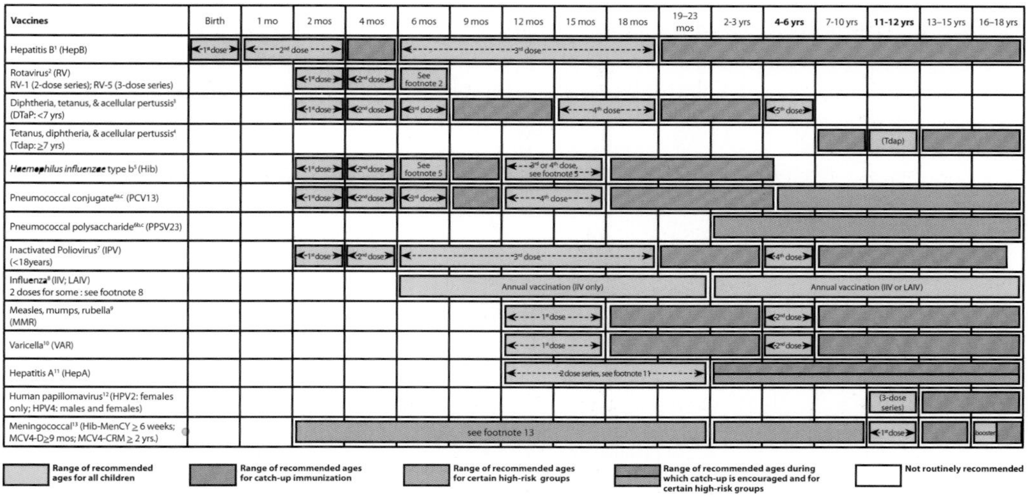

FIGURE 12.28. Recommended immunization schedule for persons ages 0 through 6 years. (From the Department of Health and Human Services, Centers for Disease Control and Prevention, 1600 Clifton Road, Atlanta, GA 30333.)

   2. Safety concerns:
      a. Live attenuated vaccines include insufficient attenuation, reversion to wild type, contamination by live organisms or toxins, and unsuspected immunodeficient patients.
      b. Killed vaccines include contamination by live organisms or toxins, autoimmune or allergic reactions, or incomplete killing.
      c. Recombinant vaccines to date are associated with few safety concerns.
      d. Plasmid DNA vaccines' continuous stimulus may lead to tolerance or autoimmunity.
   3. Description of the individual bacterial and viral vaccines in use are recorded in their respective chapters.

Review Test

Directions: Each of the numbered items or incomplete statements in this section is followed by answers or completions of the statement. Select the ONE lettered answer that is BEST in each case.

1. A cell expressing CD3$^+$, CD25$^+$, and FoxP3+ is a

(A) ($\gamma\delta$) T cell
(B) Helper T cell
(C) Cytotoxic T cell
(D) Regulatory T cell
(E) Natural killer T cell

2. A T cell located at the epithelial barrier of the gut is a

(A) ($\gamma\delta$) T cell
(B) Helper T cell
(C) Cytotoxic T cell
(D) Regulatory T cell
(E) Natural killer T cell

3. A CD3$^+$ cell that is CD1 restricted to glycolipids is a

(A) ($\gamma\delta$) T cell
(B) Helper T cell
(C) Cytotoxic T cell
(D) Regulatory T cell
(E) Natural killer T cell

4. A CD3$^+$ cell that secretes perforin and granzyme is a

(A) ($\gamma\delta$) T cell
(B) Helper T cell
(C) Cytotoxic T cell
(D) Regulatory T cell
(E) Natural killer T cell

5. A CD3$^+$ cell that secretes IL-2 when activated is a

(A) ($\gamma\delta$) T cell
(B) Helper T cell
(C) Cytotoxic T cell
(D) Regulatory T cell
(E) Natural killer T cell

6. A product of vaccination is

(A) B-1 cells
(B) Naïve mature B cells
(C) Centrocytes
(D) Memory B cells
(E) Plasma cells

7. A cell that secretes antibodies that recognize polysaccharides is a

(A) B-1 cell
(B) Naïve mature B cell
(C) Centrocyte
(D) Memory B cell
(E) Plasma cell

8. A cell performing somatic hypermutation is a

(A) B-1 cell
(B) Naïve mature B cell
(C) Centrocyte
(D) Memory B cell
(E) Plasma cell

9. A cell that secretes large quantities of antibody but does not express surface immunoglobulin is a

(A) B-1 cell
(B) Naïve mature B cell
(C) Centrocyte
(D) Memory B cell
(E) Plasma cell

10. A cell that expresses both IgM and IgD on the cell surface is a

(A) B-1 cell
(B) Naïve mature B cell
(C) Centrocyte
(D) Memory B cell
(E) Plasma cell

11. A cell that resides in the liver and is a part of the reticulo-endothelial system is a

(A) M1 macrophage
(B) M2 macrophage
(C) Kupffer cell
(D) Foam cell
(E) Giant cell

12. A cell directed by IL-4 to promote tissue repair, angiogenesis, and tumor growth is a

(A) M1 macrophage
(B) M2 macrophage
(C) Kupffer cell
(D) Foam cell
(E) Giant cell

13. A cell derived from monocytes that attach to the arterial intima and accumulate lipids is a

(A) M1 macrophage
(B) M2 macrophage
(C) Kupffer cell
(D) Foam cell
(E) Giant cell

14. A cell directed by IFNγ to promote ROS production and cytolysis is a

(A) M1 macrophage
(B) M2 macrophage
(C) Kupffer cell
(D) Foam cell
(E) Giant cell

15. A syncytial cell found within granuloma is a

(A) M1 macrophage
(B) M2 macrophage
(C) Kupffer cell
(D) Foam cell
(E) Giant cell

16. A cell that secretes IL-4, temporarily resides in draining lymph nodes, and promotes the T_h2 response is a

(A) Neutrophil
(B) Basophil
(C) Eosinophil
(D) Plasmacytoid cell
(E) Mast cell

17. A short-lived phagocytic cell recruited to inflammatory sites by macrophage secretion of CCL8 is a

(A) Neutrophil
(B) Basophil
(C) Eosinophil
(D) Plasmacytoid cell
(E) Mast cell

18. A tissue resident cell that responds to PAMPs and releases histamine and eicosanoids is a

(A) Neutrophil
(B) Basophil
(C) Eosinophil

(D) Plasmacytoid cell
(E) Mast cell

19. A cell found in the circulation that secretes INFα and INFβ is a

(A) Neutrophil
(B) Basophil
(C) Eosinophil
(D) Plasmacytoid cell
(E) Mast cell

20. A cell expressing Fcε receptors and recruited to sites of helminth infections is a

(A) Neutrophil
(B) Basophil
(C) Eosinophil
(D) Plasmacytoid cell
(E) Mast cell

21. A pro-inflammatory cytokine with a major role in asthma is a

(A) INF-γ
(B) IL-4
(C) IL-6
(D) IL-10
(E) IL-17

22. A cytokine that promotes humoral immunity and is produced by T_h2 cells is a

(A) INF-γ
(B) IL-4
(C) IL-6
(D) IL-10
(E) IL-17

23. A cytokine that promotes cell-mediated immunity and is produced by T_h1 cells is a

(A) INF-γ
(B) IL-4
(C) IL-6
(D) IL-10
(E) IL-17

24. An anti-inflammatory cytokine is a

(A) INF-γ
(B) IL-4
(C) IL-6
(D) IL-10
(E) IL-17

25. A cytokine produced by macrophage to induce liver production of acute phase proteins is a

(A) INF-γ
(B) IL-4

(C) IL-6

(D) IL-10

(E) IL-17

26. A cell producing cytotoxic compounds following T_h1 cell activation is a(n)

(A) Immature myeloid-derived dendritic cell

(B) Mature myeloid-derived dendritic cell

(C) Follicular dendritic cell

(D) B cell

(E) Macrophage

27. A cell expressing cell surface MHC Class II, CD80/88 and secretes IL-12 is a(n)

(A) Immature myeloid-derived dendritic cell

(B) Mature myeloid-derived dendritic cell

(C) Follicular dendritic cell

(D) B cell

(E) Macrophage

28. A cell captured by endocytosis using transmembrane immunoglobulin is a(n)

(A) Immature myeloid-derived dendritic cell

(B) Mature myeloid-derived dendritic cell

(C) Follicular dendritic cell

(D) B cell

(E) Macrophage

29. A cell with a majority of MHC Class II located within intracellular compartments is a(n)

(A) Immature myeloid-derived dendritic cell

(B) Mature myeloid-derived dendritic cell

(C) Follicular dendritic cell

(D) B cell

(E) Macrophage

30. An epithelial-derived cell expressing cell surface C3-antigen is a

(A) Immature myeloid-derived dendritic cell

(B) Mature myeloid-derived dendritic cell

(C) Follicular dendritic cell

(D) B cell

(E) Macrophage

Answers and Explanations

1. **The answer is D.** All T cells express CD3, and activated T cells and regulatory T cells express CD25$^+$. FoxP3 is unique to regulatory T cells.

2. **The answer is A.** A characteristic of γδ T cells is to surface on the mucosal barrier of the gut.

3. **The answer is E.** The invariant T-cell receptor of natural killer cells recognizes glycolipids expressed on CD1 molecules.

4. **The answer is C.** Several leukocytes use perforin and granzyme to perform cell-mediated cytotoxicity, but only cytotoxic T cells express this activity from the given choices.

5. **The answer is B.** The committing step for helper T cell activation is the simultaneous expression of the high affinity IL-2 receptor subunit CD25 and the release of IL-2 to provide autocrine stimulation of proliferation.

6. **The answer is D.** Vaccinations are used to establish immunological memory to a particular pathogen.

7. **The answer is A.** B-1 lymphocytes search and produce antibodies to recognize polysaccharides found on bacteria.

8. **The answer is C.** Centrocytes are located in the germinal center at a site populated with helper T cells that promote antibody editing by somatic hypermutation and class switching.

9. **The answer is E.** Plasma cells are terminal and dedicated to producing immunoglobulin; no surface receptor is needed to direct further development.

10. **The answer is B.** Both IgD and IgM are expressed on mature B cells when exiting the bone marrow. The IgD expression is lost when the B cell begins development in the germinal center.

11. **The answer is C.** The liver plays a vital role in clearance of immune complexes from the circulation using a resident macrophage called a Kupffer cell.

12. **The answer is B.** IL-4 produced by T_h2 cells or basophils during inflammation promotes macrophage development into the M2 phenotype.

13. **The answer is D.** Monocytes attaching to the arterial intima are influenced by chronic inflammation to accumulate lipids, in particular the LDL particle containing cholesterol.

14. **The answer is A.** T_h1 lymphocytes recognize non–self-antigen expressed in MHC Class II molecules on the surface on the macrophage. The T cell then triggers macrophage activation of cytolytic mechanisms.

15. **The answer is E.** Syncytial cells are commonly found in granulomas as a result of macrophage fusion to form giant cells.

16. **The answer is B.** Basophils are short-lived cells in the circulation but will take longer term residence in draining lymph nodes and will direct inflammatory responses.

17. **The answer is A.** The initial recruitment of neutrophils to an inflammatory site requires CCL8 release by resident macrophage or mast cells to initiate cellular extravasation.

18. **The answer is E.** Mast cells express toll-like receptors to recognize the initial stages of infection. Recognition of a PAMP results in a degranulation to release histamines and lipolysis to release eicosanoids.

19. **The answer is D.** Both INFα and INFβ are produced by viral infected cells infected as a localized event, but the plasmacytoid cell is responsible to produce large quantities during a viral infection to enhance MHC Class I expression on a broader scale.

20. **The answer is C.** Eosinophils are the principal agent for responding to reaginic antibody.

21. **The answer is E.** IL-17 promotes inflammatory action such as the development of M2 macrophage and recruitment of eosinophils.

22. **The answer is B.** IL-4 regulates humoral defenses.

23. **The answer is A.** INF-γ regulates cell-mediated defenses.

24. **The answer is D.** IL-10 is produced by regulatory T cells to suppress immunity.

25. **The answer is C.** IL-6 stimulates hepatocytes to secrete acute phase proteins.

26. **The answer is E.** Cell-mediated immunity is regulated by T_h1 cells secreting INFγ when engaging macrophages that display intracellular non–self-antigen on MHC Class II molecules.

27. **The answer is B.** Immature dendritic cells at the infection site are triggered to mature and migrate to the lymph node. Immature dendritic cells have low expression of MHC Class II, but mature cells have high expression levels of both MHC Class II and CD80/88.

28. **The answer is D.** Only B cells express transmembrane immunoglobulins.

29. **The answer is A.** Immature myeloid-derived dendritic cells are positioned in tissues to continuously sample extracellular debris for PAMPs and loading of intracellular MHC Class II.

30. **The answer is C.** Follicular dendritic cells are the only choice to not be bone marrow derived.

Comprehensive Examination: Block 1

Directions: *Each of the numbered items or incomplete statements in this section is followed by answers or completions of the statement. Select the ONE lettered answer that is BEST in each case.*

1. A 6-month-old infant is brought to the emergency department (ED) having woken up from a nap with a weak cry, ptosis, unreactive pupils, and the inability to lift her arms. She has had routine well-baby care. There is no sign of physical abuse or rash, and she is afebrile. The physician puts the child on a respiration monitor and calls the infectious disease consultant. What is most likely causing the problem?

(A) Viral meningitis
(B) Infant botulism
(C) Botulism from canned goods that were improperly heated
(D) Bacterial meningitis—*Listeria monocytogenes*
(E) Bacterial meningitis—*Streptococcus pneumoniae*

2. What is the mechanism of action of the toxin?

(A) Cleavage of terminal neuronal docking proteins preventing the release of acetylcholine
(B) Blocking the transport of choline into neurons
(C) Inhibition of choline acetyltransferase
(D) Inhibition of acetylcholinesterase
(E) Blocking the synapse of acetylcholine at the ganglia

3. Five children in Mrs. Thompson's third grade class develop a disease which begins as a bright red rash on the face, turns violet after a few days, then disappears; then, a maculopapular rash appears on the trunk, buttocks, and extremities. It soon fades from the trunk but persists on the thighs and forearms. Two children have also had a slight fever and a sore throat, but none were terribly sick. The genetic material of the most likely causative infectious agent is

(A) Double-stranded DNA
(B) Single-stranded DNA
(C) Double-stranded RNA

(D) Single-stranded RNA
(E) Segmented single-stranded RNA

4. If one were to create a single antigen vaccine to have prevented the outbreak and for use as a vaccine in women prior to pregnancy, what viral molecule would be most likely to lead to the production of successful neutralizing antibodies?

(A) Matrix protein
(B) Capsid protein
(C) Surface glycopeptide
(D) Polymerase

5. Which of the following bacterial compounds is important in colonization?

(A) Diaminopimelic acid
(B) Calcium dipicolinate
(C) "O" antigens
(D) Pilin
(E) Porins

6. What is the function of the cyclic AMP binding proteins in facultative bacteria?

(A) To decrease levels of elongation factors
(B) To enhance RNA polymerase activity
(C) To facilitate binding of repressor proteins
(D) To increase transcription initiation
(E) To suppress the Pasteur effect

7. An 18-year-old male college student came to the Student Health Services complaining of a sore throat, fatigue, and difficulty in swallowing. A physical examination showed an enlarged spleen; a palpable, tender liver; and swollen cervical lymph nodes. His blood is positive for heterophile antibody. What would you expect to see in a blood smear?

(A) Atypical T cells called Downey cells
(B) Gram-positive rods
(C) Gram-negative rods
(D) Mononuclear cells with Cowdry type A inclusions
(E) Multinucleated giant cells

8. A 17-year-old girl presents to your gynecology clinic with complaints of recurring pelvic pain. A probable diagnosis of pelvic inflammatory disease is made. She is a senior at a suburban high school, is involved in orchestra, and has been on the honor roll most years. She does not do drugs. She has had an equally "squeaky clean" type of boyfriend since last fall, and 6 months ago they had unprotected sex on three occasions. What is the most likely causative agent?

(A) *Candida albicans*
(B) *Chlamydia trachomatis*
(C) *Neisseria gonorrhoeae*
(D) *Haemophilus ducreyi*
(E) *Treponema pallidum*

9. A 26-year-old man presents with cellulitis two days after he is bitten by his girlfriend's cat. What is the most likely dominant organism involved in the infection?

(A) *Bartonella henselae*
(B) *Calymmatobacterium granulomatis*
(C) *Pasteurella multocida*
(D) *Toxoplasma gondii*
(E) *Clostridium tetani*

10. What compound is only found in Gram-positive bacteria?

(A) Capsule
(B) Lipopolysaccharide
(C) Outer membrane
(D) Peptidoglycan
(E) Teichoic acid

11. The parents of an 18-month-old girl appear at the emergency department of a hospital with their daughter, who had an abrupt onset of vomiting and incidences of watery diarrhea. The symptoms began 2 days previously at her day care center. She refuses to eat or drink and is very lethargic. What property of the infectious agent causing these symptoms allowed the preparation of a vaccine that could have prevented them?

(A) Ability to survive as a temperature-sensitive mutant
(B) Identification of an enterotoxin
(C) Loss of colonization factors
(D) Manipulation of "O" antigens
(E) Segmented genetic material

12. A 22-year-old female student complains of excessive fatigue for the past 2 months. Polyarthralgia and vasculitis is noted on examination. Lab tests reveal multiple auto-antibodies including antidouble-stranded DNA. The most logical diagnosis is

(A) Hashimoto's thyroiditis
(B) Multiple myeloma
(C) Sjögren's syndrome
(D) Lupus erythematosus

13. A 29-year-old woman with acquired immunodeficiency syndrome has severe, nonresolving watery diarrhea. It is not gray or greasy. Acid-fast oocysts are seen in the stools. What is the most likely causative agent?

(A) Enterohemorrhagic *Escherichia coli*
(B) *Cryptosporidium*
(C) Enterotoxic *Escherichia coli*
(D) *Giardia*
(E) *Salmonella*

14. An elderly woman presents with chronic fatigue, difficulty sleeping, a rapid heartbeat, and bulging eyes. Lab tests revealed auto-antibodies to thyroid-stimulating hormone. The most likely diagnosis is

(A) Hashimoto's disease
(B) Cancer of the thyroid
(C) Graves' disease
(D) Pernicious anemia

15. A 50-year-old woman from Key West presents with a mosquito-borne viral disease in which her antiviral antibodies from an infection nearly a decade ago were thought to have an "enhancing" effect so that the current reinfection with the virus caused a more serious bleeding disease. What is the causative agent?

(A) Coxsackie A virus
(B) Dengue virus
(C) Hanta virus
(D) Rubella virus
(E) West Nile virus

16. A 22-year-old woman presents with vaginal itching and erythema as well as a discharge which is thick and white. External erythema is also present with discrete pinpoint lesions off the edge. The discharge pH is 4.7 (normal). Amine test is negative as is the genetic probe test for *Neisseria*. What is the most likely cause?

(A) Bacterial vaginosis
(B) Overgrowth of *Gardnerella vaginalis*
(C) *Trichomonas vaginalis*
(D) *Chlamydia trachomatis*
(E) *Candida albicans*

17. An antibiotic that has a β-lactam ring in its structure is

(A) Tetracycline
(B) Cephalosporin
(C) Streptomycin
(D) Erythromycin
(E) Griseofulvin
(F) Bacitracin

18. Which bacterial gene transfer process would be inhibited by free extracellular exonucleases?

(A) Conjugation
(B) Generalized transduction
(C) Specialized transduction
(D) Transformation
(E) Transposition

19. After a trip to Peru to adopt a 6-month-old baby, a 32-year-old woman and her new baby both develop profuse, watery diarrhea with flecks of mucus. Both are hospitalized because of the severity and rapidity of the dehydration, but neither one is febrile. What is the most likely causative agent?

(A) *Campylobacter jejuni*
(B) *Escherichia coli* O157
(C) *Salmonella typhi*
(D) *Vibrio cholerae*
(E) *Shigella dysenteriae*

20. A 19-year-old pregnant student presents at her health service allergy clinic with rhinorrhea, sneezing, itching, and conjunctivitis. A RAST test finds IgE antibodies to ragweed antigens. A characteristic of this condition is

(A) IL-4 mediated IgE synthesis has increased
(B) Desensitization can occur with repeated injection of small doses of IgE
(C) Drugs that elevate cGMP can reduce symptoms
(D) Placental transfer of ragweed antibody can sensitize her unborn child

21. IgA is largely responsible for protection of the respiratory and intestinal mucosal tract. Effective protection is dependent on the action of a secretory piece which

(A) Facilitates the passage of IgA out of the plasma cell
(B) Facilitates the formation of the IgA dimer
(C) Is released by IgA causing an inflammatory response
(D) Is a poly Ig transport receptor on mucosal epithelial cells

22. A noncompliant 70-year-old HIV-positive man with a CD4$^+$ cell count of 40/mm^3 presents with a pulmonary infection caused by an organism that requires 4 weeks to grow on Lowenstein-Jensen medium. What is the best descriptor of the most likely causative agent?

(A) Acid-fast organism
(B) Dimorphic fungus
(C) Filamentous fungus
(D) Gram-positive coccus
(E) Gram-negative coccus
(F) Gram-negative rod

23. An individual is known to have chronic hepatitis B disease. Which serological marker should be monitored to determine if the blood contains the infectious virus?

(A) HBcAg
(B) HBeAg
(C) HBsAg
(D) IgG HBs
(E) IgM HBc

24. The individual most likely to progress to chronic liver disease following an acute infection is

(A) A 50-year-old who becomes HBsAg positive
(B) A baby born to a chronically active infected HBV mother
(C) A liver transplant patient infected with HCV
(D) A recent immigrant who is HEV positive
(E) A young adult coinfected with HBV and HDV

25. HLA II molecules play an important role in the immune response. One of their functions is

(A) To present peptidic epitopes to CD4$^+$ T helper cells
(B) To present peptidic epitopes to CD8$^+$ T helper cells
(C) To interact with an epitope on the membranes of most nucleated cells
(D) To interact with the gene regions: DP, DQ, DR

26. One of the hallmarks of viral infections of the temporal lobe of the brain is

(A) Holes in the parenchyma
(B) Koplik spots
(C) Maculopapular rash along dermatomes
(D) Perivascular cuffing

27. A 63-year-old alcoholic presents complaining of chest pain, fever, shaking chills, cough, and myalgia. She was very cold two nights ago and says she has felt "poorly" ever since. Her cough is producing rust-colored, odorless, mucoid sputum. Her temperature on admission is 40°C. Her white blood cell count is 16,000 cells/mm³ and is predominantly neutrophils with an overall left shift. An α-hemolytic, lancet-shaped, Gram-positive diplococcus is isolated on blood agar. What is the most likely causative agent?

(A) *Legionella pneumophila*
(B) *Klebsiella pneumoniae*
(C) *Mycoplasma pneumoniae*
(D) *Neisseria meningitidis*
(E) *Streptococcus pneumoniae*

28. Pepsin digestion of the IgG antibody against tetanus toxoid will

(A) Result in loss of the ability to form a lattice with the toxoid
(B) Produce two Fab molecules and one Fc fragment
(C) Result in a (Fab) 2 molecule and destruction of the Fc fragment
(D) Result in the loss of the Ch 1 heavy chain constant domain

29. A 33-year-old Mexican fruit picker presents to a free clinic with subcutaneous nodular lesions along the lymphatics from the initial site of trauma 3 weeks ago caused by a plum thorn puncture. What is the nature of the most likely causative agent?

(A) Acid-fast organism
(B) Dimorphic fungus
(C) Filamentous fungus
(D) Gram-positive coccus
(E) Gram-negative rod
(F) Helminth

30. The Pap smear of a 19-year-old female college soccer player contains koilocytotic cells. The disease associated with the appearance of the cells could most likely have been prevented by previous administration of a(n)

(A) Inactivated virus vaccine
(B) Inactivated whole cell vaccine
(C) Live attenuated virus vaccine
(D) Recombinant vaccine containing viruslike particles
(E) Toxoid vaccine

31. A 9-year-old girl presents with bloody diarrhea following a neighborhood barbeque. Her mother said the hamburgers were undercooked. Ultimately, a diagnosis of O157 strain of *E. coli* is made. Where are the O antigens found? In

(A) Capsule
(B) Lipopolysaccharide
(C) Lipoprotein
(D) Mesosome
(E) Peptidoglycan
(F) Teichoic acid

32. What is transferred when an F⁺ cell is crossed with an F⁻ cell?

(A) Only some bacterial chromosomal genes
(B) Generally the whole bacterial chromosome
(C) Only the fertility factor DNA
(D) Both the plasmid and chromosomal genes
(E) No genes

33. Goodpasture's syndrome is characterized by glomerulonephritis in genetically susceptible individuals. The responsible antigen is

(A) A glycoprotein dispersed uniformly on the glomerular basement membrane
(B) A circulating antigen-antibody complex
(C) Rheumatoid factor
(D) A complement (C'5a) induced influx of neutrophils

34. A 35-year-old male AIDS patient is hospitalized with a serious pneumonia. His x-ray shows an interstitial pattern of infection, and lab analysis of his sputum indicates the presence of giant cells. Which drug is the best one to be utilized to treat this infection?

(A) Foscarnet
(B) Ganciclovir
(C) Ribavirin
(D) Trifluridine
(E) Zidovudine

35. In March, a nursery school reports an outbreak among the children of a disease characterized by a high-grade (38.8°C to 40°C) fever that starts suddenly and rapidly falls. The children develop a short-lived (1 to 2 days) maculopapular rash that begins on the trunk and spreads to the extremities; the face is spared. The children have mild malaise, but otherwise do not appear ill. The most likely causative agent is

(A) Coxsackie A16 virus
(B) HHV-6
(C) Parvovirus B19
(D) Rubella virus
(E) VZV

36. A receptor for the human immunodeficiency virus (HIV) is

(A) CD2
(B) CD3
(C) CD4
(D) CD8
(E) CD25

37. A patient with hay fever switches from IgG formation to IgE production via

(A) Interleukin (IL)-1
(B) IL-2
(C) IL-3
(D) IL-4
(E) IL-5

38. An outbreak of respiratory disease that leads to pneumonia occurs in a nursing home. It is characterized by an interstitial x-ray pattern and both amantadine and zanamivir are effective treatments. What is the causative agent?

(A) Influenza A virus
(B) Influenza B virus
(C) *Legionella pneumonia*
(D) Metapneumovirus
(E) *Mycoplasma pneumonia*

39. Which of the following is the principal immunoglobulin (Ig) in exocrine secretions?

(A) IgA
(B) IgG
(C) IgM
(D) IgD
(E) IgE

40. A 3-year-old child develops acute glomerulonephritis following impetigo. The bacterium is a catalase-negative, Gram-positive coccus that has M12 surface protein. What is the most likely causative agent?

(A) *Enterococcus faecalis*
(B) *Staphylococcus aureus*
(C) *Staphylococcus epidermidis*
(D) *Streptococcus agalactiae*
(E) *Streptococcus pneumoniae*
(F) *Streptococcus pyogenes*

41. After extensive oral surgery, a 68-year-old patient who had rheumatic fever as a child and who did not take the prescribed perioperative prophylactic antibiotics subsequently developed subacute infective endocarditis. Which of the following is the most likely causative agent?

(A) *Enterococcus faecalis*
(B) *Staphylococcus aureus*
(C) *Viridans streptococci*
(D) *Streptococcus agalactiae*
(E) *Streptococcus pneumoniae*
(F) *Streptococcus pyogenes*

42. A 37-year-old woman who is on chemotherapy is admitted in respiratory distress. She had signs of focal central nervous system (CNS) lesions early in the day and is now in a comatose state. Both the CNS and pulmonary biopsies show dichotomously-branching (at an acute angle), septate hyphae. What is the most likely underlying condition?

(A) $CD4^+$ cell count less than 200
(B) Ketoacidotic diabetes
(C) Multiple myeloma
(D) Severe neutropenia
(E) Sickle cell disease

43. What bacteria can use fermentation pathways but also contain superoxide dismutase?

(A) Obligate aerobes
(B) Obligate anaerobes
(C) Facultative anaerobes
(D) Aerobic heterotrophs

44. When IgG is cleaved by papain, which of the following fragments appear?

(A) Two monovalent antigen-binding fragments (Fab)
(B) Two Fab fragments that contain only the variable section of the heavy chain
(C) Two Fab fragments that contain only the variable section of the light chain
(D) Two Fc (crystallizable) fragments and one Fab fragment

45. A non-vaccinated 5-year-old British child just returning from Africa presents with a severe sore throat but little fever. The throat has a grayish exudate on the sides of the pharynx and the child has a swollen neck. Clinical suspicion is of a disease with a circulating toxin inhibiting protein synthesis. What additional tissues are frequently involved?

(A) Skin
(B) Kidneys
(C) Heart and nerves
(D) Liver and kidneys
(E) Ears and sinuses

46. N-acetylmuramic acid is located in

(A) Lipopolysaccharide
(B) Lipoprotein
(C) Outer membrane
(D) Peptidoglycan
(E) Teichoic acid

47. A 24-year-old Peace Corps worker is sent back to the United States from East Africa because he has had a very high fever. African sleeping sickness is diagnosed. How is it transmitted?

(A) Tsetse fly bite
(B) Invasion of skin in water
(C) Respiratory droplets and direct mucosal contact
(D) Mosquito bite
(E) Reduviid bug bite
(F) Sandfly bite

48. A 48-year-old woman who presents with muscle weakness and a thymoma is suspected of having myasthenia gravis. If correct, lab tests should show autoantibody against

(A) Thyroid-stimulating hormone
(B) Acetylcholine receptor
(C) Intrinsic factor
(D) Rheumatoid factor

49. A patient who is diabetic and has been in the hospital twice in the last year presents with a boil on his neck. You drain it, but because of his hospitalizations you realize that there is a good chance that it could be a drug-resistant strain and order direct Gram stain cultures, as well as susceptibility testing and anaerobic culture. The preliminary report comes back with Gram-negative cocci in clusters. This puzzles you, so you call the lab supervisor who realizes the stain was done by a new lab person. It turns out to be *Staphylococcus aureus*.

What mistake in the Gram stain did the new person most likely make to produce pink cocci with no hint of purple?

(A) She left the safranin on too long
(B) She decolorized a bit too long
(C) She forgot the decolorization completely
(D) She forgot the Gram's iodine
(E) She forgot the safranin

50. An asymptomatic 35-year-old male Catholic missionary has returned to the United States following 12 years in rural Mexico. His routine physical examination shows elevated transaminases. His medical history in Mexico was unremarkable except for an auto accident requiring a blood transfusion of 3 pints of blood. What definitive lab test should be performed to determine what effective treatment should be prescribed?

(A) Blood culture on MacConkey media
(B) Differential cytology of the blood
(C) Electron microscopy for Dane particles
(D) Molecular genotyping of circulating virus
(E) Serology for levels of IgG HEV

51. Which of the following virulence factors is produced by several genera of bacteria that are notable mucosal colonizers including *S. pneumoniae*?

(A) Elastase
(B) Hemagglutinin
(C) Immunoglobulin A protease
(D) Mucinase

52. A sexually transmitted disease with no genital signs or symptoms is

(A) Epstein-Barr virus
(B) Hepatitis B virus
(C) Human T-cell lymphotropic virus
(D) Parvovirus B19

53. A live attenuated vaccine is not available for protection from HPV-associated cancer because

(A) The virus does not survive in the mouth and oropharynx
(B) E6 and E7 viral proteins are associated with oncogenesis
(C) Viral membrane receptor glycoprotein is very unstable
(D) The virus only grows in human cells

Comprehensive Examination: Block 1
Answers and Explanations

1. **The answer is B.** The symptoms are classical for botulism. Common sources of botulinum toxin include canned home goods, and, in cases of infant botulism, household dust or honey. It is most likely that this is from the ingestion of environmental spores (dust or honey) rather than from canned goods, although that is a possibility. *Listeria* meningitis would be very uncommon this long after birth, and the child would probably be febrile and not have the descending paralysis. She should not have *Streptococcal meningitis* as she is vaccinated, and it would present as a febrile disease with a stiff neck. It is also not typical for viral meningitis.

2. **The answer is A.** Botulinum toxin (a metalloprotease) cleaves docking proteins and blocks exocytosis of acetylcholine from storage vesicles, producing a flaccid paralysis. Choline acetyltransferase, choice C, is an enzyme catalyzing synthesis of acetylcholine from an acetate and choline. Sodium-dependent transport of choline can be blocked by hemicholinium (choice B). Enzyme acetylcholinesterase is responsible for catalyzing hydrolysis of acetylcholine (choice D). Acetylcholine synapses at the ganglia of many neurons and tissues, and this step is not blocked by botulinum toxin (choice E).

3. **The answer is B.** The disease is most probably erythema infectiosum (slapped cheek syndrome) caused by parvovirus B19, a single-stranded DNA virus.

4. **The answer is B.** The disease is most probably erythema infectiosum (slapped cheek syndrome) caused by parvovirus B19, a single-stranded DNA virus. Parvovirus B19 is naked, so protective neutralizing antibodies would be to the viral capsid. It does not carry a polymerase but uses cellular polymerases, which is why it requires replicating cells. It is not enveloped, so it has no glycoproteins or any matrix proteins.

5. **The answer is D.** Pilin is the main protein component of the pili involved in bacterial adherence.

6. **The answer is B.** Cyclic AMP binding proteins bind to specific DNA sequences near promoters, which facilitate RNA polymerase binding to the promoters, thus enhancing transcription of genes associated with those promoters.

7. **The answer is A.** The young man has infectious mononucleosis caused by EBV, which produces a heterophile antibody that is the basis of the Monospot test, and the Downey cells, which are reactive T cells.

8. **The answer is B.** *Chl. trachomatis* and *N. gonorrhoeae* are the only two choices listed commonly causing PID. However, *Chl. trachomatis* is about 4 times more common; in fact, it is the most common bacterial STD in the general population at large. *N. gonorrhoeae* is more likely to be seen in economically disadvantaged urban teens.

9. **The answer is C.** *Pasteurella multocida* is a dominant organism in the cat's mouth. Choice A, *Bartonella,* is the causative agent of cat scratch fever and is less common in bites. Choice B, *Calymmatobacterium,* causes a sexually transmitted infection, and *Toxoplasma* (choice D) is associated with cats but transmitted by their feces, not bites. Choice E, tetanus, is not likely unless the man has not been vaccinated.

10. **The answer is E.** Teichoic and teichuronic acids, which are polymers containing ribitol or glycerol, are found in the cell walls or cell-wall membranes of Gram-positive bacteria.

11. **The answer is E.** Rotaviruses (which are segmented, dsRNA viruses) are the most frequent cause of diarrheas in infants. RotaTeq and Rotarix vaccines are available for prevention.

12. **The answer is D.** These signs and symptoms are characteristic of lupus erythematosus, with antibodies to double-stranded DNA being selective for SLE. Although autoantibodies are present in Hashimoto's thyroiditis, anti-dsDNA is absent.

13. **The answer is B.** Oocysts are only formed by protozoans, eliminating A, C, and E. Acid-fast oocysts are only found in *Cryptosporidium, Cyclospora,* or *Isospora* infections.

14. **The answer is C.** The autoantibodies to TSH in Graves' disease compete with TSH for its receptor site and mimic TSH activity. Pernicious anemia is characterized by antibodies to the gastric parietal cell and intrinsic factor, resulting in an inability to absorb vitamin B_{12}.

15. **The answer is B.** Dengue virus is an arbovirus that causes a disease sometimes known as "break bone fever" because of the muscle and joint pain associated with it. Infection by a different virus serotype following a primary infection causes a more serious disease that is thought to be due to the enhancing effect that antibodies to the initial virus have on the second virus's infection properties.

16. **The answer is E.** The discharge is characteristic of *Candida* overgrowth. Note that no foul odor is mentioned, and the negative amine test "rules down" bacterial vaginosis and *Trichomonas.* Both yeast vaginitis and yeast diaper rash have the described satellite lesions outside the area of major erythema. *Gardnerella* is the prominent agent in bacterial vaginosis. The normal pH range is 4.5 to 5 and yeast vaginitis is usually in that range.

17. **The answer is B.** Cephalosporin drugs have the β-lactam ring, as do the penicillins. They also inhibit cell-wall biosynthesis and are inactivated by some β-lactamases.

18. **The answer is D.** In transformation, the DNA is extracellular before it is picked up by the competent cells; during this period, the DNA is subject to the extracellular exonucleases. Because the DNA in generalized and specialized transduction is protected extracellularly by the virus capsid, it is not subject to extracellular exonucleases. In conjunction, the DNA is never outside of a cell. Transposition is a mechanism of inserting a transposon into another molecule of DNA and has no extracellular transport mechanism associated with it.

19. **The answer is D.** The mention of Peru should raise suspicion of cholera. (Rotavirus would have to be ruled out for the baby, but it is not one of the choices.) The loss of fluids and electrolytes is rapid and most severe with *Vibrio cholerae.* The lack of fever and lack of pus and blood in the stools suggests that the causative agent is not *Campylobacter, Salmonella,* or *Shigella.* The lack of blood also decreases the chance of *Escherichia coli* O157. If untreated, cholera may lead to dehydration, hemoconcentration, and hypovolemic shock.

20. **The answer is A.** The cytokine IL-4 is necessary for the switch to IgE synthesis. Desensitization can occur with repeated injections of allergen, not IgE. IgE antibody does not cross the placenta. Drugs that elevate cGMP enhance symptoms.

21. **The answer is D.** The secretory piece is part of a poly Ig transport receptor facilitating transfer of IgA to mucosal epithelial cells.

22. **The answer is A.** *Mycobacterium avium*-intracellulare or *Mycobacterium tuberculosis,* both acid-fast organisms, are the most likely causes of this pulmonary infection in a patient with acquired immunodeficiency syndrome. Both can be cultured on Lowenstein-Jensen but, in general, broth systems providing a similar high lipid content for making the mycobacterial cell wall have replaced Lowenstein-Jensen. *Pneumocystis jiroveci,* now considered a fungus, cannot be cultured on any medium.

23. **The answer is B.** Levels of HBeAg are monitored to determine if blood contains infectious HBV.

24. **The answer is B.** Progression to chronic disease is inversely related to the age of infection with HBV and 90% of neonates can become chronically ill. HCV infection progression is also high, but is 70% rather than 90%.

25. **The answer is A.** HLA-2 presents epitopes to CD4$^+$ Th cells. HLA-1 presents epitopes to CD8$^+$ Th cells.

26. **The answer is D.** Lymphocytes and plasma cells surround the brain's blood vessels as they exit to combat the virus in the brain parenchyma.

27. **The answer is E.** *Streptococcus pneumoniae* is the most common causative agent of pneumonia in alcoholics. *Klebsiella pneumoniae* is less common but even more deadly because of the high incidence of abscesses. (Almost all of the patients who have pneumonia caused by *K. pneumoniae* suffer from chronic lung disease or alcoholism.) If foul-smelling sputum had been present, then anaerobes would most likely be involved. *Legionella* and *Klebsiella* are both Gram-negative rods. *Neisseria meningitidis* is a Gram-negative diplococcus. Neither *Legionella* nor *Mycoplasma* would have grown on blood agar.

28. **The answer is C.** Because an (Fab) 2 results, pepsin-digested antibody will still be able to form a lattice.

29. **The answer is B.** *Sporothrix schenckii,* a dimorphic fungus, is found in the environment on various plant materials. Subcutaneous infections begin with traumatic implantation of contaminated plant material such as slivers from mine timbers, thorns, or the combination of wires and sphagnum moss (used by floral designers). The resulting sporotrichosis is characterized by a fixed nodular subcutaneous lesion or lesions along the lymphatics from the initial trauma site. When found in tissues, the fungus grows as an oval to cigar-shaped yeast. It grows as sporulating filaments in the environment and has a worldwide distribution. Cases are most common in tropical regions because people are less likely to wear protective clothing (e.g., long pants, long-sleeved shirts).

30. **The answer is D.** Koilocytotic cells have enlarged nuclei and cytoplasmic vacuoles are produced from HPV-infected epithelial cells. The Gardasil vaccine employed to prevent HPV genital disease is a recombinant quadrivalent vaccine containing viruslike particles of types 6, 11, 16, and 18 HPV.

31. **The answer is B.** O antigen or O-specific side chains are major surface antigens in the polysaccharide component of lipopolysaccharide.

32. **The answer is C.** An F$^+$ cell contains the fertility factor in the plasmid state. In the cross between an F$^+$ cell and an F$^-$ cell, chromosomal genes are not transferred because they are not covalently linked to the plasmid. Only the plasmid genes are transferred.

33. **The answer is A.** In contrast to GLN in SLE (where circulating antigen-antibody complexes deposit randomly in the kidney in a lumpy bumpy pattern), the antigen in Goodpasture's syndrome is part of the glomerular basement membrane and its reaction with antibody produces a linear fluorescent pattern.

34. **The answer is B.** The pneumonia is caused by CMV and is best treated with the CMV antiviral ganciclovir.

35. **The answer is B.** The disease is most likely roseola caused by HHV-6 since it has a short duration and the face, palms, and soles are not affected.

36. **The answer is C.** CD4 is a prominent receptor for Gp 160.

37. **The answer is D.** IL-4 causes the switch from IgG to IgE.

38. **The answer is A.** The M2 protein of the influenza A virus forms a protein channel that facilitates uncoating of the virus. Amantadine inhibits channel function of influenza A virus, but not influenza B virus. Zanamivir inhibits the viral neuraminidase of both influenza A and B viruses.

39. **The answer is A.** IgA is the principal Ig in exocrine secretions in the oral and gastric cavities.

40. **The answer is F.** *Streptococcus pyogenes* is a group A streptococci that has an M protein on its outer cell walls that interferes with phagocytosis in the immunologically naïve individual. M12 strains are often nephritogenic.

41. **The answer is C.** *Viridans streptococci*, which are part of the normal oral flora in humans, are noted for their ability to attach to damaged heart valves when they enter the circulation after oral surgery. If you answered *Strep. pyogenes*, the original trigger for rheumatic fever was an untreated *Strep. pyogenes* pharyngitis. Each additional exposure creates the risk of additional damage. So if his school-age grandkids were coming for a week during Kwanza, then he would probably need to have prophylactic antibiotics. But the question only asks about major dental work.

42. **The answer is D.** The disease is invasive aspergillosis, which is found primarily in patients with neutrophil counts less than $500/mm^3$.

43. **The answer is C.** Facultative anaerobes grow in the presence or absence of oxygen; a respiratory mode is used when oxygen is present, and fermentation occurs when it is not. Facultative anaerobes contain the enzyme superoxide dismutase, which aids aerobic growth by preventing the accumulation of the superoxide ion. Obligate aerobes do not have fermentative pathways and require oxygen for growth; obligate anaerobes lack superoxide dismutase. The heterotrophs require preformed organic compounds for growth.

44. **The answer is A.** Papain cleaves IgG into two monovalent antigen-binding fragments containing both a heavy and light chain.

45. **The answer is C.** The disease is diphtheria. *Corynebacterium diphtheriae* remains localized to the surface of the oropharynx throat and does not invade tissues; rather, the exotoxin enters the bloodstream and affects tissues, primarily the heart and nerves, causing myocarditis and recurrent laryngeal neuropathy.

46. **The answer is D.** Peptidoglycan (mucopeptide and murein) is a complex cell-wall polymer containing *N*-acetylglucosamine and *N*-acetylmuramic acid and associated peptides.

47. **The answer is A.** African trypanosomiasis (African sleeping sickness) is transmitted by tsetse flies.

48. **The answer is B.** Autoantibodies against acetylcholine receptors are characteristic of myasthenia gravis and are not present in the other conditions.

49. **The answer is D.** It is most likely that she forgot to put the iodine on so the dye does not form the large complex; in this situation, the uncomplexed crystal violet will decolorize even Gram-positive organisms. It was also a sharp physician who realized that there are no Gram-negative cocci arranged in clusters and that abscesses are either *Staph.* or rod-shaped anaerobes or mixed infections.

50. **The answer is D.** The man was infected with HCV during his blood transfusion. Molecular genotyping of circulating virions is necessary since effective treatment with α-interferon and ribavirin occurs in only two genotypes (2 and 3) of the six genotypes.

51. **The answer is C.** Organisms that colonize mucosal surfaces such as the *Neisseria meningitidis* and *Streptococcus pneumoniae* generally produce immunoglobulin A proteases.

52. **The answer is B.** HBV infection has no genital signs or symptoms, but is considered one of the STDs.

53. **The answer is B.** HPV viral proteins E6 and E7 are involved in the normal replication of the virus, but are also associated with the oncogenic properties of the virus. This association makes a live attenuated virus an inappropriate vaccine candidate.

Comprehensive Examination: Block 2

Directions: *Each of the numbered items or incomplete statements in this section is followed by answers or completions of the statement. Select the ONE lettered answer that is BEST in each case.*

1. There is an outbreak of watery diarrhea in six members of a party of 20 who ate at a Chinese restaurant the day before. Fried rice is implicated. What is the most likely causative agent?

(A) *Bacillus cereus*
(B) *Giardia lamblia*
(C) *Norwalk agent*
(D) *Rotavirus*
(E) *Salmonella enteritidis*
(F) *Staphylococcus aureus*

2. A neonate develops meningitis at 7 days of age. Her mother is 16 years of age, single, has had multiple sexual partners without barrier protection, and lives in the United States. The baby was born 23 hours after the mother's amniotic sac ruptured. What is the most likely causative agent?

(A) *Escherichia coli*
(B) *Haemophilus influenzae*
(C) *Listeria monocytogenes*
(D) *Neisseria meningitidis*
(E) *Streptococcus agalactiae*

3. An emerging pathogen has been associated with serious lower respiratory tract disease. Both amprenavir and saquinavir have been demonstrated to be effective in treating the infection. What step in the pathogenesis of the infectious agent is affected by these drugs?

(A) Cross-linking of the agent's cell wall
(B) Inhibition of the agent's DNA replication
(C) Inhibition of the agent's reverse transcriptase
(D) Premature release of the agent's mRNA from the translation complex
(E) Processing of polyproteins

4. In January a 4-month-old girl is seen by her family physician. Her mother noted that she has been coughing and has had a slight fever for 3 days and recently developed difficulty breathing that is characterized by wheezing. She has a runny nose composed of clear fluid with some cells present. X-rays show her lungs are clear of infection. Examination of the nasal discharge is likely to show what entity to confirm diagnosis?

(A) Eosinophilic cytoplasmic inclusions in cells
(B) Gram-positive cocci
(C) Gram-negative coccobacilli
(D) Multinucleated giant cells
(E) Secretory IgA heterophile antibody

5. Mobile genetic elements that code for antibiotic resistance genes in bacteria but are incapable of self-replication are

(A) Mesosomes
(B) R factor
(C) Temperate RNA phages
(D) Transposons
(E) Virulent DNA phages

6. What is the mechanism of action of the aminoglycosides?

(A) Damage the membrane
(B) Inhibit the DNA gyrase
(C) Inhibit mycolic acid synthesis
(D) Block initiation complex
(E) Inhibit peptide chain elongation

7. Which of the individuals listed below is the most likely to develop a serious disease from West Nile virus?

(A) A 4-month-old hospitalized with a serious RSV infection
(B) A 3-year-old with croup
(C) A 21-year-old college student returning from a vacation in Costa Rica
(D) A 24-year-old tour guide in the four corners of the southwestern United States
(E) A 55-year-old camper returning from a 2-week wilderness experience in Minnesota

8. In the following pairs of organisms, which two are easiest to distinguish from each other by Gram stain?

(A) *Bacillus* and *Clostridium*
(B) *Salmonella* and *Shigella*
(C) *Haemophilus* and *Escherichia*
(D) *Corynebacterium* and *Lactobacillus*
(E) *Listeria* and *Proteus*

9. Two physicians traveling in Central America develop what they self-diagnose as ET *Escherichia coli*. What is responsible for the fluid and electrolyte disruption?

(A) Adherence causing palisade layers of the bacterium on the surface of the small intestine
(B) Exotoxin that inhibits protein synthesis by nicking 60S ribosomal subunits
(C) Entrance through intestinal M cells and migration through the tissue via actin polymerization/"jetting"
(D) Exotoxin that inhibits protein synthesis by blocking elongation factor 2
(E) Exotoxin that causes an increase in cyclic adenosine monophosphate
(F) Exotoxin that inhibits protein synthesis by nicking 60S ribosomal subunits

10. In a high-frequency recombination (Hfr) cross with an F$^-$ bacterial cell, each having a single DNA molecule, what is the most likely outcome?

(A) Bacterial genes will be transferred from the Hfr cell to the F$^-$ cell, but there will be no change in the "sex" of either cell
(B) Some genes will be transferred and the recipient cell will become Hfr
(C) Only plasmid genes will be transferred
(D) Each cell may acquire genes from the other

11. A new reverse transcriptase has been discovered. In addition to its effect on HIV disease, it should be checked for its potential in treating

(A) Infectious hepatitis
(B) Infectious mononucleosis
(C) Measles
(D) Serum hepatitis
(E) Shingles

12. A recent Asian immigrant was found to be positive for the tuberculin skin test. The positive result most likely can be attributed to

(A) Antibody against mycobacteria plus complement

(B) Previous BCG vaccination
(C) Activation of previously sensitized NK cells
(D) Niacin production by PPD

13. A 60-year-old man who traveled to Haiti and took prophylactic chloroquine but stopped just as he left the region now has developed *Plasmodium vivax* malaria. What stage(s) was/were not eliminated because he stopped taking the drug early?

(A) Erythrocytic schizonts/merozoites
(B) Sporozoites
(C) Bradyzoites
(D) Liver schizonts/merozoites
(E) Gametocytes

14. A characteristic of patients with systemic lupus erythematosus (SLE) is

(A) A linear deposition of immunoglobulin on the glomerular basement membrane
(B) Antibody against the thyroid receptor
(C) Vasculitis
(D) Absence of antibodies to double-stranded DNA
(E) Each of the above characteristics is present

15. In January, a 74-year-old woman is brought to the hospital emergency department by her husband, who states that she had complained of a fever and headache during the past week. During the last 2 days, she has been confused and cannot perform her daily chores. Her physical examination indicates some weaknesses in her left side and her head MRI shows necrosis in the right temporal lobe. What is the most likely causative agent?

(A) Coxsackie A16 virus
(B) HSV-1
(C) Rabies virus
(D) West Nile virus
(E) Western equine encephalitis virus

16. A 57-year-old man presents with paranasal swelling, hemorrhagic exudates in the eyes and nares, and mental lethargy. Nonseptate hyphae are found invading the tissues. Rhinocerebral *Mucor* infection (zygomycosis) is diagnosed. What is the most likely underlying condition?

(A) C5 to C8 deficiencies
(B) Epstein-Barr virus infection
(C) Hepatitis A infection
(D) Hepatitis B infection
(E) Ketoacidotic diabetes
(F) Severe neutropenia

17. An 18-year-old college freshman living in a university residence hall develops severe headache, neck stiffness, and fever. When he cannot be aroused, he is transported to the hospital where a Gram stain of a centrifuged cerebral spinal fluid shows Gram-negative diplococci. A latex particle agglutination test confirms the etiological cause of the bacterial meningitis.

Which causative agent is most likely?
(A) *Escherichia coli*
(B) *Haemophilus influenzae*
(C) *Listeria monocytogenes*
(D) *Neisseria meningitidis*
(E) *Streptococcus pneumoniae*

18. In question 17, the substance found in the patient's CSF that gives the positive agglutination test also plays a role in the pathogenesis. What is that role?

(A) It inhibits phagocytic uptake in the bloodstream of a nonimmune individual
(B) It promotes invasion of the bloodstream
(C) It enhances opsonization
(D) It causes a strong inflammatory response loosening tight junctions, allowing invasion of the central nervous system
(E) It allows binding to the vascular endothelium, triggering the uptake and passage into the CNS

19. Repeated *Neisseria meningitidis* septicemias in an individual should raise physician awareness of what underlying condition?

(A) C5 to C8 deficiencies
(B) Chronic hepatitis B infection
(C) Ketosis-prone diabetes
(D) Multiple myeloma
(E) Severe neutropenia

20. Which of the following interleukins is an endogenous pyrogen?

(A) IL-1
(B) IL-2
(C) IL-3
(D) IL-4
(E) IL-5

21. What is the defect in a 5-year-old boy with chronic granulomatous disease?

(A) Inability of polymorphonuclear leukocytes (PMN) to ingest bacteria
(B) Reduced levels of the fifth component of complement (C 5a)

(C) Dysgammaglobulinemia
(D) Inability of PMNs to kill already ingested bacteria

22. A 28-year-old neutropenic woman with *Pseudomonas aeruginosa* septicemia develops shock. What triggers the shock?

(A) Catalase
(B) Lipid A
(C) Flagella from Gram-negative bacteria
(D) O-specific polysaccharide side chain of endotoxin
(E) Teichoic acid-peptidoglycan fragments

23. A 5-year-old Somali immigrant girl presented to the local Family Medicine Clinic with a 2-day history of headache, earache, and swallowing difficulty. Physical examination showed bilateral swelling of the parotid glands. She had been in this country for 4 months and had started her childhood vaccinations 2 weeks ago. The genetic nature of the pathogen causing her disease is

(A) Double-stranded DNA
(B) Double-stranded RNA
(C) Negative-sense RNA
(D) Positive-sense RNA
(E) Single-stranded DNA

24. A female infant is born to a 16-year-old mother. The infant shows signs and symptoms of hepatosplenomegaly, jaundice, low birth weight, chorioretinitis, and microcephaly. The mother appears healthy and reports an unremarkable pregnancy except for a period during the third month when she developed a fever, sore throat, and became extremely fatigued for a period of 10 days. The most likely causative pathogen for the infant's disease is

(A) CMV
(B) *Listeria monocytogenes*
(C) Parvovirus B19
(D) Rubella virus
(E) *Treponema pallidum*

25. Demyelinating lesions, increased IgG in spinal fluid, and chronic relapsing occurrences are characteristic of which autoimmune disease?

(A) Ulcerative colitis
(B) Multiple sclerosis
(C) Systemic lupus erythematosus (SLE)
(D) Congenital thymic aplasia
(E) Myasthenia gravis

26. An outbreak of pneumonia occurs in a pediatric intensive care facility. A negative single-stranded RNA virus lacking hemagglutinating and neuraminidase activity is isolated. The virus is a

(A) Adenovirus
(B) Influenza A virus
(C) Parainfluenza virus
(D) Respiratory syncytial virus

27. Infection with which of the following organisms is more often noted for the production of a lymphocytosis rather than a mononucleosis?

(A) Epstein-Barr virus
(B) *Bordetella pertussis*
(C) Human immunodeficiency virus
(D) *Listeria monocytogenes*

28. A neonate is suspected to have combined immunodeficiency disease (SCID). (One previous sibling died of this.) Which of the following would confirm the diagnosis?

(A) Presence of the thymus but absence of the bursal equivalent
(B) Deficiency in the nicotinamide adenine dinucleotide phosphate (NADPH) oxidase system
(C) Deficiency in adenosine deaminase, and loss of this enzyme activity
(D) An absence of neutrophils

29. In which one of the following fungal scalp infections is hair loss most likely to be permanent?

(A) Anthropophilic tinea capitis
(B) Black-dot tinea capitis of adults
(C) Favus (tinea favosa)
(D) Zoophilic tinea capitis

30. A 7-year-old boy develops vesicular skin lesions on his trunk, which quickly spread to his extremities and appear on the scalp. Scrapings from the vesicles show multinucleated cells and Cowdry type A inclusion bodies. This disease could have been prevented with a vaccine composed of

(A) Capsid protein
(B) Inactivated virions
(C) Live attenuated virus strain
(D) Live reassortment virus
(E) Vaccinia virus carrying capsid protein gene

31. A 26-year-old woman presents with high fever, painful and frequent urination, and left flank pain. The isolate is a Gram-negative, rod-shaped, facultative anaerobe that is oxidase-negative and ferments both glucose and lactose. From these data, what genus is most likely?

(A) *Neisseria*
(B) *Proteus*
(C) *Vibrio*
(D) *Campylobacter*
(E) *Escherichia*

32. The agent in question 31, which is causing the ascending urinary tract infection and pyelonephritis, has a normal flora "fraternal twin" of the same genus and species. What virulence factor does the pathogen have and the normal flora organism lack even although both are *E coli*?

(A) Flagellum
(B) Capsule
(C) Lipoteichoic acid
(D) P-pili
(E) LT (heat labile toxin)

33. Chronic inflammatory disease confined to the rectum characterizes

(A) Ulcerative colitis
(B) Myasthenia gravis
(C) Wiskott-Aldrich syndrome
(D) Systemic lupus erythematosus (SLE)
(E) Graves' disease

34. An arthropod vector is involved in infection by

(A) Respiratory syncytial virus
(B) Parvovirus
(C) Reovirus
(D) Parainfluenza virus
(E) Bunyavirus
(F) Arenavirus

35. A 6-month-old child has had watery diarrhea for 6 days. The stools have no blood and no pus. The causative agent has double-stranded RNA as genetic material. Which of the following is the most likely causative agent?

(A) *Bacillus cereus*
(B) *Giardia lamblia*
(C) Norwalk agent
(D) Rotavirus
(E) *Salmonella enteritidis*
(F) *Staphylococcus aureus*

36. A 26-year-old man who is heterozygous for Rh factor marries an Rh– woman. What would genetic theory predict about their offspring?

(A) No offspring would be Rh+
(B) 25% of their offspring would be Rh+
(C) 50% of their offspring would be Rh+
(D) 100% of their offspring would be Rh+

37. Which immunoglobulin has the highest level in a normal 1-day-old infant?

(A) IgA
(B) IgG
(C) IgM
(D) IgD
(E) IgE

38. A 19-year-old college freshman has a sore throat, sore and enlarging cervical lymph nodes, and a fever. The student is also greatly fatigued. A diagnosis of infectious mononucleosis is made. Which of the following factors is present?

(A) Delta hemagglutinin
(B) E1A protein
(C) Large T antigen
(D) TAT protein
(E) VCA protein
(F) Matrix protein

39. Which of the following binds to class II histocompatibility antigens?

(A) CD2
(B) CD3
(C) CD4
(D) CD8
(E) CD25

40. A child presents with impetigo with bullae. A Gram-positive, beta-hemolytic, catalase-positive, coagulase-positive coccus is isolated. Which of the following is the most likely organism?

(A) Group A streptococcus
(B) Group B streptococcus
(C) *Staphylococcus aureus*
(D) *Staphylococcus epidermidis*

41. Intracellular survival and replication are the major virulence factors rather than exotoxin production for which of the following organisms?

(A) *Vibrio cholerae*
(B) *Corynebacterium diphtheria*

(C) Gastroenteritis caused by enterotoxigenic *Escherichia coli*
(D) *Bordetella pertussis*
(E) *Yersinia pestis*

42. An 18-year-old New York dirt bike racer, who recently raced for the first time in races along the Mississippi and also in the desert southwest, presents in September with cough, malaise, low-grade fever, myalgias, and chest pain. Rales are heard and respiratory infiltrates are noted on radiograph. Sputum stained with calcofluor white and viewed with an ultraviolet microscope shows hundreds of tiny yeast cells inside white cells. If cultured at room temperature, hyphae with small microconidia and tuberculate macroconidia would grow. What is the most likely causative agent?

(A) *Candida albicans*
(B) *Coccidioides immitis*
(C) *Histoplasma capsulatum*
(D) *Aspergillus fumigatus*
(E) *Mycoplasma pneumoniae*
(F) *Streptococcus pneumoniae*

43. If a series of drug resistance genes are transferred together routinely, what is the most likely method of transfer?

(A) Plasmid-mediated conjugation
(B) Generalized transduction
(C) Specialized transduction
(D) Transformation

44. What autoimmune disease is characterized by antibodies against intrinsic factor?

(A) Congenital agammaglobulinemia
(B) Pernicious anemia
(C) Wiskott-Aldrich syndrome
(D) Dysgammaglobulinemia
(E) Graves' disease

45. A patient with severe burns that have become infected with *Pseudomonas aeruginosa* has a circulating exotoxin whose activity is similar to what other organism's exotoxin?

(A) Botulinum toxin
(B) Diphtheria toxin
(C) Pertussis toxin
(D) Shiga toxin
(E) Tetanus toxin

46. A 92-year-old male presents with a cough of several months duration. He has been coughing up brownish "stuff." The man is 5'6" tall and his weight is down from 150 to 140 lbs., having lost 10 lbs. in the past 2 months without trying. His tuberculin skin test has been greater than 10 mm the three times you have tested him in the 25 years he has been your patient. The chest radiograph is consistent with reactivational TB. You order *Mycobacterium tuberculosis* testing and susceptibilities and start him on standard therapy. Luminescent real time PCR confirms *M. tuberculosis*. What has been the standard medium used to grow *M. tuberculosis* and what is the standard clue to TB in examination cases?

(A) Blood agar
(B) Buffered charcoal yeast extract agar
(C) Chocolate agar
(D) Lowenstein-Jensen medium
(E) Tellurite-containing medium such as Regan-Lowe

47. A 17-year-old male visiting his grandparents in Louisiana in August develops a severe unrelenting headache that is not relieved by analgesics. He is very sleepy and complains about an odd odor that he thinks is in the whole house. Primary amebic meningoencephalitis is diagnosed. How was it most likely acquired?

(A) Intravenous drug abuse
(B) Diving or swimming in contaminated water
(C) His grandfather's use of horse dung as vegetable fertilizer
(D) Eating undercooked crayfish (a shell fish)
(E) Handling cat litter

48. A 4-year-old boy has a yearlong history of repeated staphylococcal and streptococcal infections. He was referred to the genetic counseling unit where he was found to have depressed superoxide dismutase activity. Treatment with which of the following is most likely to be successful?

(A) Interferon gamma
(B) CD4$^+$ T helper cells
(C) Insertion of the gene for adenosine deaminase
(D) Transforming growth factor β

49. A 23-year-old who just returned from a 2-week missionary trip to rural Haiti presents with a 2-day history of watery diarrhea. What is most likely causing his problem?

(A) A bacterium producing an enterotoxin that is also an exotoxin
(B) A bacterium producing an enterotoxin that is also an endotoxin
(C) A bacterium that is invading tissue
(D) A bacterium that is invading and producing an exotoxin

50. A 43-year-old woman develops cervical carcinoma. What viral protein played a role in the development of the carcinoma?

(A) Large T antigen
(B) E1A protein
(C) E6 protein
(D) TAX protein

51. A woman who is an intravenous drug abuser and who has been a prostitute for the past 20 years now has an aortitis. She has no mucosal ulcerations or exanthems. Her VDRL (Venereal Disease Research Laboratory) test is negative and her fluorescent treponemal antibody absorption test is positive. What is the most likely diagnosis?

(A) Early primary syphilis
(B) Lyme disease
(C) Secondary syphilis
(D) Latent syphilis
(E) Tertiary syphilis

52. A strain of Influenza A virus is resistant to treatment with oseltamivir. The most likely mechanism for this resistance is

(A) Decreased affinity for the M2 protein
(B) Inability to phosphorylate the antiviral
(C) Mutation in the neuraminidase gene
(D) Synthesis of a β-lactamase

53. It is August. A 30-year-old man appears at your office complaining of difficulty in breathing, headache, and joint and lower back pain. He has a 101°F fever and a prominent cough. During your history taking, only one unusual activity, the thorough cleaning of an old hunting shack, was noted. The cleaning involved removal of old food containers, pots, and bedding, plus some rodent nests. He also deployed new mouse traps. Based on this history, what agent is most likely causing his symptoms?

(A) *Chlamydia pneumonia*
(B) Influenza A virus
(C) *Legionella pneumonia*
(D) *Pneumocystis jiroveci*
(E) Sin Nombre virus

Comprehensive Examination: Block 2 Answers and Explanations

1. **The answer is A.** *Bacillus cereus,* found in rice, is not killed by steaming. The addition of eggs and other ingredients to make fried rice encourages growth if the fried rice is not held at a high enough temperature to inhibit growth. Onset of watery diarrhea may occur within 2 hours or as long as 18 hours after consumption and is in response to the presence of toxin.

2. **The answer is E.** *Streptococcus agalactiae* (group B streptococci) is the most common cause of neonatal meningitis. It is most prevalent in young women who have had multiple partners and is most likely to infect the baby during a protracted delivery. *Escherichia coli* is the second most common cause of neonatal meningitis. *Listeria* is a less frequent cause of neonatal meningitis and other severe diseases in newborns. *Haemophilus influenzae* and *Neisseria meningitidis* rarely cause neonatal meningitis.

3. **The answer is E.** Both amprenavir and saquinavir are antivirals that inhibit the HIV protease, which is involved in the cleavage of HIV polyproteins.

4. **The answer is D.** The signs and symptoms of the little girl's infection are consistent with a bronchiolitis. The most common cause of bronchiolitis in infants is respiratory syncytial virus. Syncytia are multinucleated cells.

5. **The answer is D.** Transposons are incapable of independent replication but may contain antibiotic resistance genes as well as insertion sequences that provide for transfer of genetic information to bacterial chromosomes or plasmids.

6. **The answer is D.** Aminoglycosides bind to multiple sites on both the 30S and 50S ribosomes, thereby preventing the tRNA from forming initiation complexes. They are bactericidal for many aerobic Gram-negative bacteria.

7. **The answer is E.** West Nile virus is an arbovirus transferred to humans by a mosquito vector. The most serious consequences following infection occur in those individuals over 50 years of age who can develop a life-threatening encephalitis.

8. **The answer is E.** *Listeria* is a Gram-positive rod, whereas *Proteus* is a Gram-negative rod. *Clostridium, Lactobacillus, Corynebacterium,* and *Bacillus* are all Gram-positive rods, whereas *Haemophilus, Escherichia, Salmonella,* and *Shigella* are all Gram-negative rods.

9. **The answer is E.** Traveler's diarrhea is most frequently caused by enterotoxigenic strains of *Escherichia coli* that produce the heat-labile (LT) and heat-stable (ST) toxin. LT is an exotoxin that causes an increase in cAMP. It is not invasive, making choice C incorrect. Choice B is also incorrect; it is the mechanism of Shiga toxin and the O157 shiga-like toxin, also known as verotoxin.

10. **The answer is A.** The donor cell, which transfers part of one of the two strands of its DNA, will duplicate any areas of single-stranded DNA and so will not change genotype, including its "maleness." Only a portion of the integrated fertility factor and some bacterial genes on that strand of DNA will be transferred, so the recipient cell may pick up some new bacterial genes. But because the last thing to be transferred would be the rest of the fertility factor, the cell almost never becomes Hfr.

11. **The answer is D.** Serum hepatitis is the only disease listed in which the causative agent has a reverse transcriptase involved in replication.

12. **The answer is B.** Many Asian immigrants have been immunized against TB with BCG vaccines. Neither sensitized NK cells, niacin, nor antibody are participants in the tuberculin test.

13. **The answer is D.** Chloroquine kills only the erythrocytic schizonts/merozoites, so you must take the chloroquine for 4 weeks after leaving the malarial area to allow all stages to continue past the liver stages into the sensitive forms.

14. **The answer is C.** Vasculitis is a prominent feature of SLE.

15. **The answer is B.** Viral encephalitis in January, which localizes to the temporal lobe, is most likely HSV-1

16. **The answer is E.** Ketoacidotic diabetes is a major predisposing condition for zygomycosis, although lymphoma and leukemia also predispose the patient to zygomycosis.

17. **The answer is D.** In the specific patient (young adult, new stresses, crowded living conditions such as residence halls or, potentially, college bars), your first suspicion even before the Gram stain and LPA tests should be *Neisseria meningitidis,* which was confirmed by the Gram stain. *E. coli* would be unlikely unless he had a CNS shunt or was a neonate. *H. influenzae* would be unlikely in anyone except a 3-month-old to 5-year-old child who had not been vaccinated as a child.

18. **The answer is A.** In addition to a Gram stain of sediment of CSF, another rapid diagnostic tool for CNS infection is a panel of latex particle agglutination tests for polysaccharide of the common extracellular bacterial agents of meningitis. The capsular polysaccharide on the bacteria in the body inhibit phagocytic uptake until opsonized.

19. **The answer is A.** The killing of *Neisseria meningitidis* organisms is primarily dependent on complement-mediated cell lysis. Patients with genetic deficiencies in C5 to C8 cannot carry out complement-mediated lysis of bacterial cells and have repeated septicemias with *N. meningitidis.*

20. **The answer is A.** IL-1 is an endogenous pyrogen along with IL-6 and TNF-α.

21. **The answer is D.** Patients with CGD lack the enzyme superoxide dismutase and have depressed hydrogen peroxide levels, functional entities in eliminating already ingested bacteria.

22. **The answer is B.** *Pseudomonas* is a Gram-negative organism; therefore, the patient has a Gram-negative septicemia. Endotoxic activity is associated with lipid A. No toxicity is associated with the O polysaccharides, the flagella from Gram-negative bacteria, or catalase. If it had been a Gram-positive bacterium, teichoic acid-peptidoglycan fragments can trigger a similar process.

23. **The answer is C.** The girl is infected with the mumps virus, a single-stranded negative-sense RNA virus.

24. **The answer is A.** CMV is the most likely pathogen; it was probably passed to the infant during a primary CMV infection of the mother during her first trimester of pregnancy. The baby has congenital cytomegalovirus infection.

25. **The answer is B.** These symptoms are characteristics of multiple sclerosis. Myasthenia gravis is associated with an antiacetylcholine receptor antibody, resulting in muscle weakness. DiGeorge syndrome, SLE, and ulcerative colitis do not have a brain component.

26. **The answer is D.** Only influenza A virus, parainfluenza virus, and RSV are single-strand negative sense RNA viruses. RSV lacks a hemagglutinin and neuraminidase activity.

27. **The answer is B.** *Bordetella pertussis* is unusual among bacterial infections in that it causes a lymphocytosis. A mononucleosis-like presentation may occur during the first year of human immunodeficiency virus infection.

28. **The answer is C.** Absence of adenosine deaminase results in the accumulation of adenosine interfering with DNA synthesis. Although lymphocytes are severely depressed, myeloid cells are present in normal numbers. The thymus does not develop.

29. The answer is C. Scarring and permanent hair loss are most likely to occur with favus (tinea favosa).

30. The answer is C. The young boy has chickenpox caused by VZV; it can be prevented by immunization with the live attenuated Oka strain of the virus.

31. The answer is E. Neisseria are diplococci, vibrios are comma shaped, and campylobacteria are spiral shaped. Neisseria and vibrios are all oxidase positive. Because campylobacter is grown under unique conditions and temperature, it is identified by just growing under those conditions. It has both a poorly functioning oxidase and catalase. *Proteus* and *Escherichia* are rod shaped and both are oxidase negative. *Escherichia* is the only one of the two that is a lactose fermenter.

32. The answer is D. Common pili of *Escherichia coli* bind to the colonic mucosa but not to the uroepithelium; therefore, in order to cause ascending urinary tract infections and not just be washed out by periodic urine flow, the *E. coli* has to have either x-adhesins (not a choice) or pyelonephritis associated pili (P-pili).

33. The answer is A. Ulcerative colitis is the only syndrome listed whose chronic inflammation is confined to the rectum.

34. The answer is E. The California and LaCrosse viruses, which have mosquito vectors, are both bunyaviruses.

35. The answer is D. The patient's age, symptoms, and nucleic acid indicate that rotavirus is the primary suspect.

36. The answer is C. Since the male is heterozygous for the Rh+ gene and Rh+ is dominant, the possibility exists for Rh+ offspring. Since the father's sperm will be half Rh+ and half Rh– and the mother's eggs will be all Rh–, genetic theory predicts that 50% of the offspring will be Rh+.

37. The answer is B. A 1-day-old infant has a maternal level of IgG due to cross-placental transfer of the mother's IgG. The other Igs are slowly being synthesized by the infant.

38. The answer is E. The VCA protein, or viral capsid antigen, is the main component of the Epstein-Barr virus (EBV) capsid. EBV is the causative agent of infectious mononucleosis.

39. The answer is C. CD4 binds to class II histocompatibility antigens, resulting in humoral immunity; CD8 binds to class I histocompatibility antigens, resulting in cell-mediated immunity.

40. The answer is C. Although groups A and B streptococci and *Staphylococcus aureus* are beta-hemolytic, only the streptococci are catalase negative. Only *S. aureus* is both beta-hemolytic and coagulase positive.

41. The answer is E. The virulence of *Yersinia pestis* in humans depends on a variety of factors, the most important of which is its ability to proliferate intracellularly. Associated with this ability and virulence are Ca^{2+} dependence; V and W antigens; *Yersinia* outer membrane proteins; F1 envelope antigen; coagulase and fibrinolysin production; and pigment absorption.

42. The answer is C. This condition was probably picked up in the Midwest, most likely along the Mississippi. (They may have stirred up dried bird excreta dust from starlings, chickens, or bats that contained *Histoplasma capsulatum*.) It can only be *Histoplasma capsulatum* from the description.

43. The answer is A. Genes for drug resistance may reside individually on the bacterial chromosome or on plasmids. Clusters of multiple drug resistance genes are occasionally on chromosomes but are more commonly on plasmids. Also, in general, plasmid DNA is entirely transferred in a conjugal cross of F^+ cells with F^- cells. R-factors are like those F^+ cells with just a few extra, closely linked drug resistance genes. So the conjugal transfer of an R-factor is the process that is most likely to transfer multiple drug resistance.

44. The answer is B. Pernicious anemia patients give rise to antibodies against intrinsic factor that inhibit the transfer of vitamin B_{12} from the stomach to the bloodstream.

45. **The answer is B.** Diphtheria toxin and *Pseudomonas* exotoxin A are both adenosine diphosphate-ribosylating toxins that irreversibly inactivate elongation factor 2 and inhibit protein synthesis. Although they have similar modes of action, they differ in their cellular targets and antigenicity.

46. **The answer is D.** Standard cultures may still be set up on Lowenstein-Jensen agar. Palmitic acid-containing broths (some with anti-TB drugs) have replaced solid agars, and growth detection systems now allow more rapid diagnosis. (The mycobacteria have limited numbers of ribosomal genes slowing their growth.) Choice B (BCYE) is a clue to legionellosis; chocolate agar is required to grow either *Neisseria* spp. or *Haemophilus influenzae* from sterile sites like CSF. Thayer-Martin is a chocolate agar with antibiotics used to culture *Neisseria* spp. from any mucosal surface preventing overgrowth of the normal flora. Tellurite (choice E) is a clue to *C. diphtherias.*

47. **The answer is B.** Swimming/diving/jumping in warm contaminated waters may cause infection with *Naegleria,* which rapidly develops into primary amebic meningoencephalitis, which is generally fatal. It is thought that the organism enters through the cribriform plate.

48. **The answer is A.** Repeated infections with depressed superoxide activity characterize chronic granulomatous disease. Interferon-γ has been successful in treatment. Loss of adenine deaminase is the lesion found in SCID patients. TGF-β inhibits T-cell and B-cell proliferation.

49. **The answer is A.** No mention of high fever or vomiting is included in the case, so the disease is most likely "traveler's diarrhea," commonly caused by enterotoxic *E. coli.* ETEC produces two exotoxins (LT and ST), both acting on the intestine, so they can also be called enterotoxins. It is common that when bacteria invade the gastrointestinal tract tissue, inflammation and prostaglandins are triggered, causing higher fever, abdominal pain, and diarrhea. Choice D is type I *Shigella dysenteriae,* which is both invasive and produces the Shiga toxin.

50. **The answer is C.** Cervical carcinoma is caused by oncogenic strains of the human papillomavirus (most commonly 16, 18, and 31). The early protein E6 is associated with the oncogenic potential of human papillomavirus.

51. **The answer is E.** The FTA-abs test detects specific antitreponemal antibody. The FTA-abs remains positive for life with or without antibiotic therapy. The VDRL test detects less specific reaginic antibodies, which decline with successful treatment, but also sometimes decline without treatment in tertiary syphilis. Therefore, based on the serologic data, this patient could have very early primary syphilis or untreated tertiary syphilis. The symptoms are consistent with tertiary syphilis.

52. **The answer is C.** The most common mechanism of resistance to antivirals is a genetic mutation in the viral gene coding for the viral protein that interacts with the antiviral so that the antiviral no longer interacts and is effective.

53. **The answer is E.** Although several of the organisms could result in these clinical signs and symptoms, the interactions of the patient in an old hunting shack containing rodent feces point toward the Hantavirus, Sin Nombre, as the cause.

Comprehensive Examination: Block 3

Directions: *Each of the numbered items or incomplete statements in this section is followed by answers or completions of the statement. Select the ONE lettered answer that is BEST in each case.*

1. A 10-month-old child presents with a temperature of 39.8°C (103.6°F) and lethargy. Brudzinski's and Kernig's signs are both present. Gram stain of sediment from CSF showed Gram-negative rods. What part of the routine health care could have prevented this disease?

(A) A trivalent killed viral vaccine
(B) A polysaccharide vaccine with 23 different antigens
(C) A covalently linked protein-polysaccharide vaccine
(D) A 13-valent polysaccharide-protein conjugate vaccine
(E) A quadrivalent capsular-conjugate vaccine

2. A neonate with very low Apgar scores dies 2 hours after birth. Autopsy reveals disseminated granulomatous lesions throughout; some are caseating, but they are not calcified. During her pregnancy, the mother most likely had a septicemia caused by

(A) *Escherichia coli*
(B) Group B streptococci
(C) *Listeria monocytogenes*
(D) Parvovirus B19
(E) *Toxoplasma gondii*

3. A nonnucleoside analog that inhibits herpesvirus DNA replication is

(A) Acyclovir
(B) Amantadine
(C) Cytarabine
(D) Foscarnet
(E) Interferon

4. The *v-src* oncogene of Rous sarcoma virus is a

(A) Protein kinase
(B) Growth factor
(C) DNA-binding protein
(D) G protein
(E) GTP binding protein

5. In which of the following phases of growth is a Gram-positive bacterium most susceptible to the action of penicillin?

(A) Lag
(B) Exponential
(C) Stationary
(D) Decline
(E) Death

6. The genetic mechanism responsible for the conversion of a nontoxigenic strain of *Corynebacterium diphtheriae* to a toxigenic strain is

(A) Lysogenic phage conversion
(B) In vivo transformation
(C) Reciprocal genetic recombination
(D) Conjugation

7. Latent infection of neurons occurs with

(A) Cytomegalovirus
(B) Herpes simplex virus
(C) Measles virus
(D) Poliomyelitis virus
(E) Rabies virus

8. What respiratory infection is known to increase susceptibility to pneumonia caused by *Streptococcus pneumoniae*?

(A) Epstein-Barr virus infection
(B) *Haemophilus influenzae* type b or type d infection
(C) Influenza virus infection
(D) *Mycobacterium tuberculosis* infection
(E) *Mycoplasma pneumoniae* infection

9. A patient with sickle cell anemia is most likely to have repeated septicemias and possible osteomyelitis with which agent?

(A) *Candida albicans*
(B) Nontypeable *Haemophilus influenzae*
(C) *Mycobacterium avium*-intracellulare
(D) *Salmonella enteritidis*
(E) *Staphylococcus aureus*

10. The mother of a 9-year-old who is in the same school as another child just diagnosed with meningitis (even though the child did not know nor had any direct contact with the infected child) called the pediatrician, demanding her son be prophylactically treated. The physician suggests vaccinating the boy, doing surveillance cultures, and watching the child for symptoms. The medium that the lab will use has antibiotics in it and therefore is called a(n)

(A) Minimal medium
(B) Differential medium
(C) Selective medium
(D) Inhibitory medium

11. What characteristic of the influenza A virus allows genetic reassortment?

(A) Poor editing by the RNA-dependent RNA polymerase
(B) Presence of the *rec-A* gene product
(C) Defective chaperone proteins
(D) Poor editing function of the reverse transcriptase
(E) Segmented genome

12. Joe has been HIV positive for the past 6 years. His disease has been slowly progressing. Mike, his only partner for the past 3 years, is free of the disease. A plausible explanation for Mike's lack of infection would be

(A) His CD4/CD8 ratio is probably greater than 2
(B) He has a high concentration of NK cells that kill the virus
(C) He lacks the coreceptor CXCR4
(D) He has built up a high titer of anti-GP160 antibody

13. A Brazilian who left poverty and moved to Los Angeles 10 years ago has died suddenly of heart failure. Autopsy showed cardiomyopathy due to Chagas' disease. Which vector transferred the trypanosomes?

(A) Lice—genus *Pediculus*
(B) Mites
(C) Mosquitoes—genus *Aedes*
(D) Mosquitoes—genus *Anopheles*
(E) Reduviid bugs
(F) Sandflies

14. An autoimmune disease characterized by absence of T cells, hypocalcemia, and tetany with lowered cell-mediated immunity is

(A) Ulcerative colitis
(B) Multiple sclerosis

(C) Chronic granulomatous disease
(D) Systemic lupus erythematosus (SLE)
(E) Congenital thymic aplasia (DiGeorge syndrome)

15. Which of the following phrases best describes a prophage?

(A) Phage that lacks receptors
(B) Phage attached to the cell wall that has released its DNA
(C) Newly assembled intracellular phage particle
(D) Intracellular temperate phage DNA

16. An 18-year-old Iowan dirt bike racer, who raced for the first time in the desert southwest 3 weeks ago, presents in September with cough, malaise, low-grade fever, myalgias, and chest pain. Rales are heard and respiratory infiltrates are noted on radiograph. Sputum stained with calcofluor white and viewed on an ultraviolet microscope shows large blue-white fluorescing spherical structures (with a wall) and with numerous small round cells inside. What is the most likely causative agent?

(A) *Candida albicans*
(B) *Coccidioides immitis*
(C) *Histoplasma capsulatum*
(D) *Influenza virus* type A
(E) *Mycoplasma pneumoniae*
(F) *Streptococcus pneumoniae*

17. A 26-year-old man presents with an infected foot from stepping on a nail 2 days ago. The nail penetrated through the sole of his tennis shoe. He sprayed some antiseptic on it and did not seek medical help because he had his last tetanus booster about 1 year ago and he thought that would take care of the wound. The foot is quite inflamed around the wound with a little blue-green pus on the bandage. The organism isolated is a Gram-negative rod that is oxidase positive and does not ferment any carbohydrates. Which organism is most likely?

(A) *Clostridium tetani*
(B) *Escherichia coli*
(C) *Klebsiella pneumoniae*
(D) *Proteus vulgaris*
(E) *Pseudomonas aeruginosa*

18. In addition to IL-1, which of the following is an inflammation-inducing cytokine?

(A) IL-2
(B) IL-5

(C) TNF-α
(D) TGF-β

19. A Peace Corps volunteer who recently returned from rural Africa develops symptoms of liver damage and a blocked bile duct after general anesthesia for a knee replacement. What is the nature of the most likely causative agent?

(A) Cestode
(B) Dimorphic fungus
(C) Filamentous fungus
(D) Fluke
(E) Nematode
(F) Protozoa

20. An autoimmune state characterized by a triad of thrombocytopenia, eczema, and recurrent infections is

(A) Myasthenia gravis
(B) Severe combined immunodeficiency disease (SCID)
(C) Pernicious anemia
(D) Congenital agammaglobulinemia
(E) Wiskott-Aldrich syndrome

21. Following neonatal thymectomy, you would expect

(A) Depletion of the periarteriolar region of the spleen
(B) Elimination of germinal center formation
(C) An increase in ability to reject skin grafts
(D) An increase in autoimmunity

22. *Corynebacterium diphtheriae* is isolated from a patient with pharyngitis. What is the best predictor that the strain is pathogenic?

(A) Those producing the blackest colonies on tellurite medium
(B) Those with a plasmid with *tox+* genes
(C) Those with chromosomal *inv+* genes
(D) Those lysogenized by corynebacteriophage-β

23. An RNA tumor virus associated with the neurologic disease tropical spastic paraparesis is

(A) AKR leukemia virus
(B) Human immunodeficiency virus
(C) Human T-lymphotropic virus type 1
(D) Rous sarcoma virus

24. 2,5A synthetase is induced by

(A) Acyclovir
(B) Amantadine
(C) Cytarabine

(D) Foscarnet
(E) Interferon
(F) Ribavirin

25. When complement is fixed by antigen-antibody complexes, what chemotactic factor for neutrophils is released?

(A) C1
(B) C2
(C) C3a
(D) C4b
(E) C789 complex

26. Several workers in a turkey processing plant develop a mild conjunctivitis without corneal involvement. No bacteria can be identified. The most probable cause is

(A) Acanthamoeba
(B) Chlamydia trachomatis
(C) Herpes simplex virus
(D) Newcastle disease virus

27. A 15-year-old boy on antibiotics to clear up a community-acquired methicillin-resistant *Staphylococcus aureus* has clindamycin added to his treatment regimen to slow the production of the various toxins including Panton-Valentine leukocidin. He recovers but develops *Clostridium difficile* diarrhea. Why does *C. difficile* cause diarrhea?

(A) *C. difficile* multiplies and causes disease in a mechanism similar to that of *Listeria*
(B) *C. difficile* multiplies, secreting Shiga toxin during cell lysis
(C) *C. difficile* stacks itself on the colonic surface to cause malabsorption and the appearance of a pseudomembrane
(D) *C. difficile* exotoxins damage the cells, causing a disruption in transport and attracting polymorphonuclear cells to cause the appearance of a pseudomembrane

28. Which complement component is most closely related to anaphylatoxin?

(A) C1qrs
(B) C2b
(C) C4b2a
(D) C5a
(E) C5b

29. A 30-year-old woman presents with an inflamed, itchy, expanding cutaneous lesion on her side. She suspects she might have picked it up from her dog because it is where the dog sleeps next to her and the dog is losing fur. (The dog also needs to be treated by the vet.) You treat the woman with a topical drug from one of the major drug families commonly used to treat the infection. What is the mechanism of action of that drug class?

(A) Inhibition of ergosterol synthesis
(B) Nicking 60S ribosomes
(C) Inhibition of formation of the peptide bond and peptide chain elongation on 70S ribosomes
(D) Inhibition of chitin synthesis
(E) Inhibition of mycolic acid synthesis
(F) Inhibition of microtubule formation

30. A segmented, ambisense genome is found in

(A) Respiratory syncytial virus
(B) Parvovirus
(C) Reovirus
(D) Parainfluenza virus
(E) Bunyavirus
(F) Arenavirus

31. A 25-year-old resident presents to the emergency department with severe eye pain. She has not been home for 2 days and has had the current pair of contacts continuously in her eyes for 6 weeks. What major protective mechanism of the eye could not keep up with such contaminated contacts, resulting in infection?

(A) Lysozyme
(B) B cells
(C) NK cells
(D) T cells
(E) Teichoic acids

32. What is the most likely causative agent of the resident's eye infection in question 31?

(A) *Aspergillus*
(B) *Fusarium*
(C) *Acanthamoeba*
(D) *Pseudomonas*
(E) *Staphylococcus*

33. CD8 is a surface membrane protein on T cells, which has the following characteristic.

(A) It recognizes class I human leukocyte antigens (HLA)
(B) It recognizes class II HLA
(C) It is a marker for T helper cells
(D) It is strongly chemotactic

34. An oncogene that codes for a guanine-nucleotide-binding protein is found in

(A) Mouse mammary tumor virus
(B) Rous sarcoma virus
(C) Polyomavirus
(D) Human T-lymphotropic virus
(E) Hepatitis B virus
(F) Harvey sarcoma virus

35. A cofactor in Burkitt's lymphoma is

(A) Cytomegalovirus infection
(B) Hepatitis A virus infection
(C) Hepatitis B virus infection
(D) Influenza virus type A infection
(E) *Mycoplasma pneumoniae* infection
(F) Epstein-Barr virus infection

36. A characteristic of IL-1 is

(A) It inhibits T cells
(B) It initiates the acute phase reactant response
(C) Its synthesis is restricted to phagocytic cells
(D) It suppresses tumor necrosis factor

37. Which of the following statements characterize $\gamma 2 \kappa 2$ antibody?

(A) It contains a J chain
(B) It contains a secretory piece
(C) It is the initial antibody synthesized after antigen
(D) It contains a hypervariable region
(E) Each of the above statements is characteristic of this antibody

38. A 45-year-old man had mental degeneration after a prolonged but inapparent infection. At autopsy, a subacute spongiform encephalopathy is found. What is the nature of the most likely causative agent?

(A) Acid-fast organism
(B) Dimorphic fungus
(C) DNA virus
(D) Viroid
(E) Prion

39. Anti-A isohemagglutinins are present in persons with which one of the following blood types?

(A) Type A
(B) Type B
(C) Type AB

40. In June, an 18-year-old man develops a sore throat with a fever and a nonproductive cough that develops into pneumonia with a severe, prolonged hacking cough but little sputum production. Cryoagglutinins are present. He is treated appropriately and successfully with azithromycin. What is the nature of the most likely causative agent?

(A) Acid-fast organism
(B) *Chlamydia*
(C) DNA virus
(D) Gram-negative rod
(E) Gram-positive coccus
(F) *Mycoplasma*

41. Bacterial surface polysaccharide plays a critical role in

(A) Gonorrhea
(B) Meningitis with no underlying trauma
(C) *Mycoplasma* pneumonia
(D) Pyelonephritis
(E) Urinary tract infection

42. A 10-year-old boy presents with an itchy scalp with the underlying hair becoming lighter. The patch has expanded to 2 inches. What should you expect to see in a KOH-digested mount of skin scrapings taken at the infected margin of a lesion from this patient with tinea capitis?

(A) Yeast cells, pseudohyphae, and true hyphae
(B) Regular septate hyphae with little branching
(C) Irregular but broad, aseptate hyphae
(D) Septate hyphae regularly branching dichotomously at an acute angle
(E) Yeasts only

43. A 36-year-old female drug abuser has an abscess on her jaw where she lost a tooth from being struck in the face 2 weeks ago. She did not get medical help. You lance the lesion, express some lumpy material with difficulty, and send a swab of the organism to the lab for Gram stain, culture, and susceptibilities. The predominant organism in the Gram stain is a filamentous bacterium that is Gram positive, yet nothing grows in the lab. What is the most likely explanation for why it did not grow?

(A) It is an obligate aerobe
(B) It is microaerophilic
(C) It is a facultative anaerobe
(D) It is an obligate anaerobe
(E) The lab did not grow it on the correct medium

44. Both division and differentiation of B cells leading to production of plasma cells require

(A) CD4 and CD8 cells
(B) Interleukin (IL)-1 and IL-3
(C) Only IL-1
(D) IL-4 and IL-6

45. A patient presents with explosive, watery, noninflammatory diarrhea along with headache, abdominal cramps, nausea, vomiting, and fever. Symptoms began the day after eating raw oysters in August. What is the most likely causative agent?

(A) *Giardia lamblia*
(B) Norwalk agent
(C) Rotavirus
(D) *Salmonella enteritidis*
(E) *Staphylococcus aureus*
(F) *Vibrio parahaemolyticus*

46. A 1-year-old girl who has received no vaccines because of parental fear of autism develops *Streptococcal pneumoniae* meningitis. Which vaccine might have prevented this?

(A) A 13-valent capsular vaccine
(B) A 23-valent polysaccharide vaccine
(C) A conjugate (protein-polysaccharide) vaccine
(D) A toxoid vaccine

47. A 65-year-old female Peace Corps worker is sent back to the states from East Africa because she had had a very high fever and African sleeping sickness is suspected. What characteristic of the organism makes it a fatal infection unless treated properly?

(A) Highly sialylated surface proteins making it "invisible" to the immune system
(B) Surface antigenic variation
(C) Ability to turn on a T2 response
(D) Damage to neutrophils
(E) Polysaccharide capsule

48. A 2-year-old infant's mother reported her son has had three infections in the past 6 months. Which of his serum values (mg%) would indicate he had an immunodeficiency disease?

(A) IgA → 350
(B) IgG → 650
(C) IgM → 150
(D) IgE → 0.05

49. What organism (besides *Trypanosoma brucei*) is noted for its antigenic variation that leads to its ability to repeatedly reinfect the same person and cause disease and has led to difficulty in vaccine development? Estimates of number of different serotypes are well over 1 million.

(A) *Chlamydia trachomatis*
(B) *Neisseria gonorrhoeae*
(C) *Neisseria meningitidis*
(D) *Streptococcus pneumoniae*
(E) *Treponema pallidum*

50. A 26-year-old woman presents with diarrhea containing both blood and pus. The lab cultures on a special medium incubated at 42°C under microaerophilic conditions grow a Gram-negative spiral-shaped organism that is isolated. What is the most likely genus?

(A) *Campylobacter*
(B) *Helicobacter*
(C) *Salmonella*
(D) *Shigella*
(E) *Vibrio*

51. An otherwise healthy 23-year-old woman presents with urinary urgency and frequency along with pain on micturition. What is the most likely causative agent?

(A) *Bacteroides* species
(B) *Staphylococcus saprophyticus*
(C) *Clostridium difficile*
(D) *Clostridium perfringens*
(E) *Clostridium tetani*
(F) *Escherichia coli*

52. Viral proteins that disrupt calcium homeostasis within infected cells are

(A) Capsomeres
(B) Effluxions
(C) Matrix proteins
(D) Viroporins

53. A preschool day care has reported that the majority of the children are complaining of very sore throats. A closer examination of the situation indicates that they also have slight fevers and vesicular lesions (some of which have ulcerated) on their tonsillar and pharyngeal mucosa. The most likely cause is

(A) Adenovirus
(B) Coronavirus
(C) Coxsackie A virus
(D) Parainfluenza virus
(E) Respiratory syncytial virus

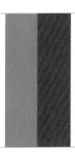

Comprehensive Examination:
Block 3
Answers and Explanations

1. **The answer is C.** Based on the description of the disease, the child has bacterial meningitis. The Gram stain suggests *Haemophilus influenzae* is the causative agent, which is confirmed by latex particle agglutination. The vaccine is a conjugate polysaccharide-protein vaccine as described in choice C. The other vaccines described belong to poliovirus (A), the adult *Strep. pneumoniae* vaccine (B), the infant *Strep. pneumoniae* vaccine (D), and the *Neisseria meningitis* vaccine.

2. **The answer is C.** *Listeria* may cause in utero infections or may infect the baby during delivery. In utero *Listeria* infections are generally severe and are characterized by caseating, granulomatous lesions. Except for *Toxoplasma* and parvovirus, the other organisms listed cause infections acquired during birth. *Toxoplasma* usually manifests with calcified central nervous system lesions in the baby. Parvovirus B19 can cause anemia and hydrops fetalis when it crosses the placenta.

3. **The answer is D.** Foscarnet inhibits herpesvirus DNA polymerase directly.

4. **The answer is A.** The *v-src* oncogene associated with the Rous sarcoma virus codes for a tyrosine protein kinase with a biologic activity that results in cellular transformation.

5. **The answer is B.** Gram-positive bacteria would be most susceptible to penicillin in the exponential phase, because this is the phase in which cell-wall synthesis is greatest.

6. **The answer is A.** A toxigenic strain of *Corynebacterium diphtheriae* is produced as a result of lysogenic phage conversion after a temperate bacteriophage infects a nontoxigenic strain of the organism.

7. **The answer is B.** Herpes simplex viruses have the ability to become latent in neurons and reactivate (replicate) under certain conditions that are not well understood.

8. **The answer is C.** Pneumococcal pneumonia is most frequent in patients with some damage to mucociliary elevators in the upper respiratory tracts. Antecedent measles, influenza virus infections, and alcoholism predispose patients to pneumococcal pneumonia.

9. **The answer is D.** Sickle cell anemia patients have problems with septicemias with encapsulated organisms, such as pneumococcus and *Klebsiella*. Of those listed, *Salmonella enteritidis* has a prominent capsule and it is noted for causing repeated infections in sickle cell carriers. *Staphylococcus aureus* (often unencapsulated but sometimes with a microcapsule) is also a cause of osteomyelitis but is much less common as a causative agent of osteomyelitis in SCD than *Salmonella*.

10. **The answer is C.** A selective medium permits growth in the presence of agents that inhibit other bacteria, in this case the normal oropharyngeal flora. A minimal medium contains the minimum quantity and number of nutrients capable of sustaining growth of the organism. A differential medium differentiates among organisms on the basis of color due to different fermentation or pH. Although you are inhibiting some bacteria, this name is not used as you are setting conditions to selectively grow the *Neisseria*.

11. **The answer is E.** Influenza A virus, which causes a localized respiratory infection, has a segmented genome composed of eight pieces of negative-sense, single-stranded RNA, which can "reassort" when two different strains infect the same cell.

12. **The answer is C.** The absence of the obligate coreceptor CXCR4 for HIV prevents viral entry into CD4$^+$ cells. There is no evidence that NK cells, a high CD4/CD8 ratio, or anti GP-160 antibodies is protective.

13. **The answer is E.** Chagas' disease (South American trypanosomiasis) is transmitted by reduviid bugs that defecate as they bite. The trypanosome is actually in the feces, which is scratched into the bite site. Reduviid bugs are also called kissing, assassin, or cone-nosed bugs.

14. **The answer is E.** Congenital thymic aplasia is caused by an unknown intrauterine injury to the third and fourth pharyngeal pouches around the 12th week of gestation. Failure of the parathyroid glands to develop results in tetany and hypocalcemia. Injury to the thymus accounts for the absence of T cells.

15. **The answer is D.** The integrated intracellular form of the DNA of a temperate phage is called a prophage.

16. **The answer is B.** The causative agent can only be *Coccidioides immitis* from the description of the spherules and endospores in the sputum. Note that no definitive geographic clue is given in this question. Without the results of the microscopic examination it possibly could have been *Histoplasma capsulatum* or *Blastomyces* pneumonia. The patient is also the right age group for *Mycoplasma* pneumonia, but again the microscopic data point instead to *Coccidioides*.

17. **The answer is E.** From both the genus description and the epidemiology, it is most likely *Pseudomonas aeruginosa*. The rubber soles of tennis shoes generally clean off nails as they enter, so it is the flora of the inside of the tennis shoe, frequently *Pseudomonas aeruginosa*, causing these infections.

18. **The answer is C.** Both IL-1 and TNF-α are released following tissue injury and induce inflammation.

19. **The answer is E.** Adult *Ascaris lumbricoides* is a roundworm that maintains its position in the gastrointestinal tract by continual movement "upstream," not by attaching. It is noted for migration into the bile duct, gallbladder, and liver, producing severe tissue damage. This process is often exacerbated by fever, antibiotics, or anesthetics.

20. **The answer is E.** A primary defect in the short arm of the X chromosome results in thrombocytopenia, eczema, and recurrent infections. Depressed CMI and serum Ig levels along with a poor response to capsular polysaccharide antigens complete the syndrome.

21. **The answer is A.** T cells mainly home to the periarteriolar regions of the spleen and lymph nodes. B cells and macrophages make up the major cell populations in the germinal centers.

22. **The answer is D.** Only toxin-producing strains of *Corynebacterium diphtheriae* cause diphtheria. The genes directing the production of the toxin are located on molecules of corynebacteriophage-β DNA, which may infect and lysogenize *C. diphtheriae,* causing production of the toxin. Neither plasmids nor the chromosome contain the genes to direct the synthesis of the toxin. Repressor molecules for the *tox*+ gene are on the chromosome, however. Both toxigenic and nontoxigenic strains of *C. diphtheriae* will be gray to black on tellurite medium.

23. **The answer is C.** Human T-lymphotropic virus type 1 causes adult acute T-cell leukemia, but is also associated with tropical spastic paraparesis, a slowly progressive (10 or more years) neurologic disease endemic in some areas of the Caribbean.

24. **The answer is E.** Interferon, a host-encoded glycoprotein that is produced in response to virus infection, induces the synthesis of several antiviral proteins, including 2, 5A synthetase.

25. **The answer is C.** C3a and C3b are the prime components released following the action of C3 convertase. C3a along with C5a are strong chemotactic agents.

26. **The answer is D.** Newcastle disease virus is a known occupational disease of poultry workers. It causes a mild conjunctivitis without corneal involvement.

27. **The answer is D.** *Clostridium difficile* causes the production of exotoxins, which cause diarrhea and production of the pseudomembrane.

28. **The answer is D.** C5a binds to mast cells and basophils to induce histamine, smooth muscle contraction, and other mediators, which increase vascular permeability.

29. **The answer is A.** The infection is most likely tinea corporis transferred by direct contact from the dog to the human. The drug most likely to be used is a topical imidazole, which inhibits the synthesis of ergosterol needed for fungal membranes. The other drugs commonly used include terbinafine, for which the answer would be the same, or griseofulvin, which inhibits cell division by disrupting microtubules.

30. **The answer is F.** The short genome RNA molecule of arenavirus is ambisense—that is, the 3′ half has negative sense and the 5′ half has positive sense.

31. **The answer is A.** Lysozyme found in tears is one of our major protective mechanisms of the eye. It is, in general, more effective against Gram-positive organisms.

32. **The answer is D.** Three of the causative *agents—Aspergillus, Fusarium,* and *Pseudomonas*—are involved in eye trauma. *Pseudomonas,* the most common, is associated with wearing extended wear contact lenses too long and not taking them out at night. *Aspergillus* and *Fusarium* are both fungi, so they can be eliminated on the basis of the description. *Acanthamoeba* is an ameba and does cause eye infection but is generally associated with homemade contact lens solution. *Staphylococcus* is Gram-positive and mainly associated with styes.

33. **The answer is A.** CD8 on the T-cell membrane binds to HLA class I antigens, initiating the process leading to CMI.

34. **The answer is F.** The *ras* gene of the Harvey sarcoma virus codes for a guanine-nucleotide-binding protein, which has biologic activity that causes cellular transformation.

35. **The answer is F.** Antecedent Epstein-Barr virus infection in a malarial region is associated with Burkitt's lymphoma.

36. **The answer is B.** Following tissue injury, IL-1 along with TNF-α initiates the acute phase reactant response.

37. **The answer is D.** $\gamma 2\kappa 2$ antibody describes an IgG antibody. It does not require a J chain, as do IgM and IgA, nor does it need a secretory piece, as does IgA. IgM is the initial antibody synthesized after antigen stimulation. All antibodies possess a hypervariable region.

38. **The answer is E.** Creutzfeldt-Jakob disease is an unconventional slow virus, or prion disease.

39. **The answer is B.** Type B (and type O) individuals carry anti-A antibodies.

40. **The answer is F.** *Mycoplasma* is a common cause of pneumonia in teenagers and young adults. During the course of the infection, some autoagglutinating antibodies (cold agglutinins) may be formed against red blood cells. The antibodies are inactive at normal body temperature, but agglutinate red blood cells at 4°C.

41. **The answer is B.** For all major causative agents of meningitis that are extracellular (and these are the major ones), the capsule (polysaccharide) is important for successful hematogenous survival to reach the BBB and using different mechanisms to enter the central nervous system; examples include the yeast *Cryptococcus,* meningitis-causing strains of *Haemophilus influenzae* (predominantly with type b capsule), *Neisseria meningitidis,* and *Streptococcus pneumoniae.* All of these causative agents have polysaccharide capsules that allow survival in the bloodstream in an immunologically naive individual so they can reach the blood-brain barrier. The major virulence factors in urinary tract and ascending urinary tract infections are pili or adhesions that attach to the uroepithelium. *Mycoplasma* does not have a capsule.

42. **The answer is B.** The tineas are caused by dermatophytes that generally appear in the tissue as septate hyphae with little branching. Sometimes arthroconidia are formed where large sections or the entire filament breaks up into spores.

43. **The answer is D.** Your organism is most likely an anaerobe, most probably *Actinomyces*, that did not tolerate transport aerobically. Unless you ask for specimens to be collected anaerobically or at least ask the lab to culture an abscess, it will not be cultured anaerobically, especially when you send it in on a swab. The clinical case suggests an organism from the gingival crevices and not *Staphylococcus aureus* as the cause. Large-bore needle biopsy with the specimen sent in the syringe and anaerobic culture should have been done instead. It will likely require debridement by an oral surgeon and antibiotics for several weeks.

44. **The answer is D.** IL-4 and IL-6 are required for division and differentiation of B cells. IL-1 and IL-3 appear to play no role. CD8 cells are functional in cytotoxic cell production.

45. **The answer is F.** *Vibrio parahaemolyticus* is the most likely causative agent. It is found in raw oysters from contaminated oyster beds from spring to fall.

46. **The answer is C.** Yes, the pediatric vaccine is 13-valent; however, it is a 13-valent conjugate vaccine, so the best answer is the protein-polysaccharide conjugate vaccine. The 23-valent polysaccharide (choice B) is the vaccine used for the elderly and high-risk people.

47. **The answer is B.** *Trypanosoma brucei rhodesiense* and *T. brucei rhodesiense* both have the ability to continue to change their antigenic coats so much so that if hypergammaglobulinemia is not found in the CSF of a suspected case, it rules out African sleeping sickness.

48. **The answer is B.** Only IgG values are less than normal (IgG1 approximately 900 mg%).

49. **The answer is B.** The phenomenon described is antigenic variation. It is a particular problem in *Neisseria gonorrhoeae*.

50. **The answer is A.** Both *Campylobacter* and *Helicobacter* are spiral-shaped microaerophiles requiring a special medium but only *Campylobacter* grows at 42°C. *Salmonella* and *Shigella* are facultative anaerobes, so they would grow microaerophilically, but neither will grow at 42°C. *Vibrio* is comma shaped and requires an alkaline medium and 35°C to 37°C for good growth.

51. **The answer is F.** *Escherichia coli* is a common causative agent of urinary tract infection. The strict anaerobes do not cause urinary tract infections. *Staphylococcus saprophyticus* does cause UTIs in this age group, but *E. coli* is still most common.

52. **The answer is D.** Viroporins are small hydrophobic viral-encoded proteins that form hydrophilic pores in infected cell membranes and disrupt physiological properties.

53. **The answer is C.** Coxsackie A viruses cause sore throats with discrete vesiculopapular lesions on the tongue, tonsils, and the roof of the mouth (Herpangina).

Comprehensive Examination: Block 4

Directions: *Each of the numbered items or incomplete statements in this section is followed by answers or completions of the statement. Select the ONE lettered answer that is BEST in each case.*

1. An 80-year-old woman is referred to your cardiac practice with no fever but worsening exertional fatigue. She has had a heart murmur since she was young. It appears to have worsened recently. At her 80th birthday party 4 weeks ago, two of her great nieces were sick, and she thinks she picked up their sore throat. She was sick with fever for about a week 3 weeks ago but did not have enough energy to go to the doctor. If you did standard bacterial blood cultures, what would be the most likely outcome?

(A) Growth of *Streptococcus pyogenes*
(B) Growth of viridans streptococci
(C) Growth of *Staphylococcus aureus*
(D) Growth of enterococci
(E) No growth

2. A 29-year-old woman developed an erythema at the insertion site of her intravenous line. Culture of the catheter tip indicates that a biofilm is present on the catheter. What is the most likely causative agent?

(A) *Enterococcus faecalis*
(B) *Staphylococcus aureus*
(C) *Staphylococcus epidermidis*
(D) *Streptococcus agalactiae*
(E) *Streptococcus pneumoniae*
(F) Viridans streptococci

3. Following a 12-year-old girl's birthday party, which took place in her backyard and involved summer sport games and swimming, several parents complained that their children developed red, watery, and slightly itchy eyes; a sore throat; and a slight fever. The children's eyes were examined and no petechial hemorrhages were observed, but preauricular adenopathy was present. What is the most likely causative agent?

(A) Adenovirus
(B) HSV-1
(C) Influenza virus

(D) *Moraxella catarrhalis*
(E) *Streptococcus pneumoniae*

4. What is the most important characteristic of the causative agent leading to this particular transmission?

(A) The virus is more common in the summer months
(B) Glycosylated surface proteins are less sensitive to chlorination
(C) Gram-negative bacteria are more resistant than Gram-positive bacteria
(D) Naked viruses are more resistant to chlorination

5. A 70-year-old woman presents with complaints of fatigue, nausea, fever, anorexia, and abdominal pains. Her travel history shows that she is recently back from a trip to western and central rural Mexico where she ate what everyone else was eating, including raw oysters from the coast. Physical examination shows a yellow tinge to her eyes, and her urine is dark. Lab studies show elevated liver enzymes. Blood cultures are negative for *Vibrio vulnificus*. Hepatitis serologies are:

Antibody to hepatitis A virus: positive

IgM antibody to hepatitis B core antigen: negative

IgG antibody to hepatitis B core antigen: positive

IgM antibody to hepatitis B surface antigen: negative

IgG antibody to hepatitis B surface antigen: positive

HBsAg: negative

What is most likely causing her current problems?

(A) Hepatitis A
(B) Hepatitis B
(C) Hepatitis C

(D) *Vibrio vulnificus*
(E) *Vibrio cholerae*

6. In question 5, the patient's medical records indicate she was vaccinated 2 years ago for hepatitis B. In light of this, how do you interpret the HBV serological findings?

(A) She has chronic hepatitis
(B) She is in the window phase of hepatitis B infection
(C) She had a subclinical hepatitis B infection before she was vaccinated
(D) The vaccine did not take and she has a current active infection

7. A 5-year-old girl is brought to your office by her mother who reports the child had a flu-like disease for the past week and now has developed a rash. Examination of the rash on the face and trunk shows general redness consistent with a slapped cheek. A single-stranded DNA virus that could be responsible is

(A) Coxsackie A virus
(B) Echovirus
(C) JC virus
(D) Parvovirus

8. A 7-year-old develops watery diarrhea, which becomes bloody, frightening him. He is afebrile but becoming very ill. Macroscopic examination of the feces shows no areas of pus; microscopically, there was no excess of PMNs over that expected from peripheral blood. If his disease is a result of a trip to a Wisconsin dairy farm and petting cattle, what is most likely causing the bleeding?

(A) A toxin binding to G_s, shutting off protein syntheses
(B) Invasion of M cells with shallow ulceration, resulting from actin C
(C) Polymerization, "jetting" the bacterium laterally
(D) A toxin nicking the eukaryotic ribosome, shutting down protein synthesis and damaging the mucosa
(E) Invasion of intestinal cells with transit to the bloodstream and reinvasion

9. A 25-year-old man who has recently started doing intravenous drugs presents to the emergency department with fever and evidence of mild tricuspid valve insufficiency. As far as he knows, he had no previous damage to his heart. What is the most likely causative agent?

(A) *Candida albicans*
(B) Coxsackie virus
(C) *Enterococcus faecalis*
(D) *Pseudomonas aeruginosa*
(E) *Staphylococcus aureus*

10. In the lab, a dense mixture of the above patient's isolate with plasma on a slide shows clumping. This test correlates with which early process in the pathogenesis of acute endocarditis in a healthy heart?

(A) Binding to fibronectin
(B) Binding to fibrinogen
(C) Triggering fibrin production
(D) Binding of protein A
(E) Superantigen activity

11. While playing in the forest, a 13-year-old boy was bitten in the lower left leg by a raccoon. What finding would suggest a serious neurologic disease could result from the bite?

(A) Cowdry type A inclusion bodies in skin scrapings
(B) Molluscum bodies on epithelial cells shed from raccoon's saliva
(C) Negri bodies in skin scrapings
(D) Presence of Downey cells in the boy's blood 2 weeks following the bite

12. The hospital blood bank desires to isolate stem cells from a patient with multiple myeloma for transplantation following his radiation treatment. The cell marker important for isolating and identifying human stem cells is

(A) CD3
(B) CD4
(C) CD28
(D) CD34

13. Six 18-year-old women return from a recent Canadian camping trip with abdominal cramping, gas, pain, and diarrhea that is pale, greasy, and malodorous. They drank untreated stream water on the last 2 days of the trip after losing their water filter. What is the most likely causative agent?

(A) *Baylisascaris procyonis*
(B) *Entamoeba histolytica*
(C) *Giardia lamblia*
(D) Norwalk agent
(E) *Salmonella enteritidis*
(F) *Vibrio parahaemolyticus*

14. Which of the following is the most sensitive type of serologic test?

(A) Virus neutralization
(B) Hemadsorption
(C) Enzyme-linked immunosorbent assay
(D) Nucleic acid hybridization

15. A functional virogene is missing in

(A) Mouse mammary tumor virus
(B) Rous sarcoma virus
(C) Polyomavirus
(D) Human T-lymphotropic virus
(E) Hepatitis B virus
(F) Harvey sarcoma virus

16. A patient presents with an inflamed itchy groin area. What antifungal would work as long as it is a dermatophyte but might make it worse if it is a yeast infection?

(A) Miconazole
(B) Nystatin
(C) Griseofulvin
(D) Trimethoprim-sulfamethoxazole
(E) Amphotericin B

17. Your patient presents with recurring pain suggestive of a duodenal ulcer and is positive for antibodies against *Helicobacter pylori*. What allowed *H. pylori* to survive the transit through the gastric lumen to start the infection?

(A) Buffering capacity generated by the Cag A protein
(B) Use of antacids by the patient
(C) Production of an urease
(D) The presence of a polysaccharide capsule that protects the cells
(E) The flagellum and chemotaxis that moves the organism quickly to the mucin layer

18. All Shigellae have some invasive capability limited to mucosa of the ileum and colon, but some *Shigella dysenteriae* strains cause more severe disease. Why?

(A) They produce a toxin similar to enterohemorrhagic *E. coli*
(B) These strains are motile
(C) They have greater resistance to stomach acid
(D) They produce a toxin similar to enterotoxic *E. coli*
(E) They produce a capsule (Vi antigen)

19. A 15-month-old child living in a religious community that does not vaccinate their children develops meningitis. A Gram-negative rod is seen in the cerebrospinal fluid. What is the most likely causative agent?

(A) An enterovirus
(B) *Escherichia coli*
(C) *Haemophilus influenzae*
(D) *Neisseria meningitidis*
(E) *Streptococcus agalactiae*

20. Which of the following statements characterizes idiotypic determinants?

(A) They are found in the crystallizable fragment of immunoglobulins
(B) They are found on protein antigens
(C) They can be antigenic
(D) They are responsible for rejection of transplants

21. Which of the following would be found in the urine of a patient with multiple myeloma?

(A) Bence-Jones proteins
(B) Complement components
(C) Heavy chains
(D) Fc chains

22. A burn patient has an infected area with odiferous, blue-green pus. What is the most likely causative agent?

(A) *Aspergillus fumigatus*
(B) *Pseudomonas aeruginosa*
(C) *Staphylococcus aureus*
(D) *Streptococcus pyogenes*
(E) *Staphylococcus epidermidis*

23. A 14-year-old girl has symptoms that include a low-grade fever, chills, headache, muscle aches, and malaise. A physical examination indicates an enlarged spleen. A Monospot test is negative. The laboratory finding that would confirm a diagnosis would be

(A) 10 times or greater macrophages in the blood
(B) Heterophile antibodies
(C) Koilocytotic cells in pharyngeal scrapings
(D) "Owl's eye" cells in urine

24. A 20-year-old female has signs and symptoms consistent with genital warts. What would have been the best approach to prevent this disease?

(A) Immunization with a live reassortment vaccine
(B) Immunization with recombinant-produced viruslike particles

(C) Passive immunization with antineuraminidase antibodies

(D) Prophylactic treatment with acyclovir

25. One advantage of live, attenuated vaccines is

(A) They do not produce persistent low-grade infections

(B) The viral strain does not revert to virulent forms

(C) They have an unlimited shelf life

(D) They induce a wide spectrum of antibodies

26. Which of the following childhood vaccines is most likely to prevent otitis media in young children?

(A) *H. influenzae*

(B) Measles, mumps, and rubella

(C) Meningococcal

(D) VZV

27. A patient with a chronic cough is given a tuberculin skin test, which when properly read has a zone of induration greater than 15 mm. What does this mean?

(A) Active infection with *Mycobacterium tuberculosis*

(B) Active infection with any of the nontuberculous mycobacteria

(C) Anergy

(D) Antibody titer to *M. tuberculosis*

(E) Previous infection with *M. tuberculosis*

(F) Vaccination with bacillus Calmette-Guerin (BCG) vaccine only

28. The role of macrophages in the immune response includes all of the following functions except

(A) Antigen engulfment

(B) Production of interleukin-1 (IL-1)

(C) Production of IL-2

(D) Production of endogenous pyrogen

(E) Presentation of antigen in the context of class II histocompatibility antigens

29. A patient with a cough of several weeks' duration but no fever has radiological signs of a coin lesion. The needle biopsy shows large, broad-based budding yeasts with a very thick cell wall. Most of the yeasts are extracellular. What is the most likely diagnosis?

(A) Aspergillosis

(B) Blastomycosis

(C) Coccidioidomycosis

(D) Histoplasmosis

(E) Cancer

30. A 12-day-old neonate is brought in because of parental concern about eye redness and "watering" associated with the conjunctiva of both eyes. Visual examination confirms and also detects several vesicles. Appropriate topical treatment is with

(A) Acyclovir

(B) Foscarnet

(C) Ribavirin

(D) Zanamivir

31. β-lactam drugs bind to penicillin-binding proteins to halt the synthesis of peptidoglycan. Where are these proteins located?

(A) In the cytoplasm

(B) In the cytoplasmic membrane

(C) In the periplasmic space

(D) In the peptidoglycan itself

(E) In the capsule

32. A new class of pathogen appears, causing pneumonia. It appears to be some sort of budding yeastlike organism with chitin in the cell wall, but the nucleus is not membrane bound and the protein synthetic equipment appears to be procaryotic. Which of the following antimicrobial agents is most likely to be effective?

(A) Metronidazole

(B) Penicillins

(C) Third generation cephalosporins

(D) Doxycycline

33. A typical IgG antibody molecule has all of the following characteristics except

(A) It consists of at least two identical heavy and two identical light chains

(B) It has two antigen-binding sites

(C) It has specificity for only one antigen

(D) It is a glycosylated molecule

(E) It has two constant domains on each of the heavy chains

34. A 59-year-old man presents at the emergency department with labored breathing and a sharp stabbing pain behind the breast bone. He complains of being weak and tired. He has a low-grade fever and an electrocardiogram shows elevated ST segments. The most likely infectious cause of these symptoms is

(A) BK virus

(B) Coxsackie B virus

(C) *Moraxella catarrhalis*

(D) *Nocardia asteroides*
(E) Rotavirus

35. A 27-year-old worker at a day care center has recently been feeling tired, has a slight fever, and has felt nauseated and vomited several times. Yesterday, she had abdominal pain and chills, and today she voided dark urine. Lab tests for serum enzymes indicated elevated AST and ALT. The genetic material of the virus most likely to cause her symptoms is

(A) Double-stranded DNA
(B) Double-stranded RNA
(C) Single-stranded DNA
(D) Single-stranded RNA

36. The T-cell antigen receptor is associated with which of the following characteristics?

(A) It is a monomeric immunoglobulin M
(B) It requires free antigen for triggering
(C) It is associated with CD4 or CD8
(D) It is nonspecific

37. Which of the following cells is capable of attacking a certain tumor cell spontaneously (i.e., without prior sensitization)?

(A) Monocyte-macrophage
(B) CD8$^+$ cell
(C) Mature B cell
(D) Natural killer (NK) cell
(E) Null (K) cell

38. A 40-year-old man presents to the ED with a painful and swollen jaw. Two days ago he had a tooth extraction where the gums and jaw were swollen and painful. "Nodules" are felt below the surface of the tissues which are not lymph nodes. Which member of the gingival normal flora will grow contiguously into the damaged tissues, producing tissue swelling and ultimately, if untreated, will develop sinus tracts that will erupt to the surface, liberating the "nodules"?

(A) *Actinomyces israelii*
(B) *Nocardia asteroides*
(C) *Mycobacterium kansasii*
(D) *Fusobacterium nucleatum*

39. Bacteria are protected from phagocytosis by

(A) Capsule
(B) Lipopolysaccharide
(C) Lipoprotein

(D) Outer membrane
(E) Peptidoglycan

40. Which of the following genetic mechanisms is responsible for the conversion of nontoxigenic strains of *Corynebacterium diphtheriae* to toxigenic strains?

(A) Lysogenic phage conversion
(B) In vivo transformation
(C) Reciprocal genetic recombination
(D) Conjugation

41. Parents bring in a 5-month-old who suddenly has lost developmental ground and is no longer able to hold his head up or sit up. In taking the health history, they did note constipation a couple of days before. The EEG confirms a pattern consistent with botulism. After assuring them that with monitoring and support the child will survive, the parents become terribly concerned that the loss of development might be permanent. What can you tell them about their child's prognosis?

(A) Elevated cerebrospinal fluid pressure occurs in over half of the children, resulting in some permanent neurologic defects
(B) Almost all of the children have some permanent neurologic defects
(C) There is some permanent muscle weakness following recovery that, like polio, may worsen late in life
(D) Neurological recovery, although slow, is expected to be complete in all children

42. A 28-year-old man compromised by chemotherapy now has a life-threatening meningitis caused by *Histoplasma capsulatum*. Which of the following antifungal drugs is fungicidal and appropriate for initial systemic use until the infection can be treated with maintenance therapy?

(A) Liposomal amphotericin B
(B) Chloramphenicol
(C) Ketoconazole
(D) Griseofulvin
(E) Itraconazole
(F) Nystatin

43. What microbe has both a live-attenuated vaccine and an inactivated vaccine currently in routine use? The inactivated one is used for anyone under 2 years or over 60, or for anyone who is immunocompromised in any way.

(A) *Streptococcus pneumoniae*
(B) Diphtheria, tetanus, pertussis

(C) Poliovirus

(D) Influenza virus

(E) Hepatitis B

44. Which of the following complement components attaches to the crystallizable fragment of immunoglobulin M?

(A) C2b

(B) C4b2a

(C) C2b

(D) C5b

(E) C1qrs

45. A 17-year-old develops *Neisseria meningitidis* meningitis. What was the first event?

(A) Crossing the blood-brain barrier

(B) Meningococcemia

(C) Skin lesions

(D) Upper respiratory colonization

(E) Waterhouse-Friderichsen syndrome

(F) CNS invasion directly through cribriform plate

46. A 34-year-old woman presents with abdominal pain made better by ingestion of bland food. A diagnosis of *Helicobacter pylori* is made. If the DNA had been analyzed, a region of unique DNA coding for the Cag A protein and its type VI injection-like secretion system would be found. What is this segment of DNA called?

(A) A replicon

(B) An integron

(C) A pathogenicity island

(D) A transposon

47. A pale 6-year-old girl from a poor rural area of Appalachia presents with chronic complaints of "tiredness, upset tummy and the runs." She is found to have microcytic hypochromic anemia. Bile-stained eggs with polar plugs are found in her feces. This infection can be prevented by

(A) Not swimming in contaminated water

(B) Not using human excrement as vegetable fertilizer

(C) Heating all canned foods to 60°C for 10 minutes

(D) Avoiding cat litter or taking proper care when changing litter

(E) Wearing shoes outside in endemic regions

48. A hospitalized burn patient develops toxic shock syndrome. An enterotoxin secreting *Staphylococcus* is isolated from the burn lesion. This superantigen acts by

(A) Inducing the secretion of high concentrations of cytokines

(B) Blocking the epitope-binding region of HLA molecules

(C) Decreasing the numbers of polymorpho-nuclear cells

(D) Binding to the Vβ region on multiple B cells

49. An 11-day-old neonate has been brought to his pediatrician because the infant has developed a sharp cough. Physical examination also reveals a mild conjunctivitis with some pus; a chest film confirms pneumonia. No organisms are seen on Gram stain of the pus. What is the most likely causative agent?

(A) An obligate intracellular organism unable to make its own ATP

(B) A diplococcus that has a high potential vto cause blindness as well as the pneumonia

(C) An organism that has no peptidoglycan or other cell-wall polymer

(D) An obligate intracellular organism infective vascular endothelium

(E) An organism that may be demonstrated by acid-fast stain and is largely intracellular

50. A 24-year-old man hospitalized in a coma for 2 weeks now has developed erythema around his catheter. You order the catheter to be pulled, the tip cultured, and a new line to be started on the opposite side of the body. The report comes back that it is *Staphylococcus epidermidis,* which does not surprise you, as it is noted for the production of a loose network of polysaccharide sticking to catheters. What is this layer on the cell called?

(A) Peptidoglycan

(B) Pili

(C) Teichoic acids

(D) Biofilm

(E) Glycocalyx

51. A 6-month-old infant has had watery diarrhea for 6 days; he vomited a couple of times. The stools have no blood and no pus. He is dehydrated. He has not been outside of Cincinnati.

Two other toddlers who visited for a day also are sick. What is most likely causing this?

(A) *Clostridium botulinum* toxin
(B) *Giardia lamblia*
(C) Norwalk agent
(D) Rotavirus
(E) *Salmonella enteritidis*
(F) *Staphylococcus aureus* enterotoxin

52. A mother brings her 8-year-old son to your office and reports that about 10 days ago he had a flu-like disease with a minor fever. Three days ago he had a very red face which turned normal color when touched, and now he has a red rash on his arms and legs which also blanches to touch. She states he had all the normal childhood shots. The most likely infectious cause of his symptoms is

(A) *Candida albicans*
(B) Coxsackie A virus
(C) Parvovirus B19
(D) *Staph. epidermidis*

53. A 65-year-old male appears in your office complaining of a sudden onset influenza-like illness characterized by high fever, chills, backache, headache, myalgia, and retro-orbital pain. There has also been some nausea and vomiting. Which of the following possible viral infections are you most concerned about as the cause of his symptoms?

(A) Colorado Tick Fever virus
(B) Rabies virus
(C) Varicella zoster virus
(D) West Nile virus

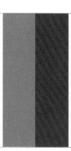

Comprehensive Examination: Block 4 Answers and Explanations

1. **The answer is E.** Without dental work or gastrointestinal or genitourinary manipulation and with the pharyngitis, the most likely explanation is that your patient had rheumatic heart disease made worse recently by an untreated strep throat. Because it is the antibodies (and, perhaps, immune cells) circulating and interacting with the heart and not bacteria, the blood cultures should be sterile. Antistreptolysin O titer should be positive.

2. **The answer is C.** *Staphylococcus epidermidis* is noted for its ability to secrete biofilms and adhere to intravenous lines. *Streptococcus mutans* (a viridans streptococcus) is also noted for the production of a dextran biofilm; however, in this case it adheres these organisms to dental surfaces leading to dental plaque and caries.

3. **The answer is A.** The given clinical symptoms suggest viral pharyngoconjunctival fever rather than bacterial conjunctivitis, where pus would have been present and preauricular nodes absent. Adenovirus frequently causes a pharyngoconjunctival fever that can be transmitted from person to person in contaminated swimming pools.

4. **The answer is D.** First you had to know that adenoviruses are naked. If chlorination is not properly maintained in pools, the virus is not sufficiently damaged to inhibit binding or viability and it leads to spread in pools. Enveloped viruses are more easily damaged by chlorination.

5. **The answer is A.** She has hepatitis A.

6. **The answer is C.** She probably had already had a subclinical infection prior to being vaccinated; otherwise, she would not have antibody to core antigen, as the vaccine has only surface antigen in it.

7. **The answer is D.** Only one virus family has single-stranded DNA as its genetic material, and that is the parvovirus family. Parvovirus B19 can cause a disease called erythema infectiosum, which produces signs and symptoms consistent with those described.

8. **The answer is D.** The symptoms are only characteristic of enterohemorrhagic *E. coli.* The toxin kills intestinal cells by shutting off protein synthesis, causing erosion of the intestinal wall. HUS may also occur.

9. **The answer is E.** With tricuspid valve insufficiency in IVDA, the most common cause is *Staphylococcus aureus,* which generally presents as an acute infection. Viridans streptococci are also common in IVDU, possibly from the practice of licking the needle to make the injection less painful.

10. **The answer is B.** The binding of surface components to the plasma fibrinogen cross-links the staphylococci. The fibrinogen binding is probably the major reason *Staphylococcus aureus* can damage the normal heart. It can also bind to fibronectin, so it is also a major causative agent of bacterial endocarditis in people with congenital defects and previously damaged hearts.

11. **The answer is C.** Intracytoplasmic inclusion bodies called Negri bodies are found in nerve cells infected by the rabies virus, which can cause a serious neurological infection unless appropriately treated. (The patient should have been immediately treated prophylactically for rabies!)

12. **The answer is D.** CD34 is selective for human stem cells. CD3 is found on all T cells. CD28 is an accessory T-cell adhesion molecule, while CD4 is a marker for T helper cells.

13. **The answer is C.** Pale, greasy, malodorous stools with malabsorption after drinking untreated stream or lake water strongly suggests a *Giardia lamblia* infection. The organisms can be detected most reliably by a fecal antigen test because they attach to the intestinal mucosa.

14. **The answer is C.** The ELISA test can measure nanogram amounts of hormones.

15. **The answer is F.** Harvey sarcoma virus, like most viruses with high oncogenic potential, is a defective virus that lacks at least one functional virogene.

16. **The answer is C.** Griseofulvin is given orally and is effective on dermatophytes, but may exacerbate yeast infections. Choice A, miconazole, works on both dermatophytes and yeasts. Choice B, nystatin, works on yeasts. Of the fungi, choice D is used orally only for pneumocystis. And choice E (AMB) is incorrect as it is not used topically on skin.

17. **The answer is C.** The production of the urease produces ammonia, which neutralizes the stomach acid in the immediate environment of each *H. pylori* as it migrates to the mucosa. Choice E is also part of the pathogenesis, but the question asks specifically about the survival during the transit.

18. **The answer is A.** The Shiga toxin-producing strains nick the 60S ribosomes of the human cells, causing severe dysentery and may also cause hemolytic uremic syndrome.

19. **The answer is C.** The only Gram-negative rods in the choices are *E. coli* and *H. influenzae*. The causative agent is more likely to be *Haemophilus influenzae* in a child this age.

20. **The answer is C.** Because idiotypic determinants on antibodies contain amino acid sequences in the (Fab') 2 variable regions that are unique to the respondent, they can be antigenic.

21. **The answer is A.** Bence-Jones proteins are light chains found in the urine of myeloma patients whose plasma cells are secreting light chains in excess.

22. **The answer is B.** Most strains of *Pseudomonas aeruginosa* produce a blue-green pigment, which is clinically notable in burn wounds infected with *Pseudomonas*. (Colonization is common but the presence of the blue-green pus is suggestive of actual presence in the tissue and infection.)

23. **The answer is D.** Symptoms are consistent with a mononucleosis disease that is usually caused by EBV or CMV. The lack of a positive Monospot test for heterophile antibodies and presence of "owl's eye" cells would indicate CMV.

24. **The answer is B.** A quadrivalent recombinant vaccine (Gardasil) containing viruslike particles of types 6, 11, 16, and 18 (these types cause 90% of genital warts) is available for prophylactic immunization to prevent genital warts and cervical cancer by types 16 and 18.

25. **The answer is D.** A live attenuated vaccine has the advantage of producing persistent infection, thus continuously stimulating the immune system with different antigens. A few viral strains in vaccines may revert to virulent form. A disadvantage is their limited shelf life.

26. **The answer is A.** Of the organisms listed, *H. influenzae* is the one most likely to cause otitis media.

27. **The answer is E.** The tuberculin test indicates previous infection with *Mycobacterium tuberculosis* or *Mycobacterium bovis* from between several weeks to 5 years. It does not provide proof of current active infection with *M. tuberculosis*. The tuberculin test detects cell-mediated immunity and not antibody. If a person is infected with a nontuberculous strain of mycobacteria, usually the skin reaction is smaller. Specific skin tests for some of these nontuberculous strains of mycobacteria are available. Vaccination with bacillus Calmette-Guérin (BCG) vaccine should not result in this large a zone of induration. The newer whole blood interferon-gamma release assays (IGRAs), which also do not distinguish latent tuberculosis infection from tuberculosis disease, are superior to distinguish infected from BCG vaccinated.

28. **The answer is C.** Macrophages do not produce IL-2.

29. **The answer is B.** The picture given is classical for the pulmonary lesions of blastomycosis, which cannot be differentiated from carcinoma without biopsy.

30. **The answer is A.** This is conjunctivitis caused by HSV-1 or -2, which should be treated by an ophthalmologist with the antiherpes drug acyclovir. But the child should also be receiving IV acyclovir for potential systemic infection.

31. **The answer is B.** The PBPs are actually in the cytoplasmic membrane, even though the substrate is the cell peptidoglycan. Thus, β-lactams must penetrate the Gram-negative outer membrane through the porins and cross the peptidoglycan to bind. In the Gram-positive bacteria, they just have to cross the peptidoglycan to bind in the membrane.

32. **The answer is D.** Metronidazole (choice A) is not likely to work, as the agent is causing pneumonia, so it is probably aerobic or a facultative anaerobe. If the cell wall does not include peptidoglycan, β-lactam drugs (choices B and C) are likely to be ineffective. However, since the ribosomes are procaryotic, doxycycline has the best chance as long as it can penetrate the pathogen's cell wall and cytoplasmic membrane.

33. **The answer is E.** The IgG molecule has three constant domains on the heavy chain.

34. **The answer is B.** Viruses are the major infectious agents that produce symptoms similar to a heart attack. The most common of these viruses is Coxsackie B virus.

35. **The answer is D.** Hepatitis A virus (HAV) is the most likely virus to cause the reported symptoms, which indicate hepatitis rather than some other disease. HAV is a positive-sense single-strand RNA virus.

36. **The answer is C.** The T-cell antigen receptor is specific, responding only to antigen fragments bound to HLA. Choice A describes the B-cell receptor.

37. **The answer is D.** Natural killer cells target cells not expressing MHC Class I antigen for cytolysis. Many transformed cells and neoplasitic cells are loose the expression of MHC class I on their cell surface.

38. **The answer is A.** *Actinomyces israelii* grows contiguously in tissues, crossing anatomic barriers and causing a lumpy jaw, which is characterized by swelling and, sometimes, sinus tract formation with sulfur granules (3D colonies). It also invades bone. *M. tuberculosis* may be hematogenously spread to any tissue but is not associated with tooth extraction. *Nocardia* can also cause a similar infection, but the source is usually environmental *nocardiae* introduced by trauma; therefore, it generally involves extremities.

39. **The answer is A.** In the immunologically naive, bacterial capsules prevent the phagocytic uptake and, therefore, the killing of the bacterium.

40. **The answer is A.** A toxigenic strain of *Corynebacterium diphtheriae* is produced as a result of lysogenic phage conversion after a temperate bacteriophage infects a nontoxigenic strain of the organism.

41. **The answer is D.** The neurotoxin involved in infant botulism, unlike bacterial meningitis, does not cause elevated cerebrospinal fluid pressure, so recovery should be complete. The use of the recombinant human antitoxin shortens hospitalization and recovery time. However, it still requires regrowth of nerve endings.

42. **The answer is A.** Both amphotericin B (the correct answer) and nystatin are fungicidal, but nystatin is not used for systemic infections. Chloramphenicol is bactericidal. Ketoconazole and itraconazole are both fungistatic, and griseofulvin is not used systemically and localizes only in keratinized tissues.

43. **The answer is D.** Besides the clues of both alive and killed vaccines in routine use, the question noted the vaccine was given across the spectrum of ages. Of the vaccines listed, only pneumococcal, DTP, and influenza fit that criterion. Two influenza vaccines are in current use.

The live (attenuated) one is given intranasally and the killed (inactivated) one is injected. *Streptococcus pneumoniae* does have two vaccines, but neither is live attenuated; the pediatric pneumococcal vaccine is 13 (used to be 7)-capsular polysaccharides chemically complexed to protein. The 23-valent polysaccharide pneumococcal vaccine is used for anyone 65 years and older. Choice C is poliovirus; in the United States, the attenuated strains were previously routinely used to vaccinate (Sabin vaccine given orally), but the incidence of vaccine-associated polio became too high. The United States then switched to an injectable, inactivated tetravalent polio vaccine. Hepatitis B vaccine is a recombinant, single component vaccine with only the HBsAg present.

44. **The answer is E.** C1q recognizes antibody attached to cell surfaces and binds the antibody. The antibody-C1q complex then initiates the classical complement pathway by activating two serine proteases C1s and C1r.

45. **The answer is D.** *Neisseria meningitidis* is transmitted by direct oral mucosal contact or direct receipt of infected respiratory droplets on another's oropharyngeal mucosa. *Nm* adheres via pili and other adhesins; additionally, IgA-protease production and the capsule allow survival in a non-immune individual, allowing upper respiratory colonization that is followed by invasion of the bloodstream. This precedes development of pneumonia or meningitis. Skin lesions develop from overproduction of outer membrane, which is excreted without being incorporated, causing endotoxic shock and petechiae that progress to frank purpura. Waterhouse-Friderichsen syndrome is late.

46. **The answer is C.** Pathogenicity islands carry virulence genes and sometimes secretion systems and are often of different GC:AT ratios than most of the organism's other DNA, suggesting it was acquired from another organism.

47. **The answer is E.** In endemic regions, hookworm filariform larvae may grow in soil contaminated with human excrement; skin contact with soil (sitting or going barefoot) allows them to penetrate skin. Wearing shoes has been shown to greatly reduce the transmission of hookworm.

48. **The answer is A.** The superantigen produced by Staphylococcus simultaneously binds the T cell receptor and the MHC class II molecule regardless of the antigen occupying the antigen-binding groove. This cross-linking between an antigen presenting cell and a T cell leads to a broad spectrum activation of effector cells resulting in a large scale production of cytokines, often referred to as a "Cytokine Storm".

49. **The answer is A.** The presentation is most likely *Chlamydia trachomatis* conjunctivitis and pneumonia. This obligate intracellular organism is unable to make its own ATP. Choice B (gonococcus) should have been eliminated on Gram stain, and most would have been intracellular but not in phagosomes. Choice C is mycoplasma, which is not intracellular and rarely causes pneumonias in neonates this young. Choice D would be a rickettsia, which is both unlikely and not a good fit for the disease. Choice E (mycobacterium) also is unlikely to cause pneumonia in someone this young and is not known to cause eye infections producing pus.

50. **The answer is E.** The layer *on the cell* could be called either a glycocalyx (choice E) or capsule (not a choice). The layer on the catheter is a biofilm, but the question asked for the name of the layer on the cell.

51. **The answer is D.** The lack of flaccid paralysis leaves out botulinum toxin, and staphylococcal toxin is also unlikely as it is a short, self-resolving illness. The most likely is rotavirus due to his age and the length of the disease.

52. **The answer is C.** The clinical signs described and the fact that childhood vaccines have been administered strongly suggest that Parvovirus B19 is the cause.

53. **The answer is D.** Given the possible answer choices, the one that is most consistent with the patient's age and the signs and symptoms is West Nile arbovirus infections.

Index

References in *italics* indicate figures; those followed by "*t*" denote tables.

335